W0261722

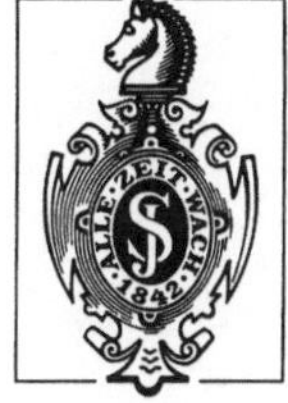

ALLZEIT·WACH
1842
S

Reinhard G. Bretzel (Hrsg.)

Diabetes mellitus

Immunologische und dynamische Aspekte
der Insulinsubstitution

Immunological and dynamic aspects of
insulin substitution

Mit 70 Abbildungen und 43 Tabellen

Springer-Verlag Berlin Heidelberg New York
London Paris Tokyo Hong Kong Barcelona

Herausgeber:
REINHARD G. BRETZEL
Klinikum der Justus-Liebig-Universität Gießen
Medizinische Klinik III und Poliklinik
Rodthohl 6, 6300 Gießen

ISBN-13:978-3-642-74611-6   e-ISBN-13:978-3-642-74610-9
DOI: 10.1007/978-3-642-74610-9

Library of Congress Cataloging-in-Publication Data
Diabetes mellitus: immunologische und dynamische Aspekte der Insulinsubstitution = immunological and dynamic aspects of insulin substitution / Reinhard G. Bretzel (Hrsg.).
p. cm.
Based on an international symposium in honour of the 60th birthday of Prof. Dr. med. Konrad Federlin, Giessen, Sept. 3, 1988. ISBN-13:978-3-642-74611-6 (U.S.)
1. Diabetes-Congresses. 2. Diabetes-Immunological aspects-Congresses. 3. Insulin-Therapeutic use-Congresses. 4. Federlin, K.-Congresses. I. Bretzel, R. G. II. Federlin, K. III. Title: Immunologische und dynamische Aspekte der Insulinsubstitution. IV. Title: Immunological and dynamic aspects of insulin substitution.
[DNLM: 1. Diabetes Mellitus-drug therapy-congresses.
2. Diabetes Mellitus-immunology-congresses. 3. Diabetes Mellitus-surgery-congresses. 4. Insulin-immunology-congresses. 5. Insulin-pharmacology-congresses. 6. Pancreas Transplantation-congresses. WK 820 D5364 1988]
RC660.A15D523 1990
616.4'62-dc20
DNLM/DLC
for Library of Congress   90-9683 CIP

Vorwort

Am 15. August 1988 beging Professor Dr. med. Konrad Federlin seinen
60. Geburtstag. Ihm zu Ehren fand ein Symposium zu den Themen statt, mit
denen sich sein wissenschaftliches Lebenswerk seit vielen Jahren verbindet: den
mannigfachen immunologischen Aspekten des Diabetes und einem möglichst
physiologischen, dynamischen Insulinersatz, der, nach seiner Hoffnung, in der
Transplantation isolierter Langerhans'scher Inseln verwirklicht werden könnte.
Diese Vorstellung hat er seit unseren gemeinsamen Anfängen noch an der Universität Ulm und seither in Gießen mit nicht nachlassender Energie verfolgt und auf
eine stets größer werdende Schar von wissenschaftlichen Mitarbeitern zu »transplantieren« verstanden.
Es bedurfte keiner großen Mühe, international anerkannte Experten zu dieser
Thematik in Gießen zusammenzuführen, sind sie doch alle seit Jahren Professor
Federlin und seiner Arbeitsgruppe eng verbunden. So tauschten Kollegen aus
Übersee, europäischen Nachbarländern und der Bundesrepublik ihre Erfahrungen aus zu Fragen der Virusaetiologie und Autoimmungenese des Typ I-Diabetes,
zur Insulinimmunologie, zu den Grundlagen der Insulinsubstitution auf konventionelle Weise und in Kombination mit oralen Antidiabetika. Diskutiert wurden
ferner die computerassistierte Therapie, die Aspekte der Diabetikerschulung und
Stoffwechselselbstkontrolle bis zur Anwendung der künstlichen Betazelle und des
Glukosesensors. Einen besonderen Platz bei der Bedeutung einer dynamischen
Insulinsubstitution für die Prophylaxe und Verlaufsbeeinflussung diabetischer
Sekundärkomplikationen nahmen die experimentellen und klinischen Erfahrungen mit dem biologischen Organersatz in Form der Pankreasorgantransplantation
oder Pankreasinseltransplantation ein.
Nahezu alle Referenten waren auch bereit, die Mühen einer Manuskriptabfassung
für diesen Band auf sich zu nehmen, wofür ich mich sehr zu bedanken habe. Mein
besonderer Dank gilt Herrn Professor Dr. med. Ernst-Friedrich Pfeiffer, dessen
langjährige Verbundenheit mit dem „Geburtstagskind" sich auf den Herausgeber
dieses Bandes übertrug und in zahlreichen Ratschägen zur inhaltlichen Gestaltung
der Tagung Ausdruck fand. Dank auch den Vorsitzenden der Sitzungen, allen
Diskutanten und Teilnehmern und schließlich den Repräsentanten der aufgeführten Firmen, ohne deren Unterstützung das Symposium und dieser Band nicht
hätten realisiert werden können.
Zu danken habe ich ferner Frau Hensler-Fritton vom Springer-Verlag für ihre
stetige geduldige Hilfe bei der Erstellung dieses Buches. Ihm möchte ich
wünschen, daß es nicht nur die zahlreichen Teilnehmer an eine hochinteressante

Tagung erinnert, sondern auch für viele weitere experimentell und klinisch tätige
Diabetologen eine aktuelle wissenschaftliche Information und Anregung darstellt.

Gießen, im Dezember 1989   REINHARD G. BRETZEL

Immunological and dynamic aspects of insulin substitution in diabetes mellitus

International Symposium in Honour of the 60th Birthday of Prof. Dr. med. Konrad Federlin
Altes Schloss, Gießen, September 3rd, 1988

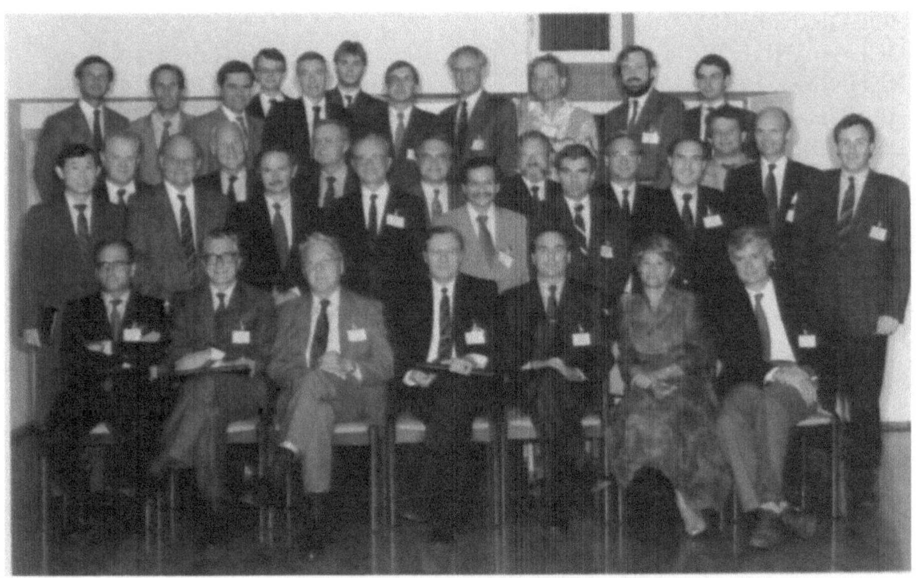

Seated left to right: D. Andreani, G. Pozza, E.F. Pfeiffer, K. Federlin, R.G. Bretzel, M. Pfeiffer, W.K. Waldhäusl

Standing first row: J.W. Yoon, G. Seidel, W. Teller, H. Mehnert, H.U. Klör, K.F. Weinges, C. Demiroglu, S. Raptis, R. Alejandro, R. Ziegler, R.V. Rajotte, J. Beyer, P. Bottermann, T. Zekorn, E. Standl, F. Becker

Standing second row: M. Woehrle, F. Melani, F. Enzmann, D. Romann, C.F. Barker, M. Brendel, C. McCullough, H. Ditschuneit, T. Deckert, R.F. Selden, B. Hering

Die Tagung wurde durch die freundliche Unterstützung
folgender Firmen ermöglicht:

ASTA PHARMA, Frankfurt
BAYER, Leverkusen
BAYROPHARM, Leverkusen
BISSENDORF, Wedemark
BOEHRINGER, Mannheim
DELALANDE, Köln
HENNING, Berlin
HOECHST, Frankfurt
LILLY, Bad Homburg
MADAUS, Köln
MERCK, Darmstadt
NORDISK, Eching
TROMMSDORFF, Aachen

Inhaltsverzeichnis

Die Bedeutung einer dynamischen Insulinsubstitution für Prophylaxe und Therapie diabetischer Sekundärkomplikationen

Pancreas and Islet Transplantation

Autorenverzeichnis

ALEJANDRO, R.
Diabetes Research Institute (R-134), University of Miami, School of Medicine, P.O. Box 016960, Miami, FL 33101, USA

ANDREANI, D.
Cattedra di Endocrinologica 1, Clinica Medica 2, Universita di Roma, I-00100 Roma

BARKER, C.F.
University of Pennsylvania, School of Medicine, 4th Floor Silverstein Pavilion, 3400 Spruce Street, Philadelphia, PA 19104, USA

BEYER, J.
III. Medizinische Klinik und Poliklinik, Innere Medizin und Endokrinologie des Klinikums der Johannes Gutenberg-Universität Mainz, Langenbeckstraße 1, D-6500 Mainz

BOTTERMANN, P.
II. Medizinische Universitätsklinik, Klinikum rechts der Isar, Technische Universität München, Ismaningerstraße 22, 8000 München 80

BRETZEL, R.G.
Klinikum der Justus-Liebig-Universität Gießen, Medizinische Klinik III und Poliklinik, Rodthohl 6, D-6300 Gießen

DAFOE, D.C.
University of Pennsylvania, School of Medicine, 4th Floor Silverstein Pavilion, 3400 Spruce Street, Philadelphia, PA 19104, USA

EVANS, M.G.
Surgical-Medical Research Institute, University of Alberta, 1074 Dentistry/Pharmacy Building, Edmonton, Alberta T6G 2N8, Canada

GRIES, F.A.
Diabetes Forschungsinstitut an der Universität Düsseldorf, Auf'm Hennekamp 65, D-4000 Düsseldorf 1

HERING, B.J.
Klinikum der Justus-Liebig-Universität Gießen, Medizinische Klinik III und Poliklinik, Rodthohl 6, D-6300 Gießen

KNETEMAN, N.M.
Surgical-Medical Research Institute, University of Alberta, 1074 Dentistry/Pharmacy Building, Edmonton, Alberta T6G 2N8, Canada

LACY, P.E.
Washington University, School of Medicine, Department of Surgery, 4960 Audubon Avenue, St. Louis, Missouri 63110, USA

LINN, T.
Klinikum der Justus-Liebig-Universität Gießen, Medizinische Klinik III und Poliklinik, Rodthohl 6, D-6300 Gießen

MARKMANN, J.F.
University of Pennsylvania, School of Medicine, 4th Floor Silverstein Pavilion, 3400 Spruce Street, Philadelphia, PA 19104, USA

MCARTHUR, R.G.
Head Department of Pediatrics, Faculty of Medicine, The University of Calgary, 3330 Hospital Drive N.W., Calgary, Alberta T2N 4Nl, Canada

MCCULLOUGH, C.S.
Washington University, School of Medicine, Department of Surgery, 4960 Audubon Avenue, St. Louis, Missouri 63110, USA

MEHNERT, H.
Städtisches Krankenhaus München-Schwabing, III. Medizinische Abteilung, Kölner Platz 1, D-8000 München 40

MINTZ, D.H.
Diabetes Research Institute (R-134), University of Miami, School of Medicine, P.O. Box 016960, Miami, FL 33101, USA

NAJI, A.
University of Pennsylvania, School of Medicine, 4th Floor Silverstein Pavilion, 3400 Spruce Street, Philadelphia, PA 19104, USA

PERLOFF, L.J.
University of Pennsylvania, School of Medicine, 4th Floor Silverstein Pavilion, 3400 Spruce Street, Philadelphia, PA 19104, USA

PFEIFFER, E.F.
Universität Ulm, Medizinische Klinik und Poliklinik, Abteilung Innere Medizin I, Oberer Eselsberg, Robert-Koch-Straße 8, D-7900 Ulm

POZZA, G.
Universita di Milano, Clinica Medica, Istituto Scientifico San Raffaele, Via Olgettina 60, I-20132 Milano, Italia

RAJOTTE, R.V.
Surgical-Medical Research Institute, University of Alberta, 1074 Dentistry/ Pharmacy Building, Edmonton, Alberta T6G 2N8, Canada

SAUER, H.
Schützenstraße 39, D-4970 Bad Oeynhausen

SCHARP, D.W.
Washington University, School of Medicine, Department of Surgery, 4960 Audubon Avenue, St. Louis, Missouri 63110, USA

SCHERBAUM, W.A.
Abteilung Innere Medizin I, Medizinische Klinik und Poliklinik der Universität Ulm, Robert-Koch-Straße 8, D-7900 Ulm

SCHERNTHANER, G.
I. Medizinische Abteilung der Krankenanstalt Rudolfstiftung, Juchgasse 25, A-1030 Wien, Österreich

SCHÖFFLING, K.
Zentrum der Inneren Medizin, Klinikum der Johann-Wolfgang-Goethe-Universität, Theodor-Stern-Kai 7, D-6000 Frankfurt/M 70

SCHREZENMEIR, J.
III. Medizinische Klinik und Poliklinik, Innere Medizin und Endokrinologie des
Klinikums der Johannes-Gutenberg-Universität Mainz, Langenbeckstraße 1,
D-6500 Mainz

SECCHI, A.
Universita di Milano, Clinica Medica, Istituto Scientifico San Raffaele, Via
Olgettina 60, I-20132 Milano, Italia

STANDL, E.
Städtisches Krankenhaus München-Schwabing, III. Med. Abteilung, Kölner Platz
1, D-8000 München 40

STRÖDTER, D.
Klinikum der Justus-Liebig-Universität Gießen, Medizinische Klinik III und
Poliklinik, Rodthohl 6, D-6300 Gießen

WALDHÄUSL, W.
Allgemeines Krankenhaus der Stadt Wien, I. Medizinische Universitätsklinik,
Lazarettgasse 14, A-1090 Wien, Österreich

WARNOCK, G.L.
Surgical-Medical Research Institute, University of Alberta, 1074 Dentistry/
Pharmacy Building, Edmonton, Alberta T6G 2N8, Canada

WIEGAND, S.
Klinikum der Justus-Liebig-Universität Gießen, Medizinische Klinik III und
Poliklinik, Rodthohl 6, D-6300 Gießen

WOEHRLE, M.
Klinikum der Justus-Liebig-Universität Gießen, Medizinische Klinik III und Poliklinik, Rodthohl 6, 6300 Gießen

YOON, J.-W.
The University of Calgary, Health Sciences Center, 3330 Hospital Drive N.W.,
Calgary, Alberta T2N 4N1, Canada

ZEKORN, T.
Klinikum der Justus-Liebig-Universität Gießen, Medizinische Klinik III und
Poliklinik, Rodthohl 6, D-6300 Gießen

ZIEGLER, D.
Diabetes Forschungsinstitut an der Universität Düsseldorf, Auf dem Hennekamp
65, D-4000 Düsseldorf 1

Vorsitzende, Referenten und Diskutanten, die nicht durch einen eigenen Beitrag vertreten sind:

DECKERT, T.
Steno-Memorial-Hospital, Niels Steensensvej 2, DK-2820 Gentofte

DITSCHUNEIT, H.
Medizinische Klinik II, Universität Ulm, Robert-Koch-Straße 8, D-7900 Ulm

DUDECK, J.
Institut für Medizinische Informatik, Universität Gießen, Heinrich-Buff-Ring 44,
D-6300 Gießen

MELANI, F.
Corso Italia 20, I-19100 Bozen

RAPTIS, S.
Evangelismos-Hospital, P.O.B. 141 27, Gr-11510 Athen

SELDEN, R.F.
Department of Molecular Biology, Massachusetts General Hospital, Wellman 11,
Boston, MA 02114, USA

TELLER, W.
Kinderklinik der Universität Ulm, Prittwitzstraße 43, D-7900 Ulm

WEINGES, K.F.
Medizinische Klinik und Poliklinik, Universität des Saarlandes, D-6650 Homburg/
Saar

ZIEGLER, R.
Medizinische Klinik I, Universität Heidelberg, Bergheimer Straße 58,
D-6900 Heidelberg

Immunologische Aspekte
der Insulinsubstitution

Viral Genesis of Type I Diabetes

J.-W. YOON and R. G. McARTHUR

Zusammenfassung

Bestimmte Viren einschließlich der D-Variante des Enzephalomyocarditis Virus und des Mengovirus 2T können pankreatische Beta-Zellen direkt infizieren und sich in den Zellen vermehren. Die Replikation der Viren in den Beta-Zellen resultiert in einer Zerstörung der Zellen innerhalb von drei Tagen und die infizierten Mäuse entwickeln in drei bis vier Tagen ein diabetes-ähnliches Syndrom, ohne daß Autoimmunmechanismen einbezogen sind. Im Gegensatz dazu erscheint das Rötelnvirus nur wenig mit dem Autoimmundiabetes (Typ I) bei Hamstern assoziiert zu sein. Aber endogenes Retrovirus, in pankreatischen Beta-Zellen exprimiert, ist eindeutig mit der Entwicklung einer Insulitis und nachfolgendem Diabetes bei non-obese diabetischen Mäusen (NOD) verbunden. Bei erstmanifestierten Typ I-Diabetikern scheint aber keine Korrelation zwischen dem Nachweis von Inselzellantikörpern und Anti-Coxsackie B Virus Antikörpern zu bestehen. Viren sind nicht nur auslösende Faktoren, sondern auch immunsupprimierende Substanzen beim Typ I-Diabetes. Eine Interferenz im Autoimmunprozeß mit Depletion von sowohl Makrophagen (z. B. Ia-positive Makrophagen) oder T-Lymphozyten (z. B. L3T4-Zellen) durch das Lactat Dehydrogenase Virus (LDV) bzw. das lymphozytische Choriomeningitis Virus (LCMV) resultiert in Verhinderung, verminderter oder verzögerter Entwicklung des Diabetes bei NOD-Mäusen und BB-Ratten. Im Gegensatz dazu ist aber eine persistierende Infektion mit Cytomegalievirus und Rötelnviren häufig mit dem Nachweis von Autoantikörpern bei Erstmanifestation eines Typ I-Diabetes in Verbindung zu bringen.

Introduction

Most patients with type I diabetes have a common pathologic picture – the near total disappearance of insulin-producing pancreatic β-cells. Genetic susceptibility appears to be a prerequisite in most, if not all, cases. If one of the parents has type I-diabetes, the risk is about 8%–10% for their offspring. If both parents have diabetes, the risk is over 23% [1, 2]. This concept is further supported by the fact that over 95% of patients with type I diabetes have HLA-DR3 or DR4, or both types [3]. However, over 50% of Caucasian nondiabetic controls also have HLA-DR3 and/or DR4 [3]. In other words, about half the Caucasian population may carry the genes conferring susceptibility to type I diabetes, but only 1 in about 200 individuals eventually develops type I diabetes. Furthermore, twin studies have clearly demonstrated a rather low concordance rate of type I diabetes in identical twins [2, 3]. Concordance for type I diabetes between monozygotic twins is only 30%–50%. Therefore, it can be concluded that genetic factors are certainly necessary but definitely not sufficient for type I diabetes. Thus, nongenetic factors clearly influence the clinical expression of genetic susceptibility [2, 3]. Studies on the interaction between diabetic susceptibility gene(s) or diabetic gene products and nongenetic factors including viruses, environmental toxins, nutrition, and various immune system alterations will be important for the understanding of the precise pathogenic mechanisms of the disease.

The hypothesis that viruses might cause type I diabetes comes from numerous case reports showing a temporal relationship between the onset of certain viral infections (e.g., rubella virus, cytomegalovirus, mumps virus, and Coxsackie B viruses) and the subsequent development of diabetes [4–7]. Recent case reports and epidemiological studies support the hypothesis by showing: (a) virus-specific antigens, lymphocytic infiltration and destruction of β-cells in the pancreatic islets from diabetic patients [8, 9]; (b) the presence of viral antibodies with rising titers in paired sera from newly diagnosed type I diabetes patients [9, 10]; (c) a high frequency of Coxsackie B virus immunoglobulin M (IgM) antibody in newly identified diabetic children [11, 12]; (d) β-cell damage in children who died of well-documented, overwhelming viral infections [13]; (e) the isolation of viruses from patients with acute-onset diabetes and the demonstration that these isolated viruses could induce diabetes in animals [9, 10]; and (f) the association of autoantibody production with certain types of viral infections (e.g., congenital rubella and cytomegalovirus) [14, 15]. In this brief review, I would like to summarize some of our studies, as well as others, regarding two possible pathogenic mechanisms for virus-induced diabetes; one is the destruction of β-cells by cytolytic viral infections and the other is autoimmune-mediated destruction of β-cells which might be triggered by persistent viral infections (Fig. 1).

Destruction of β-Cells by Cytolytic Viral Infection

Animal Models

A group of viruses including encephalomyocarditis (EMC) virus, Mengovirus 2T, and Coxsackie B viruses can directly infect pancreatic β-cells in SJL/J male mice and replicate in the cells (Fig. 2). The replication of viruses in the β-cells results in the destruction of these cells, and the infected animals subsequently develop hypoinsulinemia and hyperglycemia [16–18]. The destruction of β-cells in EMC virus-infected mice is dependent not on autoimmune responses [19, 20] but on the genetic makeup of the virus and genetic background of the host.

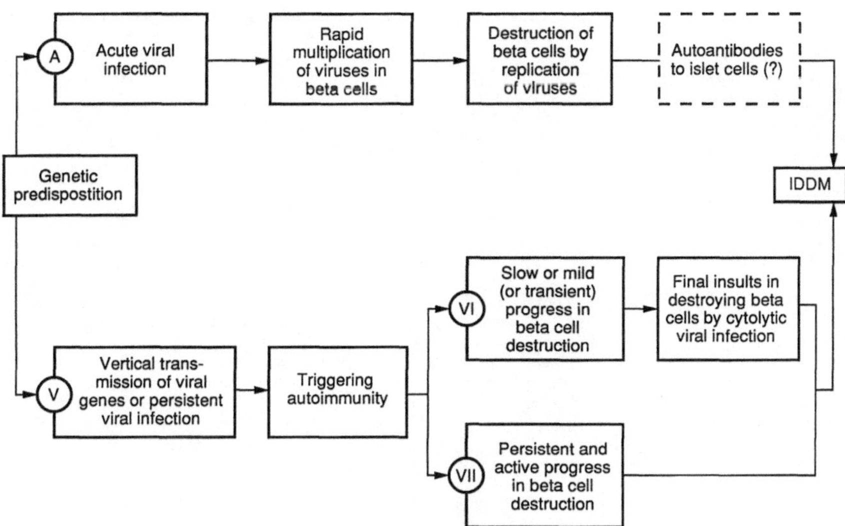

Fig. 1. Hypothesis for the role of viruses in the pathogenesis of type I diabetes, also called insulin-dependant diabetes mellitus or IDDM. Genetic predisposition is certainly necessary but definitely not sufficient for type I diabetes. Thus, nongenetic factors such as viruses influence the clinical expression of genetic susceptibility. Certain viruses (e.g., EMC-D for mice and Coxsackie B viruses for humans) can directly infect β-cells and replicate in the cells. The replication of viruses in the β-cells results in the destruction of these cells, and the infected animals (or humans) subsequently develop IDDM. Other viruses (e.g., rubella for hamsters, retrovirus for NOD mice, cytomegalovirus and rubella for humans) may trigger autoimmunity. Then, autoimmune-mediated destruction of β-cells takes place

Regarding autoimmune responses, over the last 2 years we have investigated the role of immune functions in the pathogenesis of EMC virus-induced diabetes by looking at the susceptibility of athymic nude mice, thymectomized mice, immunosuppressed mice, and the segregation of H-2 haplotypes in crosses of resistant and susceptible mice [19]. Athymic nude mice infected with EMC virus showed a diabetogenic response nearly identical to that of heterozygous littermates. Immunosuppression by antilymphocyte serum did not prevent the induction of EMC-D virus-induced diabetes. In studies on the F1 and backcross progeny of susceptible and resistant strains of mice there was no suggestion of a linkage between susceptibility and major histocompatibility locus. So far, we have found no evidence of immune involvement in the induction of diabetes mellitus by EMC-D virus [19].

Regarding the genetic makeup of the virus, two different variants (D and B) [16] isolated from the M variant of EMC virus [21] showed biological and biochemical differences [22, 23]. The D variant of EMC virus produces diabetes in over 90% of the infected animals, while none of the mice inoculated with the B variant of EMC virus developed diabetes. However, the D and B variants could not be distinguished antigenically by a sensitive plaque neutralization assay or competitive radioimmunoassay [22]. Furthermore, molecular hybridization studies with radio-labeled DNA complementary to EMC-D and EMC-B RNAs also

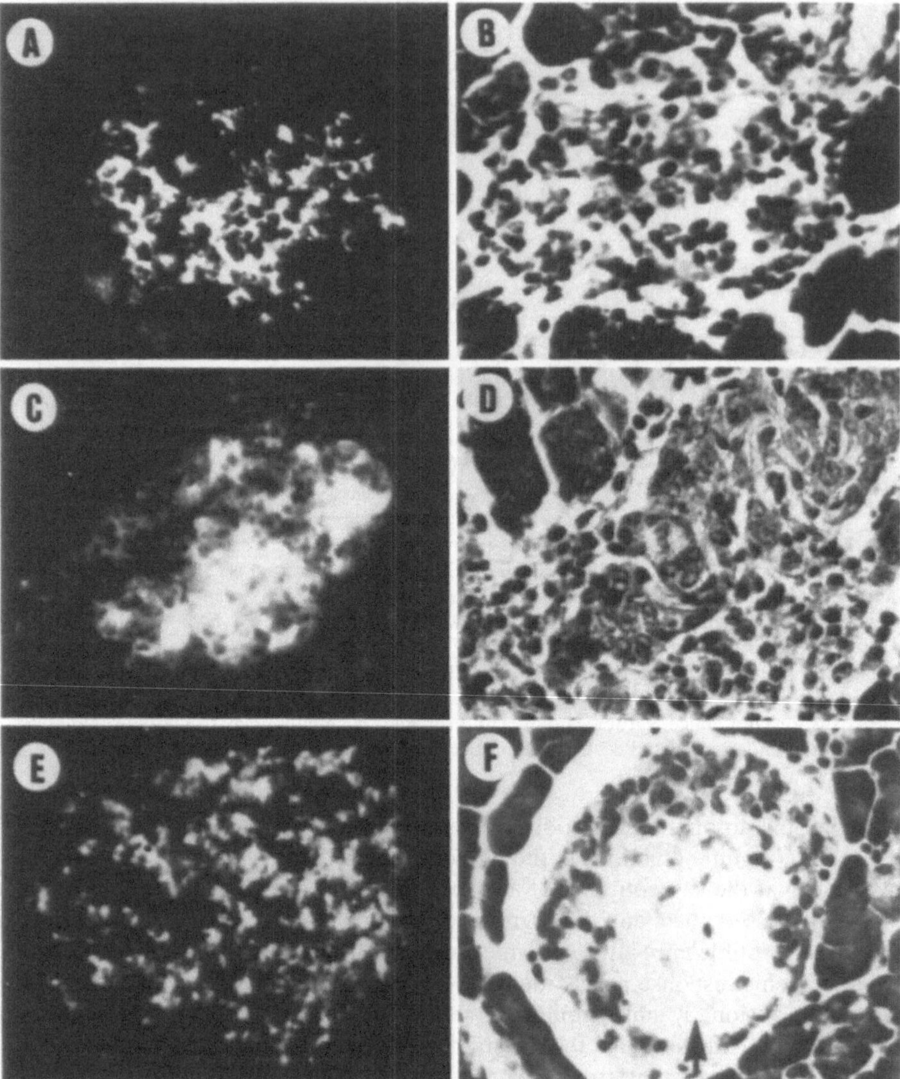

Fig. 2 A–F. Sections of pancreas from mice infected with the D variant of encephalomyocarditis (EMC) virus (**A, B**), Coxsackie B4 virus (**C, D**) or Mengovirus 2T (**E, F**). **A** Section obtained 3 days after infection with the D variant of EMC virus and stained with FITC-labelled anti-EMC virus antibody. The majority of the cells in the islets contain viral antigens. The surrounding acinar cells show little fluorescence (×350). **B** Section taken 7 days after infection with the D variant of EMC virus showing extensive inflammatory infiltrate in the islets of Langerhans and β-cell necrosis (hematoxylin-eosin stained, ×550). **C** Section obtained 4 days after infection with Coxsackie B4 virus and stained with FITC-labelled anti-Coxsackie B4 virus antibody. Most of the cells in the islets of Langerhans contained viral antigens. The surrounding acinar cells are free from viral antigen (×350). **D** Section of pancreas 5 days after infection with Coxsackie B4 virus showing extensive infiltration of islets by lymphocytes (hematoxylin-eosin, ×500). **E** Section obtained 2 days after infection with Mengovirus 2T and stained with FITC-labelled anti-Mengovirus antibody. The majority of the islets contain viral specific antigens (×550). **F** Section taken 6 days after infection with Mengovirus 2T showing complete loss of normal islet architecture and severe coagulation necrosis (hematoxylin-eosin, ×550)

failed to distinguish the D and B variants [24]. However, oligonucleotide finger-printing after T1 digestion of the RNAs from these two variants revealed a difference in one spot. An oligonucleotide was missing from the RNA of the B variant but was present in the RNA of the D variant. Recently, the oligoribonu-cleotide specific to EMC-D was isolated from a two-dimensional polyacrylamide gel and sequenced as 5'-ACAAUCUCACUUUUCCAACAACAG-3' [25]. Mo-lecular hybridizations of EMC-D and EMC-B genomic RNAs with a DNA primer complementary to the EMC-D-specific oligoribonucleotide revealed that the ab-sence of a corresponding spot in EMC-B was due to a point mutation rather that to a deletion. By sequencing a cloned cDNA of EMC-B corresponding to the EMC-D-specific oligoribonucleotide, the point mutation was identified as a G for EMC-B and a A for EMC-D transversion at base 9 of the oligonucleotide. Com-parative sequence analysis of eight randomly picked RNA segments around the EMC-D-specific oligoribonucleotide revealed that there were no base changes between EMC-D and EMC-B. Through this study it is concluded that the diabe-togenic EMC-D viral genome differs from the nondiabetogenic EMC-B viral genome by at least a point mutation [25].

The only biochemical difference found in this study was one base change in the 3'-terminal region of the I(2B) gene. The biological role of this point mutation is not known. It is unlikely to affect attachment of the virus to cells, since the site of mutation is not located in any of the outer capsid proteins. In our recent study, the antigenic differences between EMC-D and EMC-B could be identified by the EMC-D- and EMC-B-specific monoclonal antibodies [26] which were directed against the VP1 of the virus. Thus, we were particularly interested in cloning and sequencing the VP1 genes of both EMC-D and EMC-B viruses to see whether there were any differences between these two closely related variants. The genes for the major capsid protein, VP1(1D), of both diabetogenic EMC-D and non-diabetogenic EMC-B variants were cloned by using two synthetic primers which are common to both EMC-D and EMC-B. The cloned cDNAs were mapped for major restriction enzyme sites including *Acc*I, *Bam*HI, *Eco*RI, *Hinc*II, *Kpn*I, *Pvu*II, *Sst*I, *Taq*I, and *Xba*I. Among those nine restriction enzyme sites, only the *Taq*I site distinguished EMC-D genome from the counterpart of EMC-B genome. The complete nucleotide sequences (831 bases) of the VP1 genes revealed five amino acid differences between the two variants [27]. Three of the changes, at positions 41, 58, and 152, were Thr (EMC-B) to Ala (EMC-D). The additional two changes occurred at positions 63 [Gly (EMC-B) to Glu (EMC-D)] and 181 [Thr (EMC-B) to Ser (EMC-D)]. All of these amino acid changes were due to point mutations at the first base of each codon. Some of these point mutations identified in the VP1 may affect either the attachment of the virus to cells or the conformational arrangement of possible immunogenic sites. In this study, we have shown for the first time that five amino acid differences in VP1 between diabe-togenic EMC-D and nondiabetogenic EMC-B viruses result from first-base point mutations [27].

The information on the complete sequences of both viral genomes is needed to determine the functional consequences of genomic changes in both variants. Over the last year, we have determined the complete nucleotide sequences of both diabetogenic EMC-D and nondiabetogenic EMC-B viruses and identified that the EMC-D (7829 bases) differs from the EMC-B (7825 bases) by only 14 nucleotides [23]. The differences consist of two deletions of five nucleotides, one base insertion and eight point mutations. The first deletion of three nucleotides and the second deletion of two nucleotides are located in the 5' poly(C) tract and the 3'-end polyadenylation site, respectively. One base insertion in EMC-B occurs in the 5' noncoding region. The eight point mutations are located in the polyprotein coding region. Two of them are silent while the remaining six mutations, one located on the L gene and five on the VP1 gene, introduce amino acid changes. Our findings indicate that a maximum of 14 out of 7829 genomic nucleotides are critical in determining the diabetogenicity of EMC virus.

Regarding the genetic background of the host, EMC virus-induced diabetes in mice follows Mendelian inheritance and the susceptibility is primarily controlled by a single locus. When mice were infected with EMC virus (D or M variant), only certain inbred strains such as SJL/J, SWR/J, DBA/1J, and DBA/2J developed diabetes while other strains, such as C57BL/6J, CBA/J, AKR/J, and BALB/cJ, did not develop diabetes [28–31]. When diabetes-prone SWR/J mice were crossed with diabetes-resistant C57BL/6J mice, the F1 offspring were resistant to diabetes when infected with the virus. More than 20% of the F2 offspring, however, developed diabetes when exposed to the virus, indicating that susceptibility was inherited as an autosomal recessive trait. When the resistant F1 progeny were backcrossed to the resistant C57BL/6J parents, the offspring also were resistant to the development of EMC virus-induced diabetes. In contrast, when the resistant F1 progency were backcrossed to the susceptible SWR/J parents, approximately one-half of the offspring developed diabetes. Although the situation may be more complex, the data are consistent with the idea that EMC virus-induced diabetes follows Mendelian inheritance and that susceptibility is primarily controlled by a single locus [31].

Antigenically, EMC-D and Mengovirus 2T cannot be distinguished by hyper-immune sera; however, these two viruses are quite different in their tissue tropisms and mortality in mice. The D variant of EMC virus induces diabetes mellitus in strains of susceptible mice, but does not produce neuropathology or kill mice. In contrast, Mengovirus 2T produces severe brain cell damage and high mortality. By nucleic acid hybridization, these two viruses differ by about 20%; moreover, binding studies suggest that they recognize different viral receptors on the same cell [32].

The plaque-purified Mengovirus 2T infects and destroys pancreatic β-cells as demonstrated by immunofluorescence and histopathologic examination [17]. However, it has been difficult to study the tropism of the virus for β-cells because of the rapid onset of paralysis and death after infection. Therefore, the capacity of this virus to infect the β-cells and produce diabetes has to be studied early in the course of infection. It is interesting to note that the spectrum of host suscep-tibility of Mengovirus-induced diabetes is strikingly different from that produced by EMC-D virus [17]. Both viruses produced diabetes in SJL/J mice, but only Mengovirus produced abnormal glucose tolerance tests in the strains of mice which are resistant to EMC-induced diabetes such as C57BL/6J, CBA/J, C3H/J,

CE/J, and AKR/J. Immunofluorescent studies revealed that Mengovirus infected pancreatic β-cells from those mice, but EMC virus did not. Moreover, examination of islets of Langerhans from Mengovirus-infected mice revealed marked necrosis, severe inflammatory infiltration, and a decrease in the insulin content of the pancreas. To determine whether destruction of islet cells is correlated with viral replication, islets from C3H/J mice infected with either Mengovirus or EMC virus were assayed for infectious virus. At 1 and 2 days after infection, a significantly higher titer (10- to 100-fold) of the virus was observed in the mice infected with Mengovirus. These studies showed that strain differences in the induction of diabetes by EMC virus and Mengovirus could be due to the degree of virus replication in pancreatic β-cells [17].

Earlier studies showed that Coxsackie B4 virus did not produce diabetes when inoculated into mice [33]. However, by repeatedly passaging Coxsackie B4 virus in murine-enriched pancreatic β-cell cultures, it has been possible to enhance the diabetogenic capacity of this virus [18]. The capacity of Coxsackie B4 virus to induce diabetes is influenced by the genetic background of the host [18]. As in the case of EMC virus, only certain inbred strains of mice developed diabetes when exposed to Coxsackie B4 virus, and male mice developed more severe diabetes than female mice. Moreover, the strains of mice known to be susceptible to EMC-induced diabetes were also found to be susceptible to Coxsackie B4 virus-induced diabetes. Similarly, the strains of mice that were resistant to EMC-induced diabetes did not develop diabetes when exposed to Coxsackie B4 virus. The only exception thus far appears to be DBA/1J and DBA/2J mice which developed diabetes when infected with EMC virus but were resistant to the disease when exposed to Coxsackie B4 virus.

Human Type I Diabetes

The possibility that viruses might cause some cases of type I diabetes by infecting and destroying pancreatic β-cells has received considerable attention. However, it is difficult to demonstrate in vivo that viruses replicate in human β-cells and produce diabetes in man. As a practical model, an in vitro system has been developed to determine if viruses are capable of infecting and detroying human β-cells in cultures [9, 34–36]. Because the cells in these cultures were not pure β-cells, a double-label immunofluorescent antibody technique was used to show unequivocally that it was the β-cell, and not a contaminating non-β-cell, that became infected. Antibody to virus was labeled with fluorescein isothiocyanate (FITC) and antibody to insulin was labeled with tetramethyl rhodamine isothiocyanate (TRITC). By this method, it was clearly shown that several common human viruses, including mumps virus [35], Coxsackie B3 virus [34], Coxsackie B4 virus [9], and reovirus type 3 [36], could infect human β-cells. In addition, by radioimmunoassay, it was shown that the infection markedly decreased the insulin content of β-cells. Thus, at least under in vitro conditions, human β-cells are not inherently resistant to viral infection. However, there is no way to prove that these viruses actually infect and destroy human pancreatic β-cells and cause diabetes in man. It is known that some viruses will grow in cultured cells derived from animals that are resistant to infection [37]. In vitro susceptibility to β-cells may not be a true reflection of the in vivo susceptibility.

A more relevant approach is to isolate virus from the pancreas of children dying from acute-onset type I diabetes. Several years ago, we obtained material from such a case [9]. A healthy 10-year-old boy was admitted to the hospital in diabetic ketoacidosis within 3 days after the onset of a flu-like illness. Despite intensive therapy, the child's condition deteriorated and he died 7 days later. At autopsy, lymphocytic infiltration of the islets of Langerhans and necrosis of β-cells were observed. The picture was very similar to that seen in the islets of Langerhans of mice that developed diabetes after infection with EMC or Coxsackie B4 virus. Consequently, a small piece of the child's pancreas was homogenized and then inoculated into a number of different cell lines. Several days later, cytopathology was observed in several of the cultures and a variant of Coxsackie virus B4 was isolated. Studies on the patient's serum revealed a rise in the titer of neutralizing antibody to this isolate from less than 4 on the second hospital day to 32 on the day of death. In addition, when sections of the child's brain were stained with fluorescein-labeled anti-Coxsackie B4 virus antibody, a few cells were found to contain viral antigens. These findings supported the idea that the virus actually came from the child and was not an inadvertant laboratory contaminant.

However, the possibility still remained that the infection with Coxsackie B4 virus was completely unrelated to the cause of the child's diabetes. This is where our animal models proved to be invaluable. When several inbred strains of mice were inoculated with the human isolate, SJL/J male mice developed diabetes while CBA/J, C57BL/6J, and BALB/c mice did not develop diabetes. Moreover, examination of the pancreas from diabetic mice revealed extensive infiltration of inflammatory cells, destruction of β-cells, and viral antigens in the islets of Langerhans. Based on the patient's clinical picture, the virus isolation studies, and induction of diabetes in mice, it was concluded that the patient's diabetes was virus induced [9].

Support for the idea that viruses can trigger some diabetes in man has lately been strengthened by two additional case reports. The first is that of a 16-month-old child who developed a Coxsackie virus B5 infection and a few days later developed diabetes [10]. This virus was isolated from the feces of the child and produced abnormal glucose tolerance tests when inoculated into mice. The second case was a 5-year-old girl who developed myocarditis and diabetes 2–3 weeks after having open heart surgery [8]. At necropsy, her islets showed a lymphocytic infiltrate and β-cell necrosis. By means of immunofluorescent studies, Coxsackie B4 virus antigens were found in the islets and high levels of antibody to Coxsackie B4 virus were found in the serum. In other studies, pancreatic sections from four out of seven neonates who died of Coxsackie B virus infections showed insulitis and β-cell damage [13]. The insulitis and β-cell damage observed at autopsy do not prove that these children would have developed diabetes if they had survived after viral infection, but these studies provide further in vivo support for the idea that, under certain circumstances, some viruses are capable of infecting β-cells.

It is evident that diabetes is not a common consequence of Coxsackie B virus infections. Approximately 5% –20% of type I diabetes appears to be associated with the infection of Coxsackie B virus [11, 12, 38]. However, it is still unclear whether Coxsackie B virus is involved in the disease process in a primary role or as a secondary phenomenon. It is believed that immunological abnormalities can precede the onset of type I diabetes. However, about 5% –20% of type I diabetes patients failed to show immunologic abnormalities (e.g., ICA, ICSA, 64 kDa antibody, Ia-positive T cells) at the time of diagnosis [39, 40]. Therefore, it is speculated that some of those patients who fail to show immunologic abnormalities may be afflicted by a cytolytic infection of pancreatic β-cells with viruses (e.g., variants of Coxsackie B viruses).

Recent careful epidemiological studies showed that a proportion of type I diabetes is associated with Coxsackie B viral infection [11, 12, 38]. King et al. [11] detected Coxsackie B virus-specific IgM responses in 39% of children of ages 3–14 with newly diagnosed type I diabetes. In contrast, only about 6% of an age-matched control group had Coxsackie B virus-specific IgM antibody. More recently, Banatvala et al. [12] confirmed this observation in different European countries, including Austria, and in Australia. To see whether a correlation exists between the presence of anti-Coxsackie B viral antibodies and that of autoantibodies, we measured these antibodies in the same individuals and compared them (Toniolo and Yoon, unpublished data). Unfortunately, we did not find any correlation between anti-Coxsackie B viral antibodies and islet cell autoantibodies. Studies on the pathogenesis of Coxsackie B virus-induced diabetes also argue against an autoimmune component. Like other picornaviruses, Coxsackie B viruses may rapidly infect and lyse pancreatic β-cells before the development of autoimmunity. There is also no indication that Coxsackie B viruses modify the host cell surface by inserting viral antigens or that the virus triggers an autoimmune response (i.e., there is no evidence of islet cytoplasmic antibody or islet cell surface antibody). Therefore, if Coxsackie B viruses are involved in the pathogenesis of type I diabetes, the induction of diabetes by these viruses could be due to cytolytic infection of β-cells rather than to an autoimmune response. However, the possibility that chronic Coxsackie B viral infection of β-cells could result in synthesis and release of interferon-α, which in turn induces class I MHC hyperexpression on adjacent endocrine cells, cannot be excluded [41].

Destruction of β-Cells by Persistent Viral Infection Associated with Autoimmunity

Current knowledge indicates that in the major portion of type I diabetes, a rather long pathologic process might precede the onset of the disease. Thus, if viruses are involved in the pathogenesis of type I diabetes, it is important to consider the possible triggering of autoimmunity by viruses. Several candidate viruses which might be associated with triggering of autoimmune type I diabetes will be discussed in this section.

Animal Models

The congenital rubella syndrome provides one of the best documentations in man that a viral infection is associated with the subsequent development of autoimmune type I diabetes [42]. Recently, we have developed an animal model in neonatal golden Syrian hamsters infected with rubella virus passaged in β-cells which closely parallels the diabetes observed with congenital rubella [43]. Seven- to ten-day-old Syrian hamsters developed hyperglycemia, hypoinsulinemia, a mononuclear infiltrate of the islets, and positive immunofluorescence for rubella virus antigen in β-cells following inoculation with a passaged variant of rubella virus. In addition, very weak cytoplasmic islet cell antibodies were present in 8 of the 20 infected animals.

However, the mechanism of rubella virus-induced diabetes is not known. In contrast to EMC virus, rubella virus is not highly lytic. Our preliminary data showing insulitis in 34.5% of hamster islets and measurable circulating islet cell antibodies is somewhat compatible with an autoimmune process. Rubella virus belongs to the togavirus family. This enveloped virus is surrounded by a lipoprotein coat which is derived from the host cell membrane when the virus buds through it. Thus, rubella virus might insert, expose, or alter antigens in the plasma membrane of the host cell during infection. Alternatively, the virus might induce an autoimmune syndrome by disturbing T-cell subpopulations (helper or suppressor T cells) that regulate the immune response of the host [44, 45].

Since reoviruses produce a variety of lesions in newborn mice, we passaged reovirus type 3 in cultured pancreatic β-cells to see whether the virus can be adapted to the β-cells. When the β-cell-passaged virus was injected into suckling SJL/J male mice, some of the infected animals showed an abnormal response in glucose tolerance tests 10 days after infection. By immunofluorescence, specific viral antigens were found in some β-cells as well as in acinar cells. By electron microscopy, viral particles were detected in the cytoplasm of some β-cells. Surviving animals remained mildly hyperglycemic for about 3 weeks and then returned to normal [46].

However, the suckling SJL/J mice infected with β-cell-passaged reovirus type I developed transient diabetes and a runting syndrome [47]. Examination of sera from infected mice revealed autoantibodies that reacted with cytoplasmic antigens in the islets of Langerhans, anterior pituitary, and gastric mucosa of uninfected mice [47]. The administration of either anti-lymphocyte serum, anti-thymocyte serum, or cyclophosphamide reduced or prevented the development of reovirus-induced diabetes [48]. In addition, virus-infected immunosuppressed mice gained weight at almost the same rate as uninfected controls, and mortality was greatly decreased. Thus, Onodera et al., concluded that autoimmunity does play a role in the pathogenesis of reovirus-induced diabetes [47, 48].

Until now, I have discussed experimentally induced autoimmune diabetes in animals; this includes rubella virus-induced diabetes in hamsters and reovirus-induced diabetes in mice. Now, I will discuss spontaneously developed autoimmune diabetes in mice. Nonobese diabetic (NOD) mice develop a diabetic syndrome which, in many respects, resembles human type I (insulin-dependent) diabetes [49]. Diabetes in the NOD mice is characterized by the establishment of insulitis, which precedes β-cell destruction culminating in hypoinsulinemia and hyperglycemia. The precise events which trigger the onset of the disease remain largely unknown. Various effector systems including macrophages, T lymphocytes, and/or humoral mediators have been implicated as the possible effectors of immune responses.

Recent studies from our laboratory and others revealed that the administration of cyclophosphamide to NOD mice produces a rapid progression to overt diabetes with severe insulitis within 2–3 weeks [50, 51]. Cyclophosphamide significantly increases the incidence of diabetes in NOD mice either by inhibiting suppressor T cells or by activating cytotoxic T cells [52]. However, the depletion of macrophages by silica treatment resulted in the prevention of insulitis and diabetes in cyclophosphamide-treated NOD mice [50]. These findings suggested that: (a) macrophages play a major role in the initiation of organ-specific autoimmunities in NOD mice; (b) the presentation of autoantigen(s) on the specific target cells, such as β-cells, by the macrophages would be the initial step in the development of insulitis; and (c) the elimination of macrophages results in the inhibition of the immune process. Our recent investigation was initiated to determine whether there are any specific changes in the β-cells which may lead to the attraction of macrophages for the initiation of β-cell-specific autoimmune disease in the cyclophosphamide-treated NOD male mice.

The administration of cyclophosphamide to male NOD mice produced a rapid progression to overt diabetes (over 70%) with severe insulitis in 2–3 weeks while none of the untreated control NOD male mice became diabetic. When thin sections of islets from NOD male mice, which first received silica for the preservation of islets and subsequently received cyclophosphamide, were examined under the electron microscope, clusters of endogenous retrovirus particles (A type) were frequently found in the β-cells (Fig. 3). In contrast, retrovirus particles were rarely found in the β-cells from NOD male mice which received silica only. Other endocrine cells including α-, δ-pancreatic polypeptide producing (pp) cells, and exocrine acinar cells did not contain such virus particles. These virus particles were not found in spleen, liver, or kidney either in cyclophosphamide-treated or untreated NOD male mice. There was a clear correlation between the presence of retrovirus particles in the β-cells and insulitis lesions in the cyclophosphamide-treated mice. On the basis of these observations, it is concluded that the β-cell-specific expression of endogenous retrovirus is associated with the development of insulitis and diabetes in NOD mice.

The role of β-cell-specific expressed retrovirus in the pathogenesis of autoimmune type I diabetes in NOD mice has not been defined. Work in several laboratories has indicated that retrovirus (e.g. murine leukemia virus, MuLV) gp 70 may be present on the surface of cells without production of detectable infectious virus [53–55]. By immunofluorescent techniques, Lerner and his coworkers found that a protein similar or identical to the retrovirus (MuLV) gp 70 major envelope glycoprotein is on the surface of mouse (127/J) thymocytes, in lymphoid tissues, and in murine epithelial lining cells [56]. Since retroviruses (xenotropic viruses) were regularly recovered from the mouse tissues, it is believed that these immu-

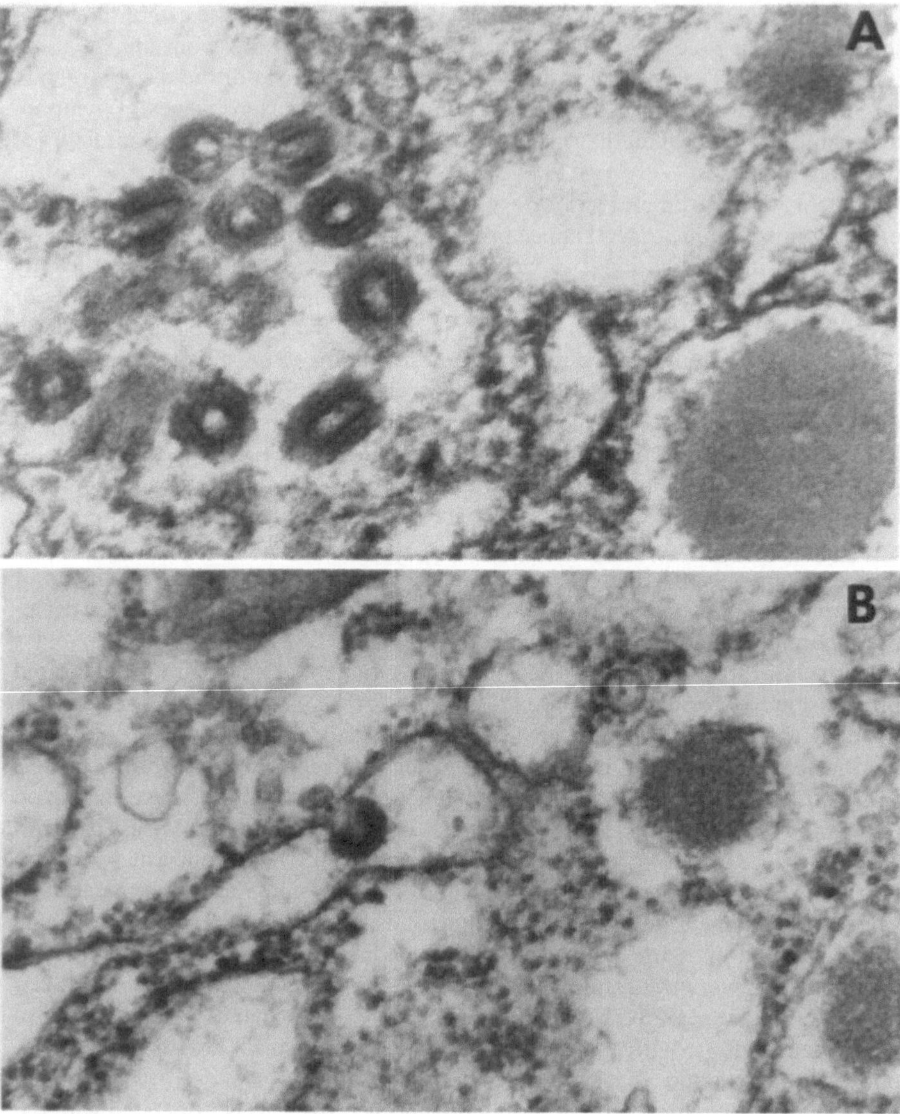

Fig. 3 A, B. Endogenous type A retrovirus particles found in the β-cells from the silica-treated NOD mice with the administration of cyclophosphamide. The cluster of virus particles is seen in the cytoplasm of β-cells (**A**) and a particle budding from the inner membrane surface of the rough endoplasmic reticulum is also seen (**B**)

nofluorescent tests could be detecting viral antigen on the cell surface. Whether the viral antigen or virus-induced autoantigen will express on the β-cells from these animals is presently under investigation.

The presentation of antigen on the target cells by antigen-presenting cells is a critical determinant for the distinction between elicitation of an immune response and immunologic tolerance [57]. The immune response to a specific antigen on the target tissue involves the activation of a T helper subset of lymphocytes. The T helper cell is activated only when it interacts with the antigen presented on the surface of a macrophage or other antigen-presenting cell (Fig. 4). In contrast, the direct exposure of lymphocytes to an antigen in the absence of antigen-presenting cells was shown to induce immunologic tolerance to the specific antigen [58]. Since the elimination of antigen-presenting cells resulted in the prevention of insulitis in NOD mice, we can hypothesize that the presentation of autoantigens on the target cells by the macrophages would be the initial step in the development of β-cell-specific autoimmune disease in NOD mice (Fig. 4). However, the amplification of immune responses by T lymphocytes (e.g., L_3T_4 and Lyt_2) should be required for the clinical expression of overt diabetes in NOD mice (Fig. 4).

Oldstone and colleagues reported that lymphocytic choriomeningitis virus (LCMV) persistently infects murine pancreatic islet cells [59]. In their studies, viral nucleoprotein was detected predominantly in the pancreatic β-cells by a

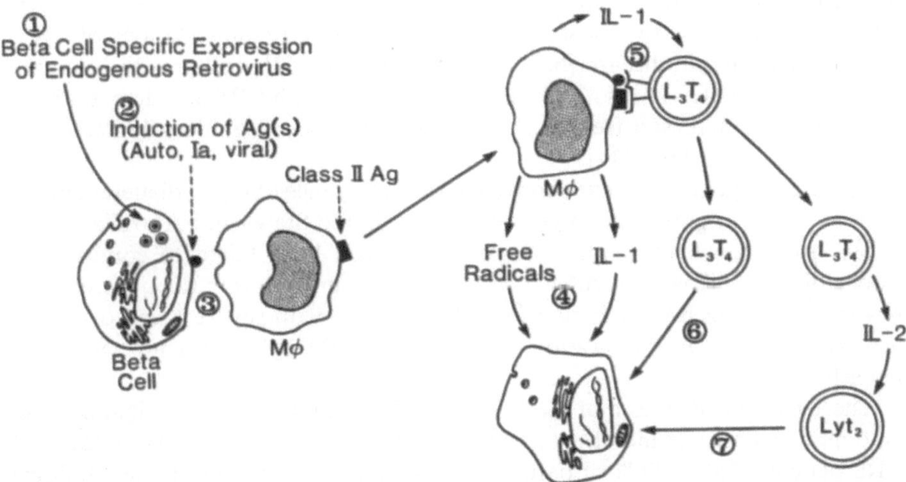

Fig. 4. Possible pathways for the destruction of β-cells in NOD mice. *1* The endogenous retrovirus may induce a β-cell-specific autoantigen, class II antigen, or viral antigen (or two of these three or all of them). *2* The expressed autoantigen(s) may attract macrophages. *3* The macrophages secrete free radical (superoxide, OH radicals) and/or interleukin-1 which may have a cytotoxic effect on β-cells. *4* During this process, the macrophages may present the processed antigen to L_3T_4 helper T lymphocytes. *5* The L_3T_4 cells may activate cytotoxic T lymphocytes and/or stimulate B-cell response to produce antibodies against islet cells. *6* A fraction of L_3T_4 cells may directly exert a cytotoxic effect on β-cells. *7* Lyt_2 cells developed during the further immune process may exert an additional cytotoxic effect to the residual β-cells, resulting in β-cell specific autoimmune disease

double-labeled immunofluorescent antibody technique. Electron microscopy confirmed these findings by showing virions budding from the β-cells. Persistent infection was associated with the chemical evidence of diabetes including hyperglycemia and abnormal glucose tolerance. However, the virus-infected islet cells showed normal anatomy and cytomorphology. Neither β-cell destruction nor lymphocytic infiltration was routinely observed. The end result is a chemical and morphologic picture similar to that observed in the early stages of adult-onset diabetes mellitus.

One of the possible mechanisms by which this virus might cause diabetes is through the establishment of an infection that might shut off the "luxury functions" of insulin-producing β-cells [59, 60]. The other possibility is that the persistent infection may also result in a gradual reduction in the number of functioning β-cells since the regenerative capacity of β-cells is thought to be poor [60]. The precise mechanism by which LCMV induces diabetes remains to be investigated. Nevertheless, this new finding is very interesting and important for studies on diabetes in humans and animals.

Human Type I Diabetes

The congenital rubella syndrome (CRS) has emerged as an important human model for type I diabetes. In CRS, diabetes takes 5–20 years to develop [61]. Although diabetes is the most common of the delayed manifestations of CRS, autoimmune thyroid disease [62]. Addison's disease [62], and growth hormone deficiency [63, 64] have also been reported. Patients with CRS and diabetes have a significantly increased frequency of HLA DR3 and a significantly decreased frequency of HLA DR2 [14].

Epidemiologic studies have shown that the prevalence of type I diabetes among CRS patients is significantly high in both the United States and Autralia (about 20%) [10, 61], whereas other studies in the UK have failed to confirm this association [65]. However, rubella virus has been isolated from the pancreas in a few cases of congenital infection [67], and insulitis with severe β-cell depletion was also reported in the case of an infant with CRS dying of acute onset diabetes [61].

There have been clues that the endocrine abnormalities in CRS might have an autoimmune basis: an increased prevalence of islet cell surface antibody (21% of CRS patients, 50%–80% of patients with abnormal carbohydrate metabolism) [42, 68], an increased prevalence of anti-thyroid microsomal and/or anti-thyroglobulin antibody (26% of CRS patients) [42, 68], and an increased prevalence of anti-insulin autoantibody (13% of CRS patients versus < 1% of controls) [69]. Although the most convincing evidence that a persistent viral infection may cause type I diabetes and produce autoantibody comes from studies of patients with CRS, it is not known how rubella virus triggers autoimmunity and type I diabetes. Animal models of rubella should be useful in elucidating underlying pathogenesis.

There was also a case report that a child with congenital cytomegalovirus infection developed diabetes mellitus at the age of 13 months [70]. At that time, he presented a 2-week history of polydipsia, vomiting, and weight loss, and was found to be severely dehydrated and ketoacidotic with a blood glucose of 50 mmol/l (900 mg/dl). In other reports, characteristic inclusion bodies have been found in the β-cells of infants and children who died with disseminated cytomegalovirus infections [13]. Insulitis and cytomegalovirus-like particles have been observed in the pancreas of a particular rodent (*Octodon degu*), which manifests spontaneous diabetes [71].

Human cytomegalovirus infection is ubiquitous and largely subclinical. In many persistent viral infections, the initial viral infection takes place before birth or very early in life, although the disease may not appear until later. The infection can be passed through the sperm or ovum if viruses integrate their genomes into the host DNA. Viral infections can also be transmitted transplacentally, perinatally, or postnatally through close contact or breast milk. The immaturity of the immune systems of infants also favors the establishment of persistent viral infections.

Nucleic acid hybridization is especially useful in studies of persistent viral infections, since it can detect even inactive or incomplete viral genomes in a cell. Since persistent viral infections are often local, in situ hybridization can be used to localize the individual cells that contain the viral genome. Our finding, with both dot and in situ hybridization techniques, that about 15 % of newly diagnosed type I diabetic patients had human cytomegalovirus-specific viral genome in their lymphocytes and islet cell autoantibodies in their sera suggests that autoimmune type I diabetes is sometimes associated with persistent cytomegalovirus infections [15].

What might be the link between persistent cytomegalovirus infection and autoimmune type I diabetes? Autoimmune disease could result from an immune response to viral antigens in the host cells or the host-cell-specific antigens that are exposed as a result of infection. If the cytomegalovirus infection persists in the β-cells and either expresses viral antigens or induces an aberrant expression of class II major histocompatibility complex (MHC) antigen on the cells, in certain circumstances – such as particular genetic background and environmental effects (e.g., drug, diet, toxins, infections) – persistent cytomegalovirus infection might trigger β-cell-specific autoimmune disease such as type I diabetes.

In addition to rubella virus and cytomegalovirus, it has been hypothesized that a preceding infection with mumps virus may also trigger at least some cases of type I diabetes. Recent reports suggested that some children may develop islet cell antibody during parotitis [72]. Gamble showed that mumps infection apparently precedes the development of diabetes in some newly diagnosed diabetic children [73]. Other epidemiologic studies do not support the hypothesis that mumps infection is associated with the onset of type I diabetes [74].

Prevention of Type I Diabetes by Virus Infection

BioBreeding (BB) rats spontaneously develop a diabetic syndrome that in many respects resembles human type I diabetes. The diabetic syndrome in BB rats results from the destruction of pancreatic β-cells by cell-mediated and/or humoral immune responses [75]. Key features supporting an autoimmune hypothesis include infiltration of islets by mononuclear cells [76–78] and the presence of circulating autoantibodies against islets [79–81]. The role of cell-mediated immunity in the pathogenesis of diabetes was further emphasized by the observation of two phenomena. First, it was shown that the development of diabetes was prevented either by performing a thymectomy neonatally [82] or by suppressing the immune system by anti lymphocyte serum [83], corticosteroid [84], and cyclosporin A [85]. The repletion of the normal cell population via neonatal bone marrow transplantation [86, 87] as well as whole blood or T-lymphocyte injection [88, 89] also resulted in the prevention of diabetes. Second, it was found that diabetes was adoptively transferred when concanavalin A-stimulated spleen cells, derived from acutely diabetic rats, were injected into nondiabetic BB or control Wistar-Furth rats [90, 91]. These experiments showed the involvement of cell-mediated immunity in the development of diabetes. The inocultion of BB rats with lymphocytic choriomeningitis virus (LCMV; Armstrong strain, clone 13) reduced the incidence of diabetes and prevented the mononuclear cell infiltration in the islets of Langerhans by somehow disordering particular lymphocyte subsets [92].

In addition to BB rats, nonobese diabetic (NOD) mice also spontaneously develop a diabetic syndrome. Diabetes in the NOD mice has been categorized as an autoimmune disease based on the involvement of various effector systems including macrophages and T lymphocytes, especially class II-restricted L_3T_4 and class I restricted Lyt_2 cells [93–95]. When newborn or 6-week-old NOD mice were infected with LCMV, they did not become diabetic [96]. This observation suggests that the prevention of diabetes by LCMV introduction is most likely due to virus-induced inactivation of potentially autoimmune reactive lymphocytes (Fig. 5).

Our recent studies showed that the depletion of macrophages in NOD mice by treatment with silica resulted in the prevention of insulitis and diabetes [97]. A preliminary observation reveals that the destruction of Ia-positive macrophages by lactic dehydrogenase virus (LDV) in NOD mice results in the prevention of diabetes (Fig. 5). Macrophages play a central role in the immune response against immunologically active molecules [66]. The key roles of macrophages include the presentation of processed antigen to helper T lymphocytes in the context of MHC class II molecules present on the surface of macrophages. Recent observations emphasized that L_3T_4-positive helper T lymphocytes play a role in the pathogenesis of diabetes in NOD mice [93, 94]. On the basis of information from these studies and our studies, I suggest that the presentation of β-cell-specific autoantigen by macrophages and the recognition of the antigen by helper T lymphocytes might be the initial steps in the development of insulitis (Fig. 4). Thus, disrupting the

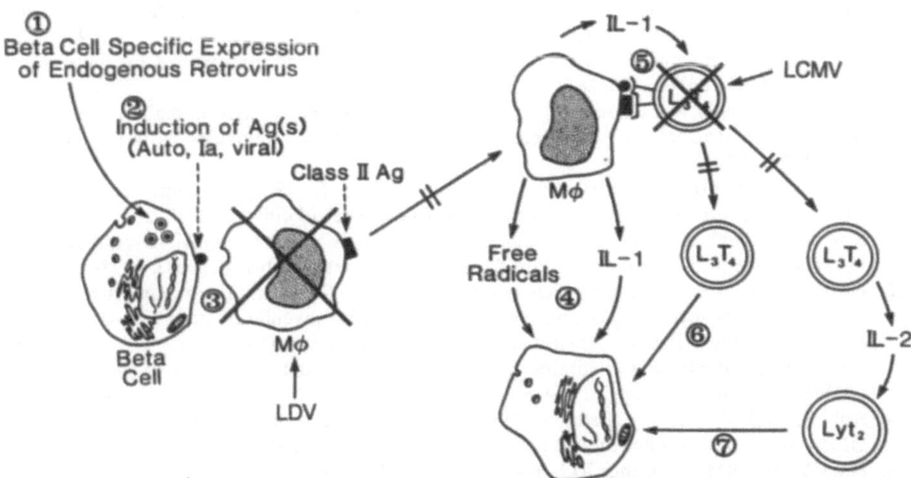

Fig. 5. Possible role of viruses in the inhibition of β-cell destruction. Lactic dehydrogenase virus (LDV) may destroy Ia-positive macrophages. The destruction of Ia-positive macrophages in NOD mice may result in the inhibition of further immune process. Lymphocytic choriomeningitis virus (LCMV) may destroy some subsets of lymphocytes, which reduces the incidence of diabetes and prevents the lymphocytic infiltration in the islets of Langerhans

immune process in either macrophages or T lymphocytes by LDV and LCMV respectively can result in the reduction or prevention of insulitis as well as diabetes (Fig. 5).

Acknowledgement. This work was supported by the Medical Research Council of Canada (MA9584), Canadian Diabetes Association and the Alberta Children's Hospital Foundation. J.W.Y. is a Heritage Medical Scientist Awardee. The secretarial help of Daphne Kwan is gratefully acknowledged.

References

1. Rossini AA, Mordes JP, Like AA (1985) Immunology of insulin-dependent diabetes mellitus. Annu Rev Immunol, 3: 289–320
2. Lernmark A (1985) Molecular biology of Type I (insulin-dependent) diabetes mellitus. Diabetologia 28: 195–203
3. Nerup J, Christy M, Platz P, Ryder LP, Svejgaard A (1984) Aspects of the genetics of insulin-dependent diabetes mellitus. In: Andreani D, Dimario U, Federlin KF, Heding LG (eds) Immunology in diabetes. Kimptom, London, pp 63–70
4. Yoon JW, Kim CJ, Pak CY, McArthur RG (1987) Enviromental factors and IDDM. Clin Invest Med 10: 457–469
5. Notkins AL, Yoon JW, Onodera T, Toniolo T, Janson AB (1981) Virus-induced diabetes mellitus. Perspect Virol 11: 141–162
6. Leiter EH, Wilson GL (1988) Viral interactions with pancreatic beta cells. In: Lefebvre PJ, Pipeleers DG (ed) The pathology of the endocrine pancreas in diabetes. Springer, Berlin, Heidelberg, New York, pp 85–105

7. Craighead JE (1975) The role of viruses in the pathogenesis of pancreatic diseases and diabetes mellitus. Prog Med Virol 19: 161–214

8. Gladisch R, Hofmann W, Waldherr R (1976) Myocarditis and insulitis in Coxsackie virus infection. Z Kardiol 65: 873–881

9. Yoon JW, Austin M, Onodera T, Notkins AL (1979) Virus-induced diabetes mellitus. Isolation of a virus from the pancreas of a child with diabetic ketoacidosis. N Engl J Med 300: 1173–1179

10. Champsaur H, Bottazzo G, Bertrams J, Assan R, Bach C (1982) Virologic, immunologic and genetic factors in insulin-dependent diabetes mellitus. J Pediatr 100: 15–20

11. King ML, Shaikh A, Bidwell D, Voller A, Banatvala JE (1983) Coxsackie-B-virus specific IgM responses in children with insulin-dependent diabetes mellitus. Lancet i: 1397–1399

12. Banatvala JE, Schernthaner G, Schober E et al. (1985) Coxsackie B, mumps, rubella and cytomegalovirus specific IgM responses in patients with juvenile-onset insulin-dependent diabetes mellitus in Britain, Austria and Australia. Lancet I: 1409–1412

13. Jenson AB, Rosenberg HS, Notkins AL (1980) Pancreatic islet cell damage in children with fatal viral infections. Lancet ii: 354–8

14. Rubinstein P, Walker ME, Fedun B, Witt ME, Cooper LZ, Ginsberg-Fellner F (1982) The HLA system in congenital rubella patients with and without diabetes. Diabetes 31: 1088–91

15. Pak CY, Eun HM, McArthur RG, Yoon JW (1988) Association of cytomegalovirus infection with autoimmune type I diabetes. Lancet II: 1–4

16. Yoon JW, McClintock PR, Onodera T, Notkins AL (1980) Virus-induced diabetes mellitus. Inhibition by a non-diabetogenic variant of encephalomyocarditis virus. J Exp Med 152: 878–892

17. Yoon JW, Morishima T, McClintock PR, Austin M, Notkins AL (1984) Virus-induced diabetes mellitus: Mengovirus infects pancreatic beta cells in strains of mice resistant to the diabetogenic effect of encephalomyocarditis virus. J Virol 50: 684–690

18. Yoon JW, Onodera T, Notkins AL (1978) Virus-induced diabetes mellitus: Beta cell damage and insulin-dependent hyperglycemia in mice infected with Coxsackie virus B4. J Exp Med 148: 1068–80

19. Yoon JW, McClintock PR, Bachurski LJ, Longstretch JD, Notkins AL (1985) Virus-induced diabetes. No evidence for immune mechanisms in the destruction of beta cells by encephalomyocarditis virus. Diabetes 34: 922–925

20. Vialettes B, Baume D, Charpin C, De Maeyer-Guignard J, Vague P (1983) Assessment of viral and immune factors in EMC virus-induced diabetes: effects of cyclosporin A and interferon. J Clin Lab Immunol 10: 35–40

21. Craighead JE, McLane MF (1968) Diabetes mellitus: induction in mice by encephalomyocarditis virus. Science 162: 913–915

22. Yoon JW, Notkins AL (1983) Virus-induced diabetes mellitus in mice. Metabolism 32 [Suppl]: 37–40

23. Bae YS, Eun HM, Yoon JW (1989) Molecular identification of diabetogenic viral gene. Diabetes 38: 316–320

24. Ray U, Aulakh G, McClintock PR, Yoon JW, Notkins AL (1983) Virus-induced diabetes mellitus: difference in the RNA fingerprints of diabetogenic and nondiabetogenic variants of encephalomyocarditis virus. J Gen Virol 64: 947–950

25. Yoon JW, Wong AKC, Bae YS, Eun HM (1988) An apparent deletion of an oligonucleotide detected by RNA fingerprint in the nondiabetogenic B variant of encephalomyocarditis virus is due to a point mutation. J Virol 62: 637–640

26. Yoon JW, Ko W, Bae YS, Pak CY, Amano K, Eun HM, Kim MK (1988) Identification of antigenic differences between the diabetogenic and nondiabetogenic variants of encephalomyocarditis virus by monoclonal antibodies. J Gen Virol 69: 1085–1090

27. Eun HM, Bäe YS, Yoon JW (1988) Amino acid differences in capsid protein, VP1, between diabetogenic and nondiabetogenic variants of encephalomyocarditis virus. Virology 163: 369–373

28. Ross ME, Onodera T, Brown KS, Notkins AL (1976) Virus-induced diabetes mellitus IV. Genetic and environmental factors influencing the development of diabetes after infection with the M variant of encephalomyocarditis virus. Diabetes 25: 190–197

29. Yoon JW, Notkins AL (1976) Virus-induced diabetes mellitus VI. Genetically determined host differences in the replication of encephalomyocarditis virus in pancreatic beta cells. J Exp Med 143: 170–185

30. Yoon JW, Lesniak MA, Fussganger R, Notkins AL (1976) Genetic differences in the susceptibility of pancreatic B cells to virus-induced diabetes mellitus. Nature 265: 178–180

31. Onodera T, Yoon JW, Brown KS, Notkins AL (1978) Evidence for a single locus controlling susceptibility to virus-induced diabetes mellitus. Nature 274: 693–695

32. Morishima T, McClintock PR, Billups LC, Notkins AL (1982) Expression and modulation of virus receptors on lymphoid and myeloid cells: relationship to infectivity. Virology 116: 605–618

33. Ross ME, Hayashi K, Notkins AL (1974) Virus-induced pancreatic disease: alterations in concentration of glucose and amylase in blood. J Inf Dis 129: 669–676

34. Yoon JW, Onodera T, Notkins AL (1978) Virus-induced diabetes mellitus. XI. Replication of Coxsackie virus B3 in human pancreatic beta cell cultures. Diabetes 27: 778–782

35. Prince G, Jenson AB, Billups L, Notkins AL (1978) Infection of human pancreatic beta cell cultures with mumps virus. Nature 271: 158–161

36. Yoon JW, Selvaggio S, Onodera T, Wheeler J, Jenson AB (1981) Infection of cultured human pancreatic B cell with reovirus type 3. Diabetologia 20: 462–468

37. McLaren LC, Holland JJ, Syverton JT (1959) The mammalian cell-virus relationship. J Exp Med 109: 475–483

38. Friman G, Fohlman J, Frisk G, Diderholm H, Ewald U, Kobbah M, Tuvemo T (1985) An incuidence peak of juvenile diabetes. Relation to Coxsackie B virus immune response. Acta Paediatr Scand [Suppl] 320: 14–19

39. Eisenbarth GS (1986) Type I diabetes mellitus. A chronic autoimmune disease. N Engl J Med 314: 1360–1368

40. Baekkeskov S, Nielsen JH, Marner B, Lernmark A (1982) Autoantibodies in newly diagnosed diabetic children immunoprecipitate specific human pancreatic islet cell protein. Nature 298: 167–169

41. Foulis AK, Farquharsaon MA, Maeger A (1987) Immunoreactive α-interferon in insulin-secreting B cells in type I diabetes mellitus. Lancet ii: 1423–1427

42. Ginsberg-Fellner F, Witt ME, Fedun B et al. (1985) Diabetes mellitus and autoimmunity in patients with congenital rubella syndrome. Rev Infect Dis 7 [Suppl 1]: 170–175

43. Rayfield EJ, Kelly KJ, Yoon JW (1986) Rubella virus-induced diabetes in hamsters. Diabetes 35: 1278–1281

44. Fauci AC (1980) Immunoregulation of autoimmunity. J Allergy Clin Immunol 66: 5–17

45. Reinherz EL, Schlossmann SF (1980) Regulation of the immune response inducer and suppressor T-lymphocytes subsets in human beings. N Engl J Med 303: 370 373

46. Onodera T, Jenson AB, Yoon JW, Notkins AL (1978) Virus-induced diabetes mellitus. Reovirus infection of pancreatic beta cells in mice. Science 301: 529–531

47. Onodera T, Toniolo A, Ray UR, Jenson AB, Knazek RA, Notkins AL (1981) Virus-induced diabetes mellitus. J Exp Med 153: 1457–1465

48. Onodera T, Ray UR, Melez KA, Suzuki H, Toniolo A, Notkins AL (1982) Virus-induced diabetes mellitus. Autoimmunity and polyendocrine disease prevented by immunosuppression. Nature 297: 66–69

49. Kataoka S, Satoh J, Fujiya H, Toyota T, Suzuki R, Itoh K, Kumagai K (1983) Immunologic aspects of the Nonobese Diabetes (NOD) mouse: abnormalities of cellular immunity. Diabetes 32: 247–253

50. Lee KU, Amano K, Yoon JW (1988) Evidence for initial involvement of macrophage in development of insulitis in NOD mice. Diabetes 37: 989–991

51. Harada M, Makino S (1982) Promotion of spontaneous diabetes in nonobese diabetes-prone mice by cyclophosphamide. Diabetologia 27: 604–606

52. Harada M, Sueishi T, Misaki R, Makino S (1987) Possible role of Lyt 2+ T cells in cyclophosphamide-enhanced diabetes in NOD mice. International research symposium "The immunology of diabetes". Oct. 27–30 1987, Woods Hole, Massachusetts

53. Ikeda H, Pincus T, Yoshiki T, Strand M, August JT, Boyse EA, Mellors RC (1974) Biological expression of antigenic determinants of murine leukemia virus proteins gp 69/71 and p. 30. J Virol 14: 1274–1280
54. Del Villano BC, Nave B, Croker BP (1975) The oncornavirus glycoprotein gp 69/71: a constituent of the surface of normal and malignant thymocytes. J Exp Med 141: 172–187
55. Kennel SJ, Feldman JD (1976) Distribution of viral glycoprotein gp 69/71 on cell surfaces of producer and nonproducer cells. Cancer Res 36: 200–208
56. Lerner RA, Wilson CB, Del Villano BC, McCohahey PJ, Dixon FJ (1976) Endogenous oncornaviral gene expression in adult and fetal mice: quantitative histologic, and physiologic studies of the major viral glycoprotein, gp 70. J Exp Med 143: 151–166
57. Unanue ER, Allen PM (1987) The basis for the immunoregulatory role of macrophages and other accessory cells. Science 236: 551–557
58. Toews GB, Bergstresser PR, Streilein JW (1980) Epidermal Langerhans cell density determines whether contact hypersensitivity or unresponsiveness follows skin painting with DNFB. J Immunol 124: 445–453
59. Oldstone MBA, Southern P, Rodriguez M, Lampert P (1984) Virus persists in B cells of islets of Langerhans and is associated with chemical manifestations of diabetes. Science 224: 1440–1443
60. Notkins AL, Yoon JW (1984) Virus-induced diabetes. In: Notkins AL, Oldstone MBA (eds) Concepts in viral pathogenesis. Springer, New York, pp 241–247
61. Menser MA, Forrest JM, Bransby RD (1978) Rubella infection and diabetes mellitus. Lancet i: 57–60
62. Schopfer K, Matter L, Flueler U, Werder E (1982) Diabetes mellitus, endocrine autoantibodies and prenatal rubella infection. Lancet ii: 159
63. Underwood LE, Van Wyk JJ (1981) Hormones in normal and aberrant growth. In: Williams RH (ed) Textbook of endocrinology, 6th edn. Saunders, Philadelphia pp 1149–1184
64. Preece MA, Kearney PJ, Marshall WC (1977) Growth-hormone deficiency in congenital rubella. Lancet ii: 842–844
65. Smithsells RW, Sheppard S, Marshall WC, Peckham C (1978) Congenital rubella and diabetes mellitus. Lancet i: 439
66. Unanue ER (1984) Antigen-presenting function of the macrophages. Annu Rev Immunol 2: 395–428
67. Patterson K, Chandra RS, Jenson AB (1981) Congenital rubella, insulitis and diabetes mellitus in an infant. Lancet i: 1048–1049
68. Ginsberg-Fellner F, Witt ME, Yagihashi S et al. (1984) Congenital rubella-syndrome as a model for type I (insulin-dependent) diabetes mellitus: increased prevalence of islet cell surface antibodies. Diabetologia 27: 87–89
69. Ginsberg-Fellner F, Fedun B, Cooper Z et al. (1987) Interrelationships of congenital rubella and type I insulin dependent diabetes mellitus. In: Jaworski MA, Molnar GD, Rajotte RV, Singh B (eds) The immunology of diabetes mellitus. Elsevier, Amsterdam, pp 279–286
70. Ward KP, Galloway WH, Auchterlonie IA (1979) Congenital cytomegalovirus infection and diabetics. Lancet i: 497
71. Fox JG, Murphy JC (1979) Cytomegalic virus-associated insulitis in diabetic Octodon degus. Vet Pathol 16: 625–628
72. Helmke K, Otten A, Willems W (1980) Islet cell antibodies in children with mumps infection. Lancet ii: 211–212
73. Gamble DR (1980) Relation of antecedent illness to development of diabetes in children. Br Med J 2: 99–101
74. Ratzman KP, Strese J, Witt S, Berling H, Keilacker H, Michaelis D (1984) Mumps infection and insulin-dependent diabetes mellitus (IDDM). Diabetes Care 7: 170–3
75. Marliss EB (ed) (1983) The Juvenile Diabetes Foundation workshop on the spontaneously diabetic BB rat: its potential for insight into human juvenile diabetes. Metab Clin Exp 32 [Suppl 1]: 1–166
76. Nakhooda AF, Like AA, Chappel CI, Wei CN, Marliss EB (1978) The spontaneously diabetic Wistar rat (the "BB" rat): studies prior to and during development of the overt syndrome. Diabetologia 14: 199–207

77. Seemayer TA, Tannenbaum GS, Goldman H, Colle E (1982) Dynamic time course studies of the spontaneously diabetic BB Wistar rat. III. Light microscopic and ultrastructural observations of pancreatic islets of Langerhans. Am J Pathol 106: 237–249

78. Logothetopoulos J, Valiquette N, Madura E, Cvet D (1984) The onset and progression of pancreatic insulitis in the overt, spontaneously diabetic, young adult BB rat studied by pancreatic biopsy. Diabetes 33: 33:36

79. Pollard DR, Gupta K, Manchino L, Hynie I (1983) An immunofluorescence study of antipancreatic islet cell antibodies in the spontaneously diabetic BB Wistar rat. Diabetologia 25: 56–59

80. Dyrberg T, Nakhooda AF, Baekkeskov S, Lernmark A, Poussier P, Marliss EB (1982) Islet cell surface antibodies and lymphocyte antibodies in the spontaneously diabetic BB Wistar rat. Diabetes 31: 278–281

81. Laborie C, Sai P, Feutren G, Debray-Sachs M, Quiniou-Debrie MC, Pousier P, Marliss EB, Assan R (1985) Time course of islet cell antibodies in diabetic and nondiabetic BB rats. Diabetes 34: 904–910

82. Like AA, Kislauskis E, Williams RM, Rossini AA (1982) Neonatal thymectomy prevents spontaneous diabetes mellitus in the BB/W rat. Science 216: 644–646

83. Like AA, Rossini AA, Appel MC, Guberski DL, Williams RM (1979) Spontaneous diabetes mellitus: reversal and prevention in the BB/W rat with antiserum to rat lymphocytes. Science 206: 1421–1423

84. Like AA, Anthony M, Guberski DL, Rossini AA (1983) Spontaneous diabetes in the BB/W rat: effects of glucocorticoids, cyclosporin-A, and antiserum to rat lymphocytes. Diabetes 32: 326–330

85. Laupacis A, Stiller CR, Gardell C, Keown P, Dupre J, Wallace AC, Thibert P (1983) Cyclosporin prevents diabetes in BB Wistar rats. Lancet i: 10–12

86. Naji A, Silvers WK, Bellgrau D, Barker CF (1981) Spontaneous diabetes in rats: destruction of islets is prevented by immunological tolerance. Science 213: 1390–1392

87. Scott J, Engelhard VH, Curnow RT, Benjamin DC (1986) Prevention of diabetes in BB rats. I. Evidence suggesting a requirement for mature T cells in bone marrow inoculum of neonatally injected rats. Diabetes 35: 1034–1040

88. Rossini AA, Mordes JP, Pelletier AM, Like AA (1983) Transfusions of whole blood prevent spontaneous diabetes mellitus in the BB/W rat. Science 219: 975–977

89. Rossini AA, Faustmann D, Woda BA, Like AA, Szymanski I, Mordes JP (1984) Lymphocyte transfusions prevent diabetes in the Bio-Breeding/Worcester rat. J Clin Invest 74: 39–46

90. Koevary SB, Rossini A, Stoller W, Chick WL (1983) Passive transfer of diabetes in the BB/W rat. Science 220: 727–728

91. Koevary SD, Williams DE, Williams RM, Chick WL (1985) Passive transfer of diabetes from BB/W to Wistar-Furth rats. J Clin Invest 75: 1904–1907

92. Dyrberg T, Schwimmbeck PL, Oldstone MBA (1988) Inhibition of diabetes in BB rats by virus infection. J Clin Invest 81: 928–931

93. Koike T, Itoh Y, Ishii T, Ito I, Takabayashi K, Maruyama N, Tomioka H, Yoshida S (1987) Preventive effect of monoclonal anti-L3T4 antibody on development of diabetes in NOD mice. Diabetes 36: 539–541

94. Wang Y, Hao L, Gill RG, Lafferty KJ (1987) Autoimmune diabetes in NOD mouse is L3T4 T-lymphocyte dependent. Diabetes 36: 535–538

95. Miyazaki A, Hanafusa T, Yamada K, Miyagawa J, Nakajima H, Nonaka K, Tarui S (1985) Predominance of T lymphocytes in pancreatic islets and spleen of pre-diabetic non-obese diabetic (NOD) mice: a longitudinal study. Clin Exp Immunol 6: 622–627

96. Oldstone MBA (1988) Prevention of Type I diabetes in nonobese diabetic mice by virus infection. Science 239: 500–502

97. Lee KU, Amano K, Yoon JW (1988) Evidence for initial involvement of macrophage in development of insulitis in NOD mice. Diabetes 37: 989–991

Autoimmunität beim Typ I-Diabetes

W. A. SCHERBAUM

Summary

Type I (insulin-dependent) diabetes mellitus is brought about by a chronic autoimmune process directed towards the islets of Langerhans, finally leading to a specific destruction of the beta cells. It has been shown that there exists a genetic susceptibility which is mainly linked with genes of the major histocompatibility complex, namely HLA-DR3, -DR4, and combinations of these HLA specificities, and that distinct DQß chain alleles confer protection from the disease. The initiating event leading to the autoimmune process still remains unclear. Infiltration of the islets with mononuclear cells is seen in the early stages of the desease and aberrant expression of HLA class II antigens as well as gamma-interferon immunostaining can be exclusively demonstrated on beta cells.

While T cells probably play the key role in the pathogenesis of beta cell destruction, islet cell specific autoantibodies are the most useful markers of autoimmunity in type I diabetes. Cytoplasmic islet cell antibodies (ICA) and/or autoantibodies to the 64-kDa islet cell antigen are positive in 80% – 100% of newly diagnosed cases. ICA are directed towards a glycolipid component of all endocrine islet cells whereas antibodies to the 64-kDa antigen as well as ICA detected by an ELISA recognize a protein. Autoantibodies to insulin (IAA) and/ or proinsulin may also be detected in 40–60% of cases before the initiation of insulin therapy.

The above mentioned antibodies may be detected months or years before the abrupt onset of clinical symptoms. This notion has enabled prospective studies of the natural course of the disease in predisposed 1st degree relatives of type I diabetic patients and in epidemiological screening programmes. In otherwise healthy relatives high levels of ICA, the presence of complement-fixing ICA, and the detection of IAA by radioimmunoassays indicate a high risk for future development of type I diabetes. A blunted first-phase insulin response to i.v. glucose appears to be the most sensitive marker for an irreversible metabolic deterioration. By a better understanding of the natural course of the disease and the associated immune process it will be possible to proceed with early immune intervention trials aiming at interruption of the autoimmune beta cell destruction.

Einleitung

Der Typ I-Diabetes wird durch einen Prozeß hervorgerufen, der zu einer Destruktion der insulinproduzierenden Betazellen der Langerhans'schen Inseln des Pankreas führt. Im folgenden soll gezeigt werden, daß es sich dabei um einen spezifischen chronischen Autoimmunprozeß handelt, der sich auf einer genetischen Grundlage entwickelt und bei dessen Entstehung äußere Faktoren eine Rolle spielen dürften. Die Analyse der dabei auftretenden Autoimmunphänomene läßt Aussagen über den Krankheitsverlauf zu und ermöglicht neue Einsichten in pathogenetische Zusammenhänge, die unter anderem für therapeutische Interventionen von Bedeutung sind [36]. Einige Fakten, die auf die Rolle autoimmuner Reaktionen bei der Entstehung des Typ I-Diabetes hinweisen, sind in Tabelle 1 zusammengestellt.

Immungenetik des Typ I-Diabetes

Zwillingsuntersuchungen bieten eine gute Möglichkeit, den Einfluß der genetischen und der Umweltkomponenten für die Entwicklung des Typ I-Diabetes abzuschätzen. Von eineiigen Zwillingen, bei denen einer an einem Typ I-Diabetes erkrankt ist, entwickeln 35 % ihrer zunächst nichtdiabetischen Geschwister die Erkrankung in einem Beobachtungszeitraum von 30 Jahren [3]. Heute ist bekannt, daß dieses genetische Risiko überwiegend an HLA-Gene gekoppelt ist. Am engsten ist die Beziehung zu bestimmten HLA-Klasse II (DR, DP, DQ)-Allelen. Über 90 % der Typ I-Diabetiker tragen das HLA-Merkmal DR3 und/oder DR4. Charakteristisch ist ein heterozygoter DR3/DR4-Genotyp, während DR2, DR5 und DR7 negativ mit dem Typ I-Diabetes assoziiert sind [4].

Tabelle 1. Hinweise für eine autoimmune Genese des Typ I-Diabetes

Infiltrat der Pankreasinseln mit mononukleären Zellen (initial)

Nachweis humoraler Autoimmunreaktionen
- Zytoplasmatische Inselzellantikörper (ICA)
- Antikörper gegen das 64 KD-Inselzellprotein
- Inselzelloberflächenantikörper (ICSA)
- Autoantikörper gegen Insulin (IAA)/Proinsulin

Zelluläre Autoimmunreaktionen gegen Inselzellbestandteile

Assoziation mit anderen Autoimmunerkrankungen und Autoantikörpern

Wirksamkeit einer Cyclosporin A-Therapie beim Typ I-Diabetes

Wirksamkeit von Immuninterventionen bei Tiermodellen des insulinpflichtigen Diabetes

Tabelle 2. Ethnische Variationen der HLA-Assoziation des insulinpflichtigen Diabetes

Ethnische Gruppe	Gehäufte HLA-Assoziation		
	DR3	DR4	DRw9
Europäer	+	+	−
Chinesen	+	−	+
Japaner	−	+	+

Neuere Daten weisen darauf hin, daß der Typ I-Diabetes stärker mit DQ- als mit DR-Genen assoziiert ist. Faszinierende Ergebnisse erbrachte die Sequenzanalyse der DQβ-Kette. Bei HLA DR4-positiven Kaukasiern ist die Aminosäure in Position 57 entscheidend: Eine Asparaginsäure in Position 57 „schützt" vor dem Erwerb eines Typ I-Diabetes [49]. Diese Befunde erlauben nun individuelle DNA-Analysen zur Abschätzung des Diabetesrisikos mit Hilfe von Gensonden [27]. Für die weitere Forschung auf der Suche nach „dem Empfänglichkeitsgen" für den Typ I-Diabetes ist aber immer noch die Analyse des gesamten HLA-Komplexes wichtig [41]. Neuere Daten weisen darauf hin, daß die Empfänglichkeit für den Typ I-Diabetes durch eine Kombination bestimmter DR- und DQ-Gene signifikant gesteigert wird. Die Untersuchungsergebnisse von HLA-Assoziationen bei Typ I-Diabetikern verschiedener ethnischer Gruppen zeigen, daß wir mit den bisher bekannten Markern nicht die Krankheitsgene definieren, sondern daß man lediglich damit assoziierte Gene erkennt (Tabelle 2).

HLA-Klasse II-Moleküle stellen Zelloberflächenrezeptoren dar, die in der Lage sind, Peptidfragmente fremder oder eigener Proteine zu binden und sie so den T-Lymphozyten zu präsentieren. Die Struktur eines HLA-Klasse II-Allels hat einen wesentlichen Einfluß auf die Bindung eines bestimmten Peptids, was seinerseits die Immunantwort gegen dieses Peptid bestimmen kann [50]. Rezeptoren auf T-Helferzellen erkennen fremde Proteine nur dann, wenn sie an ein körpereigenes HLA-Klasse II-Molekül gebunden sind. Darüber hinaus ist ein bestimmter T-Lymphozyt sowohl peptidspezifisch als auch HLA restringiert und erkennt ein definiertes Peptid nur dann, wenn es an ein ganz bestimmtes HLA-Klasse II-Molekül gebunden ist [25].

Pathologie und Immunpathologie des Typ I-Diabetes

Die Pankreasinseln des Typ I-Diabetikers sind verarmt an Betazellen, während die übrige endokrine Zellmasse der Inseln nicht reduziert ist. Diese ursprünglichen Beobachtungen von Gepts [19] konnten in umfangreichen Untersuchungen von Foulis [15] bestätigt werden. Einige wenige Betazellen können jedoch auch nach längerer Diabetesdauer übrigbleiben. In den ersten sechs Monaten nach Beginn der Krankheit findet man in der Regel eine Insulitis, die besonders ausgeprägt ist, wenn der Diabetes vor dem 15. Lebensjahr auftritt. Bei den zellulären Inselinfiltraten handelt es sich um ein buntes Bild mononukleärer Zellen [8] einschließlich Makrophagen [18]. Das exokrine Pankreas ist nicht von dem entzündlichen Prozeß betroffen, zeigt aber eine Verarmung an Zymogengranula periinsulärer Zellen, die wahrscheinlich auf einen fehlenden trophischen Effekt des Insulins zurückzuführen ist.

Aberrante Expression von HLA-Klasse II-Molekülen auf Betazellen

In einer Serie von Untersuchungen konnte gezeigt werden, daß Inselzellen von Patienten mit frisch manifestiertem Typ I-Diabetes im Gegensatz zu normalen Inselzellen HLA DR-Moleküle exprimieren [8, 16, 30]. Ein weiteres auffälliges Phänomen ist die auf die Betazellen begrenzte immunhistochemische Nachweisbarkeit von alpha-Interferon in Pankreata von Patienten mit frisch manifestiertem Typ I-Diabetes [17]. Diese Befunde weisen auf eine chronische Auseinandersetzung der Betazellen mit einem Virus, am ehesten mit Retroviren hin.

In vitro konnte zwar durch Inkubation mit gamma-Interferon + Tumor-Nekrose-Faktor alpha eine aberrante Expression von HLA DR-Molekülen auf Inselzellen induziert werden; diese ist jedoch nicht auf Betazellen beschränkt [32], so daß die Initiierung des Betazell-spezifischen destruktiven Prozesses nicht alleine auf einen Einfluß dieser Interleukine zurückgeführt werden kann.

Zelluläre Autoimmunreaktionen

In den ersten drei bis sechs Monaten nach Beginn des Typ I-Diabetes ist die Zahl der im peripheren Blut nachweisbaren aktivierten T-Lymphozyten erhöht [1, 21, 26], was auf eine allgemeine Stimulation des Immunsystems hinweist. Des weiteren wurde beim Typ I-Diabetes eine vermehrte zytotoxische Aktivität gegen Inselzellen [9] und eine erhöhte Killerzellaktivität [31] beschrieben.

Die Angaben über Störungen zellvermittelter Immunreaktionen bezüglich der Verteilung zirkulierender T-Suppressorzellen und T-Helferzellen sowie über die Ergebnisse der gemischten Lymphozytenkultur und eine Mitogenstimulation von Lymphozyten sind zum Teil sehr widersprüchlich [13]. Dies hängt unter anderem damit zusammen, daß unterschiedliche Patientengruppen gewählt wurden, die Reagenzien zum Teil nicht standardisiert sind und daß in verschiedenen Tests unterschiedliche immunologische Parameter gemessen werden. Das wesentliche Hindernis für die Gewinnung eines einheitlichen Bildes liegt jedoch in der Nichtverfügbarkeit des Inselzellantigens begründet, das für den in vitro Nachweis einer betazellspezifischen zellulären Autoimmunreaktion unabdingbar ist.

Humorale Autoimmunreaktionen

Ebenso wie die zellulären Immunphänomene, so ist auch die Nachweisbarkeit von Typ I-Diabetes-spezifischen Autoantikörpern eng mit dem Vorhandensein residualer Betazellen verbunden. Beim frisch manifestierten Typ I-Diabetes können die konventionellen Inselzellantikörper (ICA) im indirekten Immunfluoreszenztest in 70 bis 90 % der Fälle gefunden werden. Ihre Prävalenz geht nach einem Jahr Diabetesdauer auf 50 % zurück und bei längerem Bestehen der Krankheit finden sich ICA nur noch in etwa 10 % der Fälle [23]. Bei gesunden Kontrollpersonen sind diese Autoantikörper in weniger als 1 % positiv.

Die im indirekten Immunfluoreszenztest nachgewiesenen Inselzellantikörper reagieren wahrscheinlich mit einem Gangliosid [28]. Entsprechend läßt sich die ICA-Reaktivität durch Präinkubation der Seren mit einem Glykolipidextrakt von menschlichem Pankreas blockieren [11]. Während ICA ausschließlich vom IgG-Typ sind, können Inselzelloberflächenantikörper (ICSA) auch der IgM-Klasse angehören. ICSA schließen insbesondere die zytotoxischen ICSA ein, die bisher allerdings nur im Rahmen begrenzter Studien untersucht worden sind [51]. Seren von Patienten mit Typ I-Diabetes enthalten neben den oben genannten Spezifitäten auch Antikörper gegen ein Inselzellprotein. In den bisher durchgeführten Untersuchungen konnte gezeigt werden, daß diese Antikörper gegen ein 64 KD-Inselzellantigen gerichtet sind und in über 70 % der frisch manifestierten Fälle von Typ I-Diabetes nachzuweisen sind [2]; sie korrelieren aber nicht mit den Ergebnissen der ICA-Bestimmung [10]. Ähnlich korrelieren die mit dem ELISA bestimmten Inselzellantikörper [40] und die Antikörper gegen das sogenannte polare Antigen der RIN m 38-Zellen nicht streng mit den ICA-Befunden. Die biochemischen Eigenschaften dieser Antikörper sind in Tabelle 3 wiedergegeben.

Bei 30 bis 50 % der Typ I-Diabetiker können Insulin-Autoantikörper (IAA) im Serum nachgewiesen werden, auch wenn noch kein exogenes Insulin verabreicht worden ist [29, 53]. Es hat sich gezeigt, daß mit den ELISA's (Festphasentests) und mit Radioimmunoassays (Flüssigphasentests) verschiedene Spezifitäten und Affinitäten gemessen werden [43]. Während der ELISA auch bei

Tabelle 3. Einfluß einer biochemischen Vorbehandlung auf verschiedene Inselzellantikörper-Reaktivitäten

Vorbehandlung	Ergebnis des Antikörpertests		
	ICA-IFL	ICA-ELISA	„Polare" Ak
Aceton	+	+	+
Neuraminidase-Verdauung	−	+	+
Methanol-Extraktion	−	−	−
Pronase-Verdauung	+	−	−
Glycolipid-Absorption	−	+	+

einem Drittel der gesunden Familienangehörigen und der Fälle mit polyendokrinen Autoimmunerkrankungen oder von zystischer Fibrose ohne Diabetes positiv ausfällt, ist der RIA spezifischer für die Insulitis des Typ I-Diabetes, insbesondere im Kindesalter.

Neben dem oben beschriebenen inselspezifischen Autoimmunphänomen können beim Typ I-Diabetes vermehrt Autoimmunerkrankungen anderer endokriner Organe, wie z. B. ein Morbus Basedow oder eine Perniziöse Anämie und/oder die dazugehörigen Autoantikörper nachgewiesen werden [5]. Eine interessante neue Spezifität stellen die Autoantikörper gegen Nebennierenmarkzellen dar, die zwar überwiegend bei ICA-positiven Typ I-Diabetikern vorkommen, aber nicht auf eine Kreuzreaktion der ICA zurückzuführen sind [38]. Autoantikörper gegen sympathische Ganglien sind bei Typ I-Diabetikern eventuell für eine Beeinträchtigung der orthostatischen Blutdruckregulation verantwortlich [33].

Wer ist gefährdet?

Als Risikogruppen für den Typ I-Diabetes können zunächst Patienten angesehen werden, bei denen polyendokrine Autoimmunerkrankungen bekannt sind [6, 12]. Insbesondere betrifft dies Patienten mit einem autoimmunen Morbus Addison. Bei diesen kommt in 20 % der Fälle ein Typ I-Diabetes assoziiert vor. Die Hintergründe für diese Assoziationen wurden andernorts im Detail besprochen [35]. Weitere Risikogruppen betreffen Frauen, bei denen ein Schwangerschaftsdiabetes diagnostiziert wurde [14]. Die am besten untersuchte Gruppe betrifft erstgradig Verwandte von Typ I-Diabetikern; etwa 10 % der Fälle von Typ I-Diabetes haben eine entsprechende Familienanamnese, die restlichen 90 % treten sporadisch auf [22]. Diese Tatsache unterstreicht die Bedeutung epidemiologischer Untersuchungen, wenn man das Gros der prädiabetischen Individuen erfassen will. Prospektive Untersuchungen erstgradig Verwandter von Typ I-Diabetikern haben gezeigt, daß schon Jahre vor der klinischen Manifestation des Typ I-Diabetes Inselzellantikörper im Serum nachgewiesen werden können [37]. Auch die immunpräzipitierenden Antikörper gegen das 64 KD-Inselzellprotein sind schon vor Ausbruch der Krankheit vorhanden [2]. Dies weist auf einen längeren subklinischen Verlauf der Insulitis hin [47].

Der „Pseudo-Typ II"-Diabetes

Die oben genannten serologischen Autoimmunphänomene erlauben zusammen mit der HLA-Typisierung und der DNA-Analyse eine ätiologische Zuordnung zur autoimmunen Form des Diabetes, auch wenn er sich in atypischer Weise im höheren Lebensalter erstmals manifestiert oder wenn der Diabetes zunächst mit oralen Antidiabetika einstellbar ist [7, 20]. In diesen Fällen kann ein rasches Sekundärversagen prognostiziert werden.

Metabolische Frühzeichen

Insbesondere aus Verlaufsuntersuchungen nichtdiabetischer identischer Zwillinge und Drillinge von Typ I-Diabetikern ist bekannt, daß die Insulitis und die Entwicklung des Insulinmangels in der Regel einen längeren präklinischen Verlauf nehmen [44]. Dabei können insbesondere bei Kindern das Blutzuckertagesprofil und der orale Glukosetoleranztest (OGTT) bis kurz vor Krankheitsmanifestation normal ausfallen. Dagegen spielt der i.v. GGT bei der Früherkennung einer eingeschränkten Insulinsekretion eine besondere Rolle. Eine Reduktion der ersten Phase der Insulinausschüttung unter die erste Perzentile von Normalpersonen ist mit einem hohen Risiko verbunden, innerhalb der nächsten sechs Monate an einem Typ I-Diabetes zu erkranken. Dies trifft allerdings nur für ICA-positive Individuen zu; auch dem Typ II-Diabetes geht nämlich ein Verlust der frühen Insulinsekretionsphase voraus [52]. Bisher wurde kein Fall beschrieben, in dem sich eine solche frühe, voll ausgeprägte Sekretionsstörung im Spontanverlauf oder unter Therapie wieder normalisiert hätte. Ob sich die erste Phase der Insulinausschüttung kontinuierlich verschlechtert [46] oder einen sprunghaften Verlauf nimmt, ist wegen der starken inter- und intraindividuellen Varianz des Tests [42] und der limitierten Zahl der beobachteten Fälle noch strittig.

Voraussagemöglichkeiten des Typ I-Diabetes

Die ICA spielen für die Erkennung der prädiabetischen Phase eine herausragende Rolle [24]. Hohe ICA-Spiegel scheinen prognostisch ebenso relevant zu sein, wie der Nachweis einer komplementbindenden Eigenschaft der ICA. Alle nichtdiabetischen erstgradig Verwandten von Typ I-Diabetikern, bei denen in den englischen Familienuntersuchungen die ICA-Titer bei 80 JDF-Einheiten oder darüber lagen, entwickelten im Laufe von acht Jahren einen Diabetes. Niedrigere Titer sind mit einem geringeren Risiko verbunden. Schließlich können niedrigtitrige ICA auch nur vorrübergehend nachweisbar sein und haben dann weniger Bedeutung [45]. ICA-negative Verwandte hatten in Verlaufsuntersuchungen über fünf bis acht Jahre ein kumulatives Risiko von unter 1 % [48].

In jüngster Zeit ist die Wertigkeit der IAA für die Voraussage des Typ I-Diabetes näher untersucht worden. Verwandte, die sowohl ICA- als auch IAA-positiv sind, tragen ein höheres Risiko für den Typ I-Diabetes als solche mit nur einem der Marker. Im Gegensatz zu den in Radioimmunoassays nachgewiesenen IAA sind die mit dem ELISA-Test bestimmten IAA für sich alleine nicht sicher mit einem erhöhten Diabetesrisiko verbunden. Die Bestimmung von Antikörpern gegen das 64 KD-Inselzellprotein wird für die Voraussage des Typ I-Diabetes insbesondere bei Kindern und Jugendlichen eine größere Bedeutung erlangen [34], sobald vereinfachte Detektionsmethoden für diese Spezifität zur Verfügung stehen [39].

Literatur

1. Alviggi L, Hoskins PJ, Pyke DA, Johnston C, Tee DEH, Leslie RDG, Vergani D (1984) Pathogenesis of insulin-dependent diabetes: a role for activated T lymphocytes. Lancet II: 4–6
2. Baekkeskov S, Landin M, Kristensen JK, Srikanta S, Bruining GJ, Mandrup-Poulsen T, de Beaufort C, Soeldner JS, Eisenbarth G, Lindgren F, Sundquist G, Lernmark Å (1987) Antibodies to a 64,000 Mr human islet cell antigen percede the clinical onset of insulin-dependent diabetes. J Clin Invest 79: 926–934
3. Barnett AH, Eff C, Leslie RDG, Pyke DA (1981) Diabetes in identical twins: a study of 200 pairs. Diabetologia 20: 87–93
4. Bertrams J, Baur MP (1984) Disease reports: Insulin-dependent diabetes mellitus. In: Albert ED, Baur MP, Mayr WR (eds) Histocompatibility Testing. Springer, Berlin, Heidelberg, New York, pp 348–358
5. Betterle C, Zanette F, Pedini E, Presotto F, Rapp LB, Monciotti CM, Rigon F (1984) Clinical and subclinical organspecific autoimmune manifestations in type I (insulin-dependent) diabetic patients and their first-degree relatives. Diabetologia 620: 431–436
6. Betterle C, Presotto F, Pedini B, Moro L, Slack RS, Zanette F, Zanchetta R (1987) Islet cell and insulin autoantibodies in organ-specific autoimmune patients. Their behaviour and predictive value for the development of type I (insulin-dependent) diabetes mellitus. A 10-year follow-up study. Diabetologia 30: 292–297
7. Böhm BO, Schifferdecker E, Kuehnl P, Scherbaum WA, Schöffling K (1989) Linkage of type I (insulin-dependent) diabetes mellitus and "pseudo type II" diabetes with HLA DRw52 subtype. Molecular heterogeneity of the HLA DRß3 gene in HLA DR3 containing haplotype. Horm metab Res (in press)
8. Bottazzo GF, Dean BM, McNally JM, MacKay EH, Swift PGF, Gamble DR (1985) In situ characterization of autoimmune phenomena and expression of HLA molecules in the pancreas in diabetic insulitis. N Engl J Med 313: 353–360
9. Charles MA, Suzuki M, Waldeck N, Dodson LE, Slater L, Ong K, Kershnar A, Buckingham B, Golden M (1983) Immun islet killing mechanisms associated with insulin-dependent diabetes: in vitro expression of cellular and antibody-mediated islet cell toxicity in humans. J Immunol 130: 1189–1194
10. Christie M, Landin-Olsson M, Sundquist G, Dalquist G, Lernmark Å, Baekkeskov S (1988) Antibodies to a Mr-64,000 islet cell protein in Swedish children with newly diagnosed type I (insulin-dependent) diabetes. Diabetologia 31: 597–602
11. Colman PG, Nayak RC, Campbell IL, Ramesh C, Jain L, Eisenbarth GS (1988) Binding of cytoplasmic islet cell antibodies is blocked by human pancreatic glycolipid extracts. Diabetes 37: 645–652
12. Doniach D, Bottazzo GF (1981) Polyendocrine autoimmunity. In: Franklin EC, Buckley RH, Doniach D, Fahey JL, Parker CW, Rosse WS (eds) Clinical immunology update. Elsevier, New York, pp 95–121
13. Drell DW, Notkins AL (1987) Multiple immunological abnormalities in patients with type I (insulin-dependent) diabetes mellitus. Diabetologia 30: 132–143
14. Freinkel N, Metzger BE, Phelps RL, Simpson JL, Martin AO, Radvany R, Ober C, Dooley SL, Depp RO, Belton A (1986) Gestational diabetes mellitus: a syndrome with phenotypic and genotypic heterogeneity. Horm metab Res 18: 427–430

15. Foulis AK, Liddle CN, Farquharson MA, Richmond JA, Weir RS (1986 a) The histopathology of the pancreas in type I (insulin-dependent) diabetes mellitus: a 25-year review of deaths in patients under 20 years of age in the United Kingdom. Diabetologia 29: 267–274
16. Foulis AK, Farquharson MA (1986 b) Aberrant expression of HLA-DR antigens by insulin-containing β-cells in recent-onset type I diabetes mellitus. Diabetes 35: 1215–1224
17. Foulis AK, Farquharson MA, Meager A (1987) Immunoreactive alpha-interferon in insulin-secreting β-cells in type I diabetes mellitus. Lancet II: 1423–1427
18. Foulis AK (1988) Does a non-cytopathic viral infection of β-cells initiate the disease process leading up to their autoimmune destruction? Session 4: Viral Mechanisms. The Immunology of Diabetes. IXth International Workshop. Satellite Symposium at Melbourne, Australia
19. Gepts W (1965) Pathologic anatomy of the pancreas in juvenile diabetes mellitus. Diabetes 14: 619–633
20. Groop L, Miettinen A, Groop PH, Meri S, Koskimies S, Bottazzo GF (1988) Organ-specific autoimmunity and HLA-DR antigens as markers for β-cell destruction in patients with type II diabetes. Diabetes 37: 99–103
21. Jackson RA, Morris MA, Haynes BF, Eisenbarth GS (1982) Increased circulating Ia-antigen-bearing T cells in type I diabetes mellitus. N Engl J Med 306: 785–788
22. Jarett L, Soeldner JS, Lernmark A, Rizza R, Santiago J (1986) Panel discussion I: diagnosis, classification, and value of screening for diabetes mellitus. Clin Chem 32: B 30–B 36
23. Lendrum R, Walker G, Cudworth AG, Theophanides C, Pyke DA, Bloom A, Gamble DR (1976) Islet-cell antibodies in diabetes mellitus. Lancet II: 1273–1276
24. MacLaren NK (1988) How, when, and why to predict IDDM. Diabetes 37: 1591–1594
25. Marrack P, Kappler J (1988) T cells can distinguish between allogeneic major histocompatibility complex products on different cell types. Nature 332: 840–843
26. Mascart-Lemone F, Delespesse G, Dorchy H, Lemière B, Servais G (1982) Characterization of immunoregulatory T lymphocytes in insulin-dependent diabetic children by means of monoclonal antibodies. Clin Exp Immunol 47: 296–300
27. Morel PA, Dorman JS, Todd JA, McDevitt HO, Trucco M (1988) Aspartic acid at position 57 of the HLA-DQβ chain protects against type I diabetes: A family study. Proc Natl Acad Sci USA 85: 8111–8115
28. Nayak RC, Omar MAK, Rabizadeh A, Srikanta S, Eisenbarth GS (1985) "Cyotplasmic" islet cell antibodies: evidence that the target antigen is a sialoglycoconjugate. Diabetes 34: 617–619
29. Palmer JP, Asplin CM, Clemons P, Lyen K, Tatpaty O, Raghu PK, Pacquette TL (1983) Insulin antibodies in insulin-dependent diabetics before insulin treatment. Science 222: 1337–1339
30. Pipeleers DG, In't Veld PA, Pipeleers-Marichal MA, Gepts W, Van de Winkel M (1987) Presence of pancreatic hormones in islet cells with MHC-class II antigen expression. Diabetes 36: 872–876
31. Pozzilli P, Gorsuch A, Sensi M, Bottazzo GF, Cudworth AG (1979) Evidence for raised K-cell levels in type I diabetes. Lancet II: 173–175
32. Pujol-Borrell R, Todd I, Doshi M, Bottazzo GF, Sutton R, Gray D, Adolf GR, Feldmann M (1987) HLA class II induction in human islet cells by interferon gamma plus tumour necrosis factor or lymphotoxin. Nature 326: 304–306
33. Rabinowe SL, Brown FM, Watts M, Kadrofske MM, Vinik AI (1989) Anti-sympathetic ganglia antibodies and postural blood pressure in IDDM subjects of varying duration and patients at high risk of developing IDDM. Diabetes Care 12: 1–6
34. Riley W (1988) Epidemiological aspects of immune markers for type I diabetes XIII Congress of the Internationel Diabetes Foundation Sydney Australia, 20–25 November 1988
35. Scherbaum WA, Youinou P, Tater D, Jouquan J, Pujol-Borrell R, Bercovici JP, Bottazzo GF (1986) Polyendocrinopathies autoimmunes. Hypothèses pathogéniques. Annales d'Endocrinologie (Paris) 47: 420–428
36. Scherbaum WA (1987) Klinische Aspekte zur Immunpathogenese des Diabetes mellitus Typ I. Internist 820: 228–235
37. Scherbaum WA, Böhm BO, Schöffling K, Pfeiffer EF (1987) Diagnostik der Autoimmuninsulitis vor der klinischen Manifestation des Diabetes mellitus Typ I. Med Klin 82: 443–446

38. Scherbaum WA, Mogel H, Böhm BO, Hedderich U, Glück M, Schernthaner G, Bottazzo GF, Pfeiffer EF (1988 a) Autoantibodies to adrenal medullary and thyroid calcitonin cells in type I diabetes mellitus – a prospective study. J Autoimmunity 1: 219–230
39. Scherbaum WA, Böhm BO, Ketzler-Sasse U, Schöffling K, Pfeiffer EF (1988 b) ICA-positive sera as well as single-cell antibodies to somatostatin and glucagon cells bind to a common 64 KD islet cell protein. Diabetes Research and Clinical Practice. XIIIth Congress of the International Diabetes Federation. Suppl 1, Vol 5: S 51
40. Scherbaum WA, Seißler J, Hedderich U, Böhm BO, Specker M, Pfeiffer EF (1989) Determination of islet cell antibodies using an ELISA with a preparation of rat insulinoma (RINA2) cells. Diabetes Research 10: 97–102
41. Segall M (1988) HLA and genetics of IDDM. Holism vs. reductionism? Diabetes 37: 1005–1008
42. Smith CP, Tarn AC, Thomas JM, Overkamp D, Corakci A, Savage MO, Gale EAM (1988) Between and within subject variation of the first phase insulin response to intravenous glucose. Diabetologia 31: 123–125
43. Sodoyez-Goffaux F, Koch M, Dozio N, Brandenburg D, Sodoyez J-Cl (1988) Advantages and pitfalls of radioimmune and enzyme linked immunosorbent assays of insulin antibodies. Diabetologia 31: 694–702
44. Soeldner JS, Srikanta S, Eisenbarth GS, Gleason RE (1986) Pre-hyperglycemic diabetes mellitus. Clin Chem 32: B7–B18
45. Spencer KM, Tarn A, Dean BM, Lister J, Bottazzo GF (1984) Fluctuating islet cell autoimmunity in uneffected relatives of patients with insulin-dependent diabetes. Lancet I: 764–766
46. Srikanta S, Ganda OP, Gleason RE, Jackson RA, Soeldner JS, Eisenbarth GS (1984) Pretype I diabetes. Linear loss of beta cell response to intravenous glucose. Diabetes 33: 717–720
47. Tarn AC, Smith CP, Spencer KM, Bottazzo GF, Gale EAM (1987) Type I (insulin-dependent) diabetes: a disease of slow clinical onset? Brit Med J 294: 342–345
48. Tarn AC, Thomas JM, Dean BM, Ingram D, Schwartz G, Bottazzo GF, Gale EAM (1988) Predicting insulin-dependent diabetes. Lancet I: 845–850
49. Todd JA, Bell JI, McDevitt HO (1987) HLA-DQ beta gene contributes to susceptibility and resistance to insulin-dependent diabetes mellitus. Nature (Lond) 329: 599–604
50. Unanue ER, Allen PM (1987) The basis for the immunoregulatory role of macrophages and other accessory cells. Science 236: 551–557
51. Vardi P, Dibella EE, Pasquarello TJ, Srikanta S (1987) Islet cell autoantibodies: pathobiology and clinical applications. Diabetes Care 10: 645–656
52. Vialettes B, Mattei-Zevaco C, Badier C, Ramahandridona G, Lassmann-Vague V, Vague Ph (1988) Low acute insulin response to intravenous glucose. A sensitive but non-specific marker of early stages of type I (insulin-dependent) diabetes. Diabetologia 31: 592–596
53. Wilkin TJ, Hoskin PJ, Armitage M, Rodier M, Casey C, Dias J-L, Pyke DA, Leslie RDG (1985) Value of insulin autoantibodies as serum markers for insulin dependent diabetes mellitus. Lancet I: 480–482

Gegenwärtiger Stand und Zukunft der Immuntherapie des Typ I-Diabetes

G. Schernthaner

Summary

Worldwide efforts in research on the pathogenesis of type I diabetes mellitus have shown that this disease is caused by autoimmunological destruction of pancreatic β cells. The essential part of this destructive process occurs during the prediabetic phase. Based on this knowledge, therapeutic trials with immunosuppressive and immunomodulative substances have been performed within recent years. During the past 5 years numerous trials, for example with plasmapheresis, cortisone, levamisole, ciamexon, nicotinamide, antilymphocyte globulin, γ-globulin, azathioprine and cyclosporin A, have been done. Clear positive results have only been found with the two last-mentioned substances. Remission rates of about 30% – 50% in a Canadian pilot study with cyclosporin A were decisive in leading to two placebo-controlled double-blind studies. In the French cyclosporin A study 122 patients were followed up over a period of 9 months. Dependent on the cyclosporin A blood levels, 37% (>300 ng/ml) or 16.7% (<300 ng/ml) total remissions were observed in the treated group in contrast to 5% in the placebo group. The Canadian-European cyclosporin A study has included 188 patients – 42 in the Viennese Center – whose diagnosis was not older than 6 weeks and in whom the beginning of symptoms was not longer than 14 weeks before. In the cyclosporin A group total remissions were observed ten times more often, depending on the period of symptoms and the beginning of the therapy, than in the placebo group. Comparable side effects were found in both studies: hypertrichosis, gingival hyperplasia, a decline of the creatinine clearance of about 20%, and an increase of the serum creatinine of about 21%. At the moment it is impossible to estimate the degree of chronic nephrotoxicity. Recent studies on kidney biopsies of diabetic children in France who were only treated with a low cyclosporin A dose (blood levels below 350 ng/ml) have not shown any histological changes. These encouraging results of immunological intervention with cyclosporin A justify, further use of this substance in controlled studies – possibly in combination with other immunomodulators – as well as the search for cyclosporin A analogs with fewer renal side effects. We must keep in mind that the immunotherapy used until now represents just a nonspecific immunointervention at the end of a long disease process. The future of immunomodulation in type I diabetes must lie in a primary prevention of the disease, or in a specific immunointervention at a very early stage of the disease. Future studies must reveal whether new applications of immunomodulation such as inhibition of autoantigen expression, inhibition of antigen presentation, elimination of autoreactive T-cell clones or tolerance induction will be a solution. The final goal of this research must be long-term total remission reached using a therapy with few side effects.

Einleitung

Rapide Fortschritte in der Pathogeneseforschung des Typ I-Diabetes mellitus der letzten 15 Jahre haben eindeutig gezeigt, daß es sich beim Insulinmangeldiabetes (Typ I-Diabetes) um eine Erkrankung handelt, die auf eine immunologische Destruktion der insulinproduzierenden β-Zellen zurückzuführen ist [1–5]. Nach dem gegenwärtigen Stand unseres Wissens dürften exogene Faktoren (Viren, Toxine) bei Personen mit immungenetisch mediierter Krankheitsempfänglichkeit (HLA DR 3/ HLA DR 4) eine Autoimmunerkrankung (Abb. 1) auslösen, die über im Detail noch ungeklärte Mechanismen (zytotoxische T-Zellen, Lymphokine etc.) zur Insulinmangelkrankheit führt [6–8]. Im Gegensatz zur früheren Lehrmeinung handelt es sich beim Typ I-Diabetes nicht um eine akut einsetzende Erkrankung. Vielmehr findet sich bei der Mehrzahl der Patienten eine sich über Monate bis Jahre erstreckende prädiabetische Vorphase der Erkrankung [9, 10], in der immunologische Phänomene (Inselzellantikörper etc.) bereits nachweisbar sind, während die metabolischen Befunde der Patienten klinisch lange Zeit unauffällig sind.

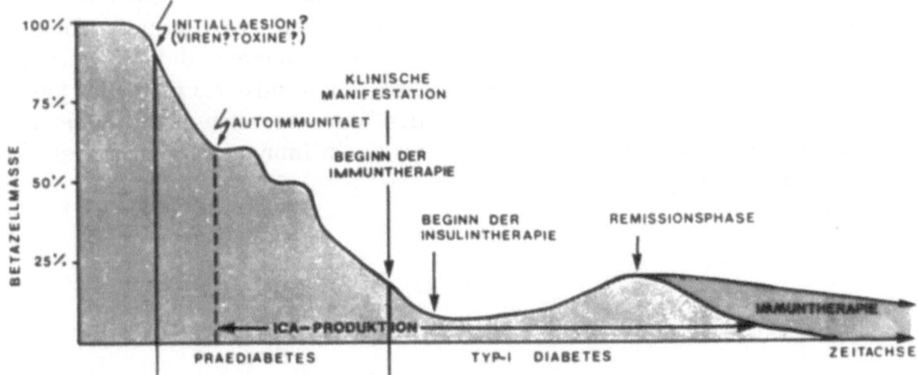

Abb. 1. Zeitlicher Ablauf der Krankheitsentstehung des Typ I-Diabetes

Argumente für die Immuntherapie

Die prinzipiellen Argumente, die für eine wissenschaftliche Erprobung der Immuntherapie in der Frühphase des Typ I-Diabetes sprechen, wurden vor kurzem an anderer Stelle ausführlich zusammengefaßt [11]. Obwohl viele Beobachtungen eindeutige Indizien für eine Autoimmunpathogenese des Typ I-Diabetes darstellen, stand der eindeutige Beweis – nämlich die Beeinflußbarkeit des Immunprozesses durch eine Immunintervention – bisher noch aus. Für die Bahnung und weitere wissenschaftliche Erarbeitung neuer Therapiekonzepte war es zunächst entscheidend zu beweisen, daß eine Unterbrechung des immunologischen Destruktionsprozesses zumindest bei einem Teil der Patienten eine langfristige Totalremission herbeiführen kann. Dieser entscheidende und für weitere Arbeiten grundsätzlich wichtige Nachweis war durch 2 Fakten erschwert: (a) Zum Zeitpunkt der klinischen Manifestation des Typ I-Diabetes sind bereits 80–90% der β-Zellmasse zerstört und (b) eine optimale Insulinsubstitutionstherapie mit Normoglykämie führt auch natürlicherweise in einem hohen Prozentsatz zur partiellen Remission [12, 13] der Erkrankung (Honeymoon-Periode). Aufgrund der bisher geübten Praxis eine Insulintherapie aus der Überlegung der „β-Zellschonung" möglichst nicht abzusetzen, wurde bisher nicht systematisch untersucht wie häufig eine Totalremission in der Frühphase des Typ I-Diabetes auftritt. Patientenschulung [14] und moderne Insulinbehandlungsstrategien [15, 16] haben zweifellos zu einer wesentlichen Verbesserung der Diabeteseinstellung und damit zu einem beträchtlichen Rückgang der diabetischen Nephropathie [17] geführt. Der von den Patienten im Rahmen der Basis-Bolus-Insulintherapie [15, 16] zu leistende Aufwand (Blutzuckermessung 4–5 Mal täglich, Insulininjektionen 4–5 Mal täglich, sowie präzise Abstimmung von Nahrungszufuhr und präprandialer Insulinsubstitution) ist allerdings beträchtlich. Darüber hinaus kann das Ausmaß der Blutzuckerschwankungen und der täglich wechselnde morgendliche Blutzuckeranstieg (Dawn-Phänomen) durch die Basis-Bolus-Insulintherapie zwar reduziert aber keineswegs verhindert [18] werden.

Die lebenslängliche Insulinabhängigkeit sowie die trotz aller Behandlungsfortschritte [14–16] auch heute noch beträchtlich eingeschränkte Lebensqualität und Lebenserwartung der betroffenen Patienten waren weitere Argumente – mehr als 60 Jahre nach Einführung der Insulintherapie – eine primäre und damit kausale Therapie des Insulinmangeldiabetes anzustreben. Aufgrund der aufgezeigten Fakten war es verständlich, daß man versuchte, den Wissenszuwachs auf dem Gebiet der Pathogeneseforschung des Typ I-Diabetes durch Immuninterventionsversuche therapeutisch zu nutzen.

Möglichkeiten der Immunintervention beim Typ I-Diabetes

Prinzipiell muß zwischen Maßnahmen in der prädiabetischen Phase und Interventionen nach Manifestation des Typ I-Diabetes unterschieden werden (Abb. 1). Vor klinischem Ausbruch der Erkrankung (Prädiabetesphase) sah man sich bis vor kurzem nicht berechtigt immuntherapeutisch zu intervenieren, da nicht jeder Inselzellantikörper-positive Patient zwangsläufig bis zum Insulinmangeldiabetes fortschreitet. Bei langdauernder Inselzellantikörperpersistenz und zunehmendem Verlust der akuten Insulinfreisetzung nach intravenöser Glukoseapplikation hat man aufgrund der hohen Wahrscheinlichkeit einer späteren Diabetesmanifestation bereits erste immunmodulatorische Versuche unternommen [19].

Bereits 1982 wurden beim Diabetes-Immunologiemeeting in Luxembourg [4] verschiedene zahlreiche Möglichkeiten der Immuntherapie beim Typ I-Diabetes diskutiert, die in der Zwischenzeit größtenteils erprobt wurden. Die bisher beim Typ I-Diabetes tatsächlich eingesetzten immuntherapeutischen Maßnahmen sind in Tabelle 1 zusammengefaßt. Neben dem Einsatz der Plasmapherese, von Cortison, Levamisol, Interferon, Ciamexon, Nicotinamid, Antilymphozyten-Globulin, Gamma-Globulin, Azathioprim und monoklonalen Antikörpern wurden vor allem durch die Einführung von Cyclosporin-A beträchtliche Hoffnungen erweckt.

Häufigkeit der Totalremissionen in der Präimmuntherapieaera

Wie häufig ist eigentlich eine Totalremission beim Typ I-Diabetes, definiert durch weitgehende Normoglykämie über mehrere Wochen bzw. Monate ohne Verabreichung einer Insulintherapie oder von oralen Antidiabetika? In den unkontrollierten Studien von Drash und Mitarbeitern [20] sowie von Knip und Mitarbeitern [21] konnte bei nur 3 bzw. 2 % der Patienten eine vorübergehende Totalremission

Tabelle 1. Bisher in der Immuntherapie des Typ I-Diabetes eingesetzte Pharmaka (Stand 1990)

Cortison [45, 46]	Plasmapherese [28–31]
Interferon [34, 35]	Levamisol [24]
Thymostimulin [27]	Immunglobulin [37]
Theophyllin [26]	Ciamexon [38, 39]
Nicotinamid [41, 42]	Antilymphozyten-Globulin [32, 33]
Cyclosporin-A[a] [22, 23, 46, 47, 47]	Azathioprin [43–45]

[a] auch in Kombination mit Cortison

Tabelle 2. Häufigkeit der Totalremission beim Typ I-Diabetes im Spontanverlauf (ohne Immuntherapie)

Unkontrollierte Studien

Drash et al. [20]   31   (1050)   3%
Knip et al. [21]   3   (113)   2%

Kontrollierte Studien

	6 Monate	9 Monate	12 Monate
Französische Cyclosporin-A Studie [22]	18.6%	5.8%	—
Kanadisch/Europäische Cyclosporin-A Studie [23]	19.1%	10.0%	9.8%

beobachtet werden, wobei die verwendeten Kriterien nicht sicher ausschließen lassen, ob der eine oder andere Patient nicht eher als Mody-Diabetes zu klassifizieren gewesen wäre (Tabelle 2). In den kontrollierten Cyclosporinstudien [22, 23] konnte bei den Placebo-behandelten Patienten nach 6monatiger Therapiedauer in beiden Studien in ca. 19% der Fälle eine Totalremission beobachtet werden. Dies weist darauf hin, daß in den beteiligten Diabeteszentren eine ausgezeichnete intensivierte Insulintherapie durchgeführt wurde. Bemerkenswert ist allerdings der Rückgang der Totalremissionsrate mit weiterer Krankheitsdauer auf 6% bzw. 10% nach 9- bzw. 12monatiger Krankheitsdauer.

Häufigkeit der Totalremissionen nach Immuntherapie

Die Abbildung 2 zeigt die wesentlich höhere Rate an Totalremissionen, die in der Kanadisch/Europäischen Cyclosporin-Studie durch die zusätzliche Cyclosporingabe erreicht werden konnte, nämlich 39% nach 6monatiger und 24% nach 12monatiger Therapiedauer. Bemerkenswert und bisher zuwenig berücksichtigt bei der Analyse der kontrollierten Cyclosporinstudien (Tabelle 3) ist die Tatsache, daß nicht nur in der Placebogruppe, sondern auch in der Cyclosporinbehandlungsgruppe ein deutlicher Abfall der Totalremissionen mit zunehmender Diabetesdauer zu beobachten war. Die Abbildung 3 läßt erkennen, warum Cyclosporin-behandelte Patienten wesentlich häufiger in die Totalremission kamen als Patienten ohne Immuntherapie. 3 Monate nach Krankheitsdiagnose konnte zwar auch bei Pacebo-behandelten Patienten ein geringer Zuwachs des stimulierten C-Peptids gegenüber der Ausgangssituation festgestellt werden. Die Cyclosporin-behandelten Patienten hatten zu diesem Zeitpunkt allerdings einen deutlich stärkeren C-Peptid Zuwachs und zeigten während der einjährigen Beobachtungsperiode keinen Rückgang der endogenen Insulinsekretion. Bei der Patientengruppe ohne Immuntherapie kam es hingegen zu einem deutlichen Abfall der C-Peptid Sekretion gegenüber der Ausgangssituation. Diese Beobachtung bestätigt einen früheren Bericht [24], wonach durch eine strikte glykaemische Kontrolle lediglich

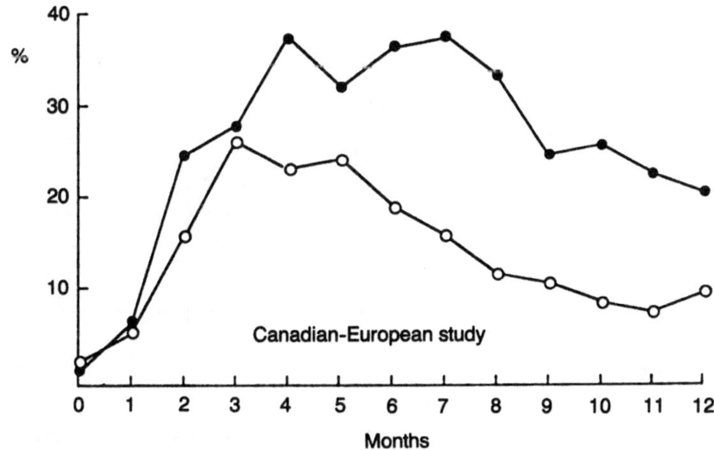

Abb. 2. Totalremissionsraten bei Cyclosporin-A (●) und Placebo (○) behandelten Patienten mit Typ I-Diabetes während des 1. Krankheitsjahres. Kanadisch/Europäische Studie [23]

Tabelle 3. Häufigkeit der Totalremissionen nach Immuntherapie mit Cyclosporin-A

		Remissionsrate (%)					
		6 Monate		9 Monate		12 Monate	
		CyA	*PLAC*	*CyA*	*PLAC*	*CyA*	*PLAC*
Französische Studie [22]	(N = 122)	25.4	18.6	24.1	5.8	—	—
Kanadisch/Europäische Studie [23]	(N = 188)	38.7	19.1	23.0	10.0	24.2	9.8

ein transienter Effekt auf die Betazellfunktion ausgeübt wird. Die Immuntherapiestudien lassen erkennen, daß für die Persistenz einer Totalremission die Aufrechterhaltung einer weitgehend normalen endogenen Betazellfunktion Voraussetzung ist.

Therapiestudien mit Immunmodulatoren

Levamisol

Die immuntherapeutischen Ergebnisse mit Levamisol bei Autoimmunerkrankungen sind bisher relativ enttäuschend gewesen. Die Erfahrungen bei Typ I-Diabetes mellitus beschränken sich auf die Anwendung bei 3 Patienten, wobei über einen Zeitraum von 6 Monaten bei keinem der mit Levamisol behandelten Patienten eine klinische Verbesserung dokumentiert werden konnte [25].

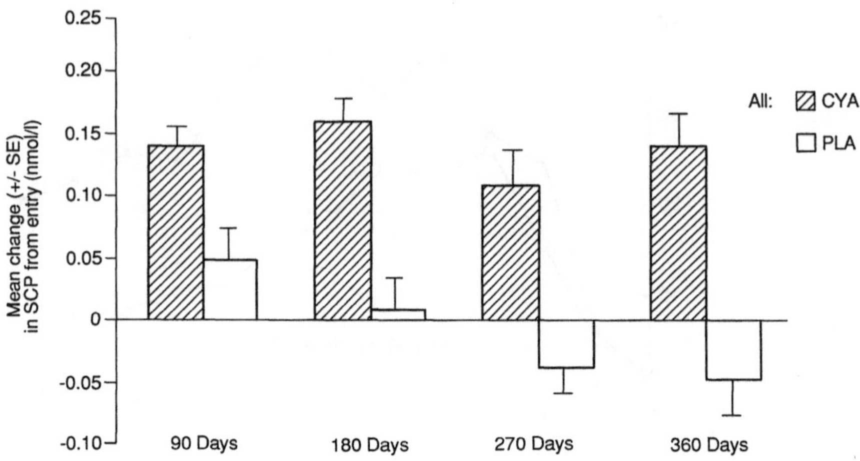

Abb. 3. Mittlere Änderung des stimulierten C-Peptids gegenüber der Ausgangssituation. Signifikanter und anhaltender Anstieg in der Cyclosporin-A-Gruppe, nur transienter und konsekutiver Abfall in der Placebo-Gruppe. Kanadisch/Europäische Studie [23]

Theophyllin

Von Theophyllin wird angenommen, daß es eine verminderte T-Suppressor-Zell-Funktion normalisieren kann. Der bei Patienten mit Typ I-Diabetes bisher erfolgte Therapieversuch mit Theophyllin (800 mg/Tag über 1 Monat verabreicht) ist allerdings nicht vielversprechend. Eine temporäre partielle Remission wurde bei 4 von 5 Theophyllin-behandelten Patienten im Vergleich zu 2 von 4 Placebo-therapierten Typ I-Diabetikern beobachtet [26].

Thymushormone

Von den verschiedenen Thymushormonen wurde beim Typ I-Diabetes bisher nur Thymostimulin (TP1) isoliert oder in Kombination mit Azathioprin eingesetzt. Die bisher bei 35 Patienten beobachteten Erfahrungen lassen einen gewissen Effekt auf die Remissionsinduktion und Remissionserhaltung erkennen, wenngleich dieser Effekt von den historischen Kontrollen nicht sehr unterschiedlich war [27].

Plasmapherese

Die Plasmapherese war eines der ersten immunmodulatorischen Verfahren, das in der Behandlung des Typ I-Diabetes eingesetzt wurde. Insgesamt liegen bisher vier Berichte vor [28–31]. Von einer Arbeitsgruppe [31] wurde die kombinierte Anwendung von Plasmapherese, Prednisolon und Antilymphozytenglobulin bei

3 Patienten getestet. Alle Patienten konnten die Insulintherapie nur vorübergehend absetzen, während im weiteren Verlauf bei allen drei Patienten ein Krankheitsrezidiv beobachtet wurde. Ludvigsson und Mitarbeiter [28] konnten nur geringe Effekte der Plasmapherese auf immunologische Parameter wie Inselzellantikörpertiter etc. feststellen, während eine Beeinflussung der basalen und stimulierten C-Peptid-Sekretion sowie der partiellen Remissiondauer und optimalen Stoffwechselkontrolle nach 18 Monaten noch erkennbar war.

Antithymocyten-Globulin

Antithymocyten-Globulin (ATG) wurde bisher bei insgesamt 10 Patienten mit Typ I-Diabetes eingesetzt [32, 33]. In einer Studie [32] erhielten 6 Patienten ATG (7–15 mg/Tag) in Kombination mit Prednison (1 mg/Kg/Tag) über einen Zeitraum von 1 bis 4 Wochen. Eine Abnahme der CD4/CD8-Ratio und eine verbesserte Stoffwechselkontrolle (trotz Insulindosisreduktion) wurden im Vergleich zu 2 Kontrollgruppen mit Prednisonmonotherapie bzw. alleiniger Insulintherapie berichtet. Zwei der sechs Patienten hatten eine Totalremission von mehr als 8 Monaten. Wesentlich schlechter sind die Therapieerfahrungen des kombinierten Einsatzes von ATG und Prednison bei 4 Kindern [33], bei denen nach 6-monatiger Beobachtungsdauer keine klinische Verbesserung festzustellen war.

Interferon

Interferon wird normalerweise nach einer Virusinfektion von infizierten Zellen produziert, wobei es weitere Zellen vor der Infektion schützt. Da Interferon NK-Zellen und Makrophagen aktiviert und da beide Zelltypen am Destruktionsprozeß der Betazellen beteiligt sein dürften, ist der Einsatz dieser Substanz in der Immuntherapie des Typ I-Diabetes nicht unproblematisch. Bei zwei neumanifestierten Kindern konnte nach dem Einsatz von Interferon kein positiver Stoffwecheleffekt nachgewiesen werden [34]. In einer größeren kontrollierten Studie an 43 Patienten konnte ebenfalls kein Effekt von Alpha-Interferon festgestellt werden [35]. Die Interferon-behandelte Gruppe und Kontrollgruppe zeigten in jeweils 42% eine partielle Remissionsphase, wobei 12 Monate nach Therapiebeginn kein Unterschied im stimulierten C-Peptid und täglichen Insulinbedarf festzustellen war. Eine durch Interferon induzierte Verstärkung des Destruktionsprozesses konnte allerdings nicht beobachtet werden. Der Einsatz von Interferon bei unselektierten Patienten ist aufgrund theoretischer Überlegungen nicht sinnvoll, vielmehr müßte die Anwendung auf Patienten mit gesicherter Virusätiologie beschränkt werden.

Gamma-Globulin

Obwohl ein günstiger Effekt von Gammaglobulin bei idiopathischer Thrombozytopenie und einigen anderen Autoimmunerkrankungen [36] bekannt ist, war der bisherige Einsatz von Gammaglobulinen beim Typ I-Diabetes nicht allzu Erfolg versprechend. Die bisher veröffentlichten Erfahrungen erstrecken sich allerdings nur auf die Gammaglobulingabe (0,4 g/kg/Tag verabreicht über 5 Tage) bei 6 Kindern. Bei 2 der 6 Kinder wurde eine Remission beobachtet, die in einem Fall 12 Monate andauerte [37]. Derzeit laufen verschiedene kontrollierte Studien zur Überprüfung eines möglichen Effektes einer parenteralen Immunglobulingabe in der Frühphase des Typ I-Diabetes.

Ciamexon

Ciamexon wirkt bevorzugt auf B-Lymphozyten und die Antikörper-abhängige zelluläre Zytotoxizität. Da eine pathogenetische Rolle von Autoantikörpern beim Typ I-Diabetes seit langer Zeit bezweifelt wird [1, 4] ist der Einsatz von Ciamexon als Immuntherapeutikum beim Typ I-Diabetes eher zweifelhaft. Überraschenderweise fand sich in einer Pilotstudie bei 8 der 11 mit Ciamexon-behandelten Patienten mit Typ I-Diabetes – hingegen nur bei 3 von 9 Kontrollpatienten eine partielle oder totale Remission [38]. Diese Ergebnisse veranlaßten zu einer Placebo-kontrollierten Ciamexon-Doppelblind-Studie, die an 169 Patienten in Deutschland und Österreich durchgeführt wurde [39]. Nach 3- bzw. 6-monatiger Therapie wurde bei 12.9 % der Ciamexon- und bei 7.6 % der Placebo-behandelten Patienten eine Totalremission beobachtet. Nach 6monatiger Therapiedauer lag die Totalremissionsrate in der Ciamexongruppe bei 17.1 % und in der Placebogruppe bei nur 1.9 %. Die nach 6-monatiger Ciamexontherapie beobachtete Totalremissionsrate von 17.1 % ist allerdings geringer als die Totalremissionsrate der Placebogruppen in den kontrollierten Cyclosporin-A-Studien [22, 23]. Im Gegensatz zur kanadisch-europäischen Cyclosporin-A-Studie [23] konnte in der Ciamexon-Studie auch kein Anstieg der C-Peptid-Sekretion gegenüber der Ausgangssituation nachgewiesen werden.

Nicotinamid

Aus tierexperimentellen Studien ist bekannt, daß Nicotinamid in der Lage ist, den diabetogenen Effekt von Alloxan und Streptozotocin abzuschwächen. Nicotinamid erhöht über eine Hemmung der Poly (ADP-Ribose) – Synthetase den NAD-Gehalt der Betazellen und damit die Insulinsynthese [40]. Bei Patienten mit Typ I-Diabetes liegen bisher 2 Studien [41, 42] über die Anwendung von Nicotinamid vor. Die hochdosierte Verabreichung (3 g/Tag) wurde bei 7 Patienten mit Typ I-Diabetes im Vergleich zu 9 Placebo-Behandlungen analysiert. Nach 6 bzw. 12 Monaten waren 5 bzw. 3 der 7 Patienten mit Nicotinamidbehandlung, hingegen nur 2 bzw. keiner der 9 Placebo-therapierten Patienten in Totalremission

[41]. Auch nach niedrigdosierter Nicotinamidtherapie (200 mg/Tag) fand sich 6 und 12 Monate nach Therapiebeginn bei 22 Patienten ein signifikanter C-Peptid-Zuwachs im Gegensatz zu einer Kontrollgruppe von 13 Patienten [42].

Azathioprin

Insgesamt liegen bisher beim Typ I-Diabetes 3 kontrollierte Studien [43–45] mit Azathioprin vor, wobei in einer [45] der 3 Studien die Kombination von Azathioprin und Glucocorticoiden bei jugendlichen Diabetikern geprüft wurde. 12 Monate nach Beginn der Azathioprinmonotherapie [43] konnte bei 7 der 13 immunsupprimierten Patienten im Gegensatz zu nur einem Patienten in der Kontrollgruppe eine klinische Totalremission mit Unterbrechung der Insulintherapie erzielt werden. Nach Absetzen von Azathioprin zeigten allerdings 5 der 7 Patienten mit klinischer Remission ein Krankheitsrezidiv, ein Befund der untermauert, daß eine Erhaltung der Totalremission ohne Fortführung der Immunsuppression nicht erreicht werden kann. Die Azathioprin-behandelten Patienten zeigten höhere C-Peptidspiegel als die Kontrollgruppe, eine Befundkonstellation, die den Zusammenhang zwischen klinischer Remission und Betazellfunktion belegt. Dieser günstige Effekt einer Azathioprinmonotherapie konnte in einer zweiten kontrollierten Studie [44] an 49 diabetischen Kindern in Australien (Altersbereich: 2–20 Jahre; mittleres Alter: 11 Jahre) nicht bestätigt werden. Eine komplette klinische Remission wurde bei keinem der mit Azathioprin behandelten Kinder beobachtet. Eine partielle Remission ($HbA_1c < 7,9\%$; Insulinbedarf $< 0,5$ U/kg/Tag) fand sich nach 6 Monaten bei 10 der 25 Placebo- und bei 7 der 24 Azathioprin-behandelten Kindern, während nach 12monatiger Therapiedauer in beiden Gruppen nur mehr bei jeweils 4 Kindern eine partielle Remission vorlag.

Unkontrollierte Cyclosporin-A-Studien bei Typ I-Diabetes

Im Vergleich zu historischen Kontrollen fand sich in der kanadischen Pilotstudie [47] bei frühzeitigem Einsatz von Cyclosporin-A eine deutlich erhöhte Remissionsrate, d. h. 1 Jahr nach Beginn waren ca. 30–50% der Patienten nicht mehr insulinbedürftig. Allerdings mußte in Perioden stärkerer Stoffwechselbelastung, z. B. bei Infektionen, häufig wieder Insulin substituiert werden. Schließlich wurde nach Absetzen der Immuntherapie nach 12–18 Monaten in der Regel ein Rezidiv, d. h. die Wiederkehr der Insulinabhängigkeit beobachtet. Die hoffnungsvollen Ergebnisse aus unkontrollierten Studien [47, 48] wurden mit Recht kritisiert, da ähnliche Resultate hinsichtlich Insulinbedarf und Remissionsdauer auch bei einzelnen Patienten mit aggressiver Insulintherapie erreicht werden konnten. Zur Sicherung des Therapieerfolges waren demnach kontrollierte Immuntherapiestudien notwendig. Ende 1984 wurden zwei multizentrische Doppelblindstudien begonnen, deren Ergebnisse nun vorliegen.

Kontrollierte Cyclosporin-A-Studien bei Typ I-Diabetes

Französische Cyclosporin-A-Studie

In der französischen Cyclosporin-A-Studie [22] wurden 122 Patienten mit Typ I-Diabetes (Manifestationsalter 15 bis 40 Jahre) zusätzlich zur Insulintherapie, entweder mit Cyclosporin-A (7,5 mg/kg Körpergewicht/Tag) oder mit Placebo behandelt. Die Cyclosporin-A (CyA) Dosis wurde entsprechend den gemessenen Vollblut-CyA-Spiegeln angepaßt, wobei eine Dosisreduktion vorgenommen wurde, wenn der CyA-Spiegel über 750 ng/ml und das Plasmakreatinin über 110 μmol/l anstieg. Nach 9monatiger Therapiedauer waren 24,1% der Cyclosporin-behandelten Patienten, hingegen nur 5.8% der Placebogrupe in Totalremission (Tabelle 3). Zwischen den CyA-Blutspiegeln in den ersten 3 Behandlungsmonaten und der Häufigkeit der Totalremissionen fand sich ein eindeutiger Zusammenhang. Patienten mit Cyclosporin-A-Blutspiegeln über 300 ng/ml waren nach 9 Monaten in 37% der Fälle in Totalremission, während die Patientengruppe mit CyA-Spiegeln unter 300 ng/ml nur in 16,7% insulinfrei wurde. Nach 6monatiger Therapiedauer fand sich auch in der Placebogruppe eine hohe Rate an Totalremissionen (20,8%). Die Remissionen waren dabei allerdings meist nur von kurzer Dauer und 3 Monate später (nach 9 Monaten) in 3/4 der Fälle nicht mehr vorhanden.

Kanadisch/europäische Cyclosporin-A-Studie

In der kanadisch/europäischen Cyclosporin-A-Studie [23] wurden insgesamt 188 Patienten (Manifestationsalter 9–35 Jahre) in 12 Zentren behandelt, davon 131 Patienten in den 5 europäischen Zentren (Helsinki, Kopenhagen, Düsseldorf, München und Wien). Im deutschsprachigen Raum wurden davon 22 Patienten in Düsseldorf, 13 Patienten in München und 42 Patienten in Wien (II. Medizinische

Tabelle 4. Signifikanter Einfluß der Dauer des Diabetes vor Beginn der Cyclosporin-A-Therapie auf die Totalremissionsrate [23]

Diabetesdauer	6 Monate		12 Monate	
	Kurz[a]	Lang[b]	Kurz	Lang
Totalremission CyA	55.3%	27.3%	31.62%	18.9%
Totalremission Placebo	13.2%	23.2%	2.73%	14.5%
p-Wert	0.001	NS	0.003	NS
p-Diff	0.003		0.06	

[a] Kurz: <6 Wochen Symptome; <2 Wochen Insulintherapie
[b] Lang: 7–14 Wochen Symptome; 3–6 Wochen Insulintherapie

Universitätsklinik) therapeutisiert. Aufgrund der Einschlußkriterien wurden lediglich jene Patienten mit Typ I-Diabetes in die Studie aufgenommen, deren Krankheitsdiagnose nicht länger als 6 Wochen und deren Symptombeginn nicht länger als 14 Wochen zurücklag. Die initiale Cyclosporindosis betrug 10 mg/kg Körpergewicht, die Dosisadjustierung erfolgte aufgrund der CyA-Vollblutspiegel in Europa (400–800 ng/ml) bzw. CyA-Serumkonzentrationen in Kanada (100 bis 200 ng/ml). Nach 6-monatiger Therapie fand sich in 38.7% der Cyclosporin-A-Behandlungsgruppe, hingegen nur in 19.2% der Placebogruppe eine Totalremission. Nach 12-monatiger Therapie betrug die Totalremissionsrate 23.4% in der CyA-Therapiegruppe und 10.8% in der Placebogruppe. Der Therapieerfolg war vor allem von der Dauer des Diabetes vor Beginn der Cyclosporintherapie abhängig (Tabelle 4). Patienten mit kurzer Krankheitsdauer vor Therapiebeginn (weniger als 6 Wochen Symptome, weniger als 2 Wochen Insulintherapie) waren nach 6 und 12 Monaten in 55.3% bzw. 32.4% der Fälle in Totalremission, während eine Insulinfreiheit in der Placebogruppe bei nur 13.5% bzw. 3.3% der Patienten zu beobachten war (p <0,01). Bei frühzeitigem Therapiebeginn trat somit in der Cyclosporin-Behandlungsgruppe 10 Mal häufiger eine Totalremission auf als in der Placebogruppe. Gegenüber der Ausgangssituation fand sich in der Cyclosporin-A-Gruppe – nicht hingegen in der Placebogruppe – 12 Monate nach Therapiebeginn eine signifikant höhere C-Peptidsekretion nach Glukagonstimulation.

Wiener Erfahrungen der Cyclosporin-A-Therapie

Die Totalremissionsrate der 42 in Wien [49] behandelten Patienten ist in Abbildung 4 dargestellt. Ab dem zweiten Behandlungsmonat wurden Totalremissionen signifikant häufiger (p <0.01) bei Patienten mit Cyclosporin-A-Therapie beobachtet als bei Patienten mit alleiniger Insulintherapie (Zugabe von Placebo). Die Insulinsubstitution wurde in beiden Gruppen nur dann schrittweise reduziert, wenn die Nüchternblutzuckerspiegel und die Blutzuckertageprofile im Normbereich lagen. In der Abbildung 5 ist die Einstellungsqualität der in Wien behandelten Patienten dargestellt, die an der Kanadisch-Europäischen Cyclosporinstudie teilgenommen hatten. Initial lagen die HbA$_1$c Werte sehr hoch und kamen nach 3–6-monatiger Therapiedauer in den Normbereich, wobei kein Unterschied zwischen Placebo- und Cyclosporin-behandelten Patienten festzustellen war. Die Patienten mit Totalremission hatten demnach eine mindestens ebensogute Stoffwechseleinstellung wie die Patienten mit Insulinbehandlung. Detaillierte Untersuchungen der Insulinsekretionsdynamik und der Insulinsensitivität bei den in Wien behandelten Patienten ergaben [50], daß zusätzlich zur Steigerung bzw. Erhaltung der β-Zellrestfunktion auch eine Normalisierung der peripheren Insulinsensitivität für die Entwicklung einer langfristigen Totalremission von Bedeutung ist. Darüberhinaus konnte gezeigt werden, daß der für die prädiabetische Phase charakteristische Verlust der frühen Insulinfreisetzung auf i.v. Glukosegabe durch Cyclosporin-A-Therapie nicht wiederhergestellt werden kann. Bemerkens-

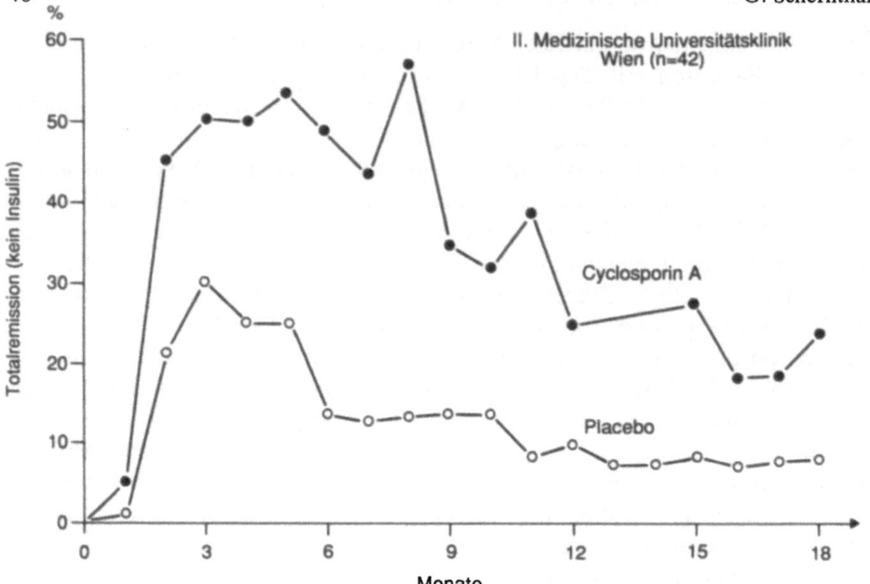

Abb. 4. Totalremissionsrate der in Wien behandelten Patienten, die an der Kanadisch/Europäischen Cyclosporin-A-Studie teilgenommen hatten [49]

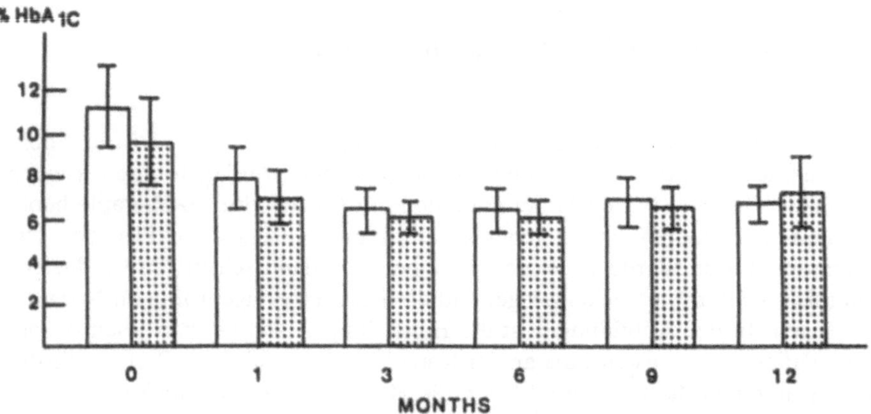

Abb. 5. Einstellungsqualität der in Wien behandelten Patienten, die an der Kanadisch/Europäischen Cyclosporin-A-Studie teilnahmen [49]
☐ Patienten mit Cyclosporin-A-Behandlung
⊞ Patienten mit Placebo-Behandlung

wert erscheint, daß Untersuchungen der natürlichen Killerzellaktivität und der Antikörper-abhängigen zellmediierten Zytotoxizität bei den in Wien mit Cyclosporin-A behandelten Patienten mit Typ I-Diabetes keinerlei Abweichungen von der Kontrollgruppe erkennen ließen [51], ein Befund der mit der sehr geringen Lymphominzidenz bei Cyclosporin-A-Monotherapie [52] in Einklang steht. Langfristige kombinierte immunsuppressive Therapiemaßnahmen – wie sie vor allem früher häufig bei Organtransplantationen eingesetzt wurden – bewirken hingegen eine signifikante Unterdrückung dieser wichtigen immunologischen Parameter [53].

Kombinierter Einsatz von Immuntherapeutika

Nach dem Einsatz zahlreicher Immunpharmaka in Form einer Monotherapie liegen bereits mehrere Studien vor, in denen die kombinierte Anwendung verschieden wirkender Substanzen in der Frühphase des Typ I-Diabetes getestet wurden.

Azathioprin und Glucocorticoide

46 Patienten mit einem mittleren Alter von 12 Jahren (Altersbereich 4–32 Jahre) wurden entweder mit kombinierter Immunsuppression (Corticosteroide für 10 Wochen, Azathioprin für die Dauer eines Jahres) oder nur mit Insulin behandelt [45]. Die Azathioprindosis betrug 2 mg/kg Körpergewicht pro Tag. Methylprednison wurde zunächst als i.v. Bolus von 30 mg/kg in vier Dosen, gefolgt von einer peroralen Prednisontherapie von 2 mg/kg/Tag, verabreicht. Die Prednisondosis wurde alle 2 Wochen reduziert und nach 10 Wochen vollkommen ausgeschlichen. In der immunsupprimierten Patientengruppe fand sich ab dem 6. Monat eine signifikante Insulindosisreduktion, wobei bei 10 Patienten die Insulintherapie sogar abgesetzt werden konnte. In der Kontrollgruppe hingegen wurden nur 2 Patienten vorübergehend insulinunabhängig. Auch die C-Peptid-Stimulation war in der immunsupprimierten Gruppe signifikant höher als in der Kontrollgruppe [45].

Cyclosporin und Glucocorticoide

Der kombinierte Einsatz von Cyclosporin-A und Methylprednisolon (1,25 g infundiert über 72 Stunden) wurde bei 38 neumanifestierten Patienten mit Typ I-Diabetes mit der Fragestellung überprüft, ob durch die zusätzliche Glucocorticoidapplikation eine raschere Remissionsinduktion erreicht werden kann [46]. 17 der 38 Patienten wurden zusätzlich mit einer Initialdosis von 10 mg Cyclosporin-A/kg/Tag und 21 mit einer Initialdosis von 7,5 mg Cyclosporin-A/kg/Tag behandelt. Eine Kontrollgruppe von 8 Patienten erhielt nur Cyclosporin-A in einer Dosis von 7,5 mg/kg/Tag. Bezüglich der klinischen Remission konnten zwischen den 3 Gruppen keine signifikanten Unterschiede festgestellt werden. Auch der C-Peptidzuwachs gegenüber der Ausgangssituation war in den 3 Gruppen ähnlich, so daß der Vorteil der zusätzlichen Prednisontherapie nicht eindeutig ersichtlich ist. Möglicherweise liegt der Vorteil der zusätzlichen Glucocorticoidgabe darin, daß trotz niedrigerer Cyclosporindosen ähnliche Remissionsraten wie mit höheren Dosen erreicht werden können.

Kritische Wertung der Immuntherapie-Studien

Mit Ausnahme von Cyclosporin-A und weniger eindrucksvoll von Azathioprin haben die bisher durchgeführten Immuninterventionsstudien beim Typ I-Diabetes keinen echten Durchbruch erreicht. Die prinzipiellen Proargumente und Kontraargumente für eine Immuntherapie mit Cyclosporin-A beim Typ I-Diabetes sind in Tabelle 5 gegenübergestellt. Als gesichert kann heute gelten, daß eine rechtzeitig einsetzende Immuntherapie mittels Cyclosporin-A bei ungefähr der Hälfte der Patienten mit Typ I-Diabetes eine Totalremission herbeiführt. Ein verzögerter Therapiebeginn (Diabetesdauer zwischen 2 und 6 Wochen, Symptomdauer 6–14 Wochen) bedeutet bereits eine weitgehende Ineffektivität der Immuntherapie, wie die Ergebnisse der kanadisch/europäischen Studie erkennen lassen. Die bessere Lebensqualität der Patienten sowie die Bahnung eines neuen Therapiekonzeptes (Primärtherapie) sind weitere Proargumente (Tabelle 5). Die bisherigen Studien (Therapiedauer nur 1–2 Jahre) lassen allerdings keine Beantwortung der wichtigen Frage zu, ob bei Patienten mit Totalremission Spätschäden gänzlich ausbleiben. Da keine komplette Stoffwechselnormalisierung erfolgt, wäre die Entwicklung von makroangiopathischen Komplikationen ähnlich wie bei Patienten mit Glukoseintoleranz prinzipiell denkbar.

Unter den Kontraargumenten ist zunächst die hohe Nonresponderrate insbesonders bei zu spätem Therapiebeginn anzuführen. Unklar ist bisher noch, weshalb auch bei frühem Therapieeinsatz bei 50 % der Patienten keine Totalremission erreicht werden kann. Überraschend ist die Tatsache, daß die Verschiebung des Immuntherapiebeginns um nur 4 Wochen eine weitgehende Unwirksamkeit zur Folge hat. Dies könnte dafür sprechen, daß der Destruktionsprozeß um die Diabetesmanifestation herum besonders rapid und progressiv verläuft, wobei zu klären bleibt, ob dabei Streßfaktoren oder bestimmten Virusinfektionen [5, 6] ein

Tabelle 5. Proargumente und Kontraargumente für eine Immuntherapie mit Cyclosporin-A beim Typ I-Diabetes

Pro-Argumente	Kontra-Argumente
• Verminderung/Abschwächung der β-Zelldestruktion	• Therapie zu spät (80 % zerstört)
• bessere Lebensqualität	• Non-Responder 20 % –60 %
• Verminderung/Verzögerung der Spätschäden?	• Therapie lebenslänglich
• Primärtherapie (Heilung?)	• Lymphom-Induktion?
• Bahnung neuer Therapiekonzepte	• Nephrotoxizität
	• β-Zell-Zytotoxizität?

Triggermechanismus zukommt. Die Notwendigkeit einer lebenslangen Therapie ergibt sich aus den Cyclosporin-A-Absetzversuchen der kanadischen Pilotstudie [52] und den vorläufigen Erfahrungen der kontrollierten Cyclosporin-A-Studien [22, 23]. Es ist anzunehmen, daß aufgrund eines „immunologischen memory" bei allen Autoimmunerkrankungen eine lebenslange Immuntherapie zur Unterdrükkung des Immungeschehens notwendig sein dürfte. Bei einer lebenslang notwendigen Therapie stellt sich immer die Fragen, welche Langzeitrisiken damit verbunden sind.

Nebenwirkungen der Cyclosporin-A-Therapie

An Nebenwirkungen wurden in der französischen Cyclosporin-A-Studie v.a. Hypertrichosen und Gingivahyperplasien beobachtet, während die Infektionsrate zwischen CyA-Gruppe (61%) und Placebogruppe (48%) nicht wesentlich unterschiedlich war. Die gefährlichste Nebenwirkung war ein Anstieg des Plasmakreatinins, wobei allerdings kein Wert über 160 μmol/l beobachtet wurde. Die Nebenwirkungen in der kanadisch/europäischen Cyclosporin-A-Studie [23] waren vergleichbar mit jenen der französischen Studie [22]. Neben den kosmetischen Nebenwirkungen war vor allem ein Abfall der Kreatininclearance um 21%, sowie ein Anstieg des Serumkreatinins um 20%, hervorzuheben [23]. Während das Lymphomrisiko bei Cyclosporin-A-Monotherapie relativ gering sein dürfte, ist die gesamte Tragweite der chronischen Nephrotoxizität heute nocht schwer zu beurteilen. Streifige interstitielle Fibrosen und Arteriolopathie stellen die Hauptveränderungen dar. Aufgrund der bisherigen Erfahrungen dürfte zwischen dem Ausmaß morphologischer Nierenveränderungen und der verwendeten Cyclosporin-A-Dosis ein relativ enger Zusammenhang bestehen, da histologische Veränderungen fehlen, wenn Cyclosporin-A in einer niedrigen Dosierung (Blutspiegel unter 350 ng/ml) eingesetzt wird.

Krankheitsrezidiv des Typ I-Diabetes mellitus

Zur Frage Rezidiv bzw. „relapse" des Typ I-Diabetes (Tabelle 6) liegen bislang keine detaillierten Untersuchungen in der Präimmuntherapieära vor. Aus der klinischen Erfahrung ist bekannt, daß das Remissionsende meist durch Infektionen ausgelöst wird. Die bisherigen Erfahrungen mit der Immuntherapie [22, 23] und der Pankreassegment-Transplantation bei eineiigen Zwillingen [54] lassen erkennen, daß ein lebenslängliches „immunologisches memory" vorliegen dürfte. Das bedeutet, daß nach Absetzen einer Immunsuppression mit einem Wiederauftreten der Insulitis bzw. des Typ I-Diabetes zu rechnen ist. Erwartungsgemäß trat bei Patienten mit Typ I-Diabetes ein Krankheitsrezidiv auf, wenn die Im-

Tabelle 6. Rezidiv („relapse") des Typ I-Diabetes mellitus

- keine detäillierten Untersuchungen in der Präimmuntherapieära
- Remissionsende durch assoziierte Infektionen (Virusinfektionen?)
- Wiederauftreten der Insulitis (bzw. des Typ I-Diabetes) nach Pankreassegment-
  transplantation bei eineiigen Zwillingen
- tritt auf nach Absetzen der Immuntherapie (Auslaß der Cyclosporintherapie)
- tritt auf trotz Cyclosporintherapie bei längerer Krankheitsdauer (nach 8–12 Mon.)

Tabelle 7. Signifikanter Einfluß des Absetzens von Cyclosporin-A auf den mittleren täglichen Insulinbedarf, die HbA_{1C}-Werte und die C-Peptid-Konzentrationen

	Vor	Nach[a]
mittlerer täglicher Insulinbedarf (kg/Tag)	0.28	0.57
HBA_{1C} (%)	8.1 ± 1.7	8.6 ± 1.8
Glukagon stimuliertes C-Peptid (nmol/ml)	0.43 ± 0.22	0.24 ± 0.14
Serumkreatinin[b] (μM)	98 ± 24	83 ± 16

[a] 6 Monate nach Absetzen von Cyclosporin-A
[b] Kontrollgruppe: 80 ± 13

muntherapie unterbrochen wurde [55]. Unklar und kritisch zu beurteilen ist das Auftreten eines Krankheitsrezidives trotz Cyclosporintherapie bei längerer Krankheitsdauer [22]. In der Tabelle 7 sehen sie den mittleren täglichen Insulinbedarf, die $HbA_{1}c$-Werte und die C-Peptid-Konzentrationen bei 24 Typ I-Diabetikern vor und 6 Monate nach Absetzen der Cyclosporintherapie. Erwartungsgemäß kam es zu einem deutlichen Anstieg des exogenen Insulinbedarfes, zu einem Abfall der endogenen Insulinsekretion sowie zu einem Anstieg des $HbA_{1}c$, während sich die Serumkreatininspiegel normalisierten.

Zukunftsentwicklungen der Immuntherapie beim Typ I-Diabetes

Aufgrund der noch ungelösten Probleme ist derzeit eine Immuntherapie mit Cyclosporin-A außerhalb von kontrollierten Studien nicht zu empfehlen. Cyclosporin-A-Analoga mit fehlender Nephrotoxizität oder Maßnahmen zur Abschwächung der renalen Nebenwirkungen von Cyclosporin-A wären Lösungsmöglichkeiten. Zu klären bleibt auch, ob der zusätzliche Einsatz von nichttoxischen monoklonalen Antikörpern in der Initialphase der Behandlung eine noch höhere Rate an Totalremissionen herbeiführen kann. Wünschenswert wäre, daß nach einer initialen aggressiven Remissionsinduktionstherapie geringer wirksame Substanzen mit weitgehend fehlenden Nebenwirkungen für die Remissionserhaltung ausreichen. In weiteren Studien muß geklärt werden, welche Cyclosporinspiegel zur Aufrechterhaltung der Totalremission notwendig sind. Wünschenswert wären Cyclosporin-A-Spiegel von weniger als 350 ng/ml, da unter diesem Grenzwert keine morphologischen Nierenveränderungen zu beobachten sind [56]. Bisher existieren auch keinerlei Erfahrungen über eine mögliche Remissionsinduktion bei neuerlichem Ausbruch des Typ I-Diabetes.

Zweifellos sind die bisher beim Typ I-Diabetes durchgeführten Immuninterventionen weitgehend „unspezifische" Maßnahmen. Es bleibt zu hoffen, daß nach weiterer Aufklärung des immunologischen Destruktionsprozesses „spezifischere" Immuntherapiestrategien (Abb. 6) gefunden werden können. Im vergangenen Jahrzehnt haben wir wesentlich neue Erkenntnisse zur Erklärung der partiellen und totalen Remissionsphase gewonnen [12, 13, 57]. Wir wissen heute, daß eine Verbesserung der peripheren Insulinsensitivität für die Induktion einer partiellen Remissionsphase ausreicht, während für das Auftreten einer Totalremission eine Kombination aus signifikant gesteigerter pankreatischer Betazellfunktion und Normalisierung der peripheren Insulinresistenz notwendig ist. Für die Remissionsinduktion ist das Ausmaß der Betazellschonung durch ausreichende Insulinzufuhr in der Initialphase des Typ I-Diabetes von großer Bedeutung. In einer experimentellen randomisierten Studie [58] konnte vor kurzem gezeigt werden, daß eine hochdosierte Insulinzufuhr (3,8 E Insulin/kg/Tag) in den ersten 14 Tagen nach Krankheitsdiagnose einen signifikanten Einfluß auf die Betazellresidualfunktion ausübt. 12 Monate nach Therapiebeginn konnte in der Gruppe mit experimenteller Insulinbehandlung eine signifikant höhere C-Peptidsekretion und eine signifikant bessere Stoffwechseleinstellung als in der Kontrollgruppe nachgewiesen werden [58].

Wir müssen uns bewußt sein, daß die bislang eingesetzte Immuntherapie nur eine unspezifische Immunintervention am Ende eines langen Krankheitsprozesses darstellt. Neue immuntherapeutische Strategien sollten zunächst in tierexperimentellen Modellen des Typ I-Diabetes wie in der BB-Rate, der NOD-Maus und

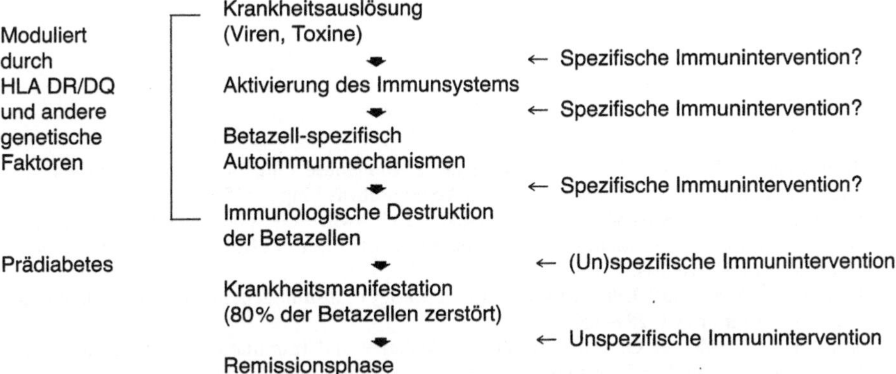

Abb. 6. Mögliche Angriffspunkte einer „spezifischen" Immunintervention im Krankheitsprozeß des Typ I-Diabetes

im low-dose-Streptozotozin-Maus-Modell erprobt werden. Aus den tierexperimentellen Modellen des Typ I-Diabetes, haben wir gelernt, daß der autoimmunologische Destruktionsprozeß stufenweise und multifaktoriell abläuft [59, 60]. Daraus resultiert, daß eine immunologische Intervention prinzipiell zu verschiedenen Zeitpunkten und an unterschiedlichen Angriffspunkten wirksam sein könnte. Im Tierexperiment haben sehr differente immunologische Interventionen wie Hemmung der Makrophagen [61, 62], Hemmung der Helfer/Inducer CD4$^+$-Zellfunktion [63, 64], Hemmung der zytotoxischen/suppressor CD8$^+$-Zellfunktion [62, 64], sowie Anwendung von monoklonalen Antikörpern, die gegen Klasse II Moleküle des Haupthistokompatibilitätskomplexes [65] oder gegen Interleukin-2 Rezeptoren [66, 67] gerichtet sind, zum Erfolg geführt. Aufgrund dieser tierexperimentellen Befunde ist nicht auszuschließen, daß nur durch eine kombinierte Intervention an verschiedenen Stellen des Destruktionsprozesses eine effektive Blockierung erreicht werden kann.

Die Zukunft der Immunmodulation bei Typ I-Diabetes muß entweder in einer primären Prävention der Erkrankung oder in einer spezifischen Immunintervention in einem sehr frühen Stadium der Erkrankung liegen. Künftige Studien müssen klären, ob neue Prinzipien der Immunmodulation wie Hemmung der Autoantigenbildung, Hemmung der Antigen-Präsentation, Elimination von autoreaktiven T-Zell Klonen oder Toleranzinduktion prinzipiell in Frage kommen. Endgültiges Ziel dieser Forschung muß es sein, eine langdauernde Totalremission mit einer nebenwirkungsarmen Therapie zu erreichen.

Abschließend kann festgestellt werden, daß die neuen Erkenntnisse auf dem Gebiet der Immunpathogenese und Immuntherapie des Typ I-Diabetes beträchtliche Hoffnungen für die zukünftige Behandlung von neumanifestierten Patienten mit Insulinmangeldiabetes erweckt haben. Die bisher vorliegenden Studien haben den Beweis erbracht, daß eine rechtzeitig eingesetzte Immuntherapie prinzipiell wirksam ist, womit die Autoimmuntheorie der Typ I-Diabetes-Pathogenese endgültig bewiesen ist. Weltweite Bemühungen und weitere Fortschritte auf dem Gebiet der Immuntherapie sind erforderlich, bevor dieses neue Therapieprinzip in die Routinebehandlung des Typ I-Diabetes eingeführt werden kann.

Literatur

1. Schernthaner G (1980) Neue Aspekte in der Pathogenese und im Krankheitsverlauf des Typ I-Diabetes mellitus. Wiener Klinische Wochenschrift [Suppl 115] 92: 1–36
2. Bottazzo GF, Dean BM, McNally JM, MacKay EH, Swift PGF, Gamble DR (1985) In situ characterization of autoimmune phenomena and expression of HLA molecules in the pancreas in diabetic insulitis. N Engl J Med, 313: 353–60
3. Rossini AA, Mordes JP, Like AA (1985) Immunology of insulin dependent diabetes mellitus. Annu Rev Immunol 3: 289–320
4. Kolb H, Schernthaner G, Gries FA (1983) Diabetes and Immunology: Pathogenesis and Immunotherapy. Huber Publishers, Bern Stuttgart Vienna, pp. 1–144
5. Schernthaner G, Banatvala JE, Scherbaum W, Bryant J, Borkenstein M, Schober E, Mayr WR (1985) Coxsackie-B-virus specific IgM responses, complement-fixing isletcell antibodies,

    HLA DR antigens, and C-peptide secretion in insulin-dependent diabetes mellitus. Lancet II: 630–632

6. Banatvala JE, Bryant J, Schernthaner G, Borkenstein M, Schober E, Brown D, DeSilva LM, Menser MA, Silinik M (1985) Coxsackie B, mumps, rubella and cytomegalovirus specific IgM responses in patients with juvenile-onset insulin-dependent diabetes mellitus in Britain, Austria and Australia. Lancet: 1409–1412

7. Mandrup-Poulsen T, Bendtzen K, Nerup J, Egeburg J, Nielsen JH (1985) Mechanisms of pancreatic islet cell destruction. Allergy 41: 249–259

8. Luger A, Schernthaner G, Urbanska A, Luger THA (1988) Cytokine production in patients with newly diagnosed insulindependent (type I) diabetes mellitus. Eur J of Clin Invest 18: 233–236

9. Eisenbarth GS (1986) Type I diabetes mellitus: a chronic autoimmune disease. Diabetes 314: 1360–1367

10. Tarn AC, Thomas JM, Dean BM, Schwarz G, Bottazzo GF, Gale EAM (1988) Predicting insulin-dependent diabetes. Lancet I: 845–850

11. Schernthaner G (1987) Immuntherapie als kausales Behandlungsprinzip des Typ I-Diabetes mellitus? In: Bergis K (Hrsg) Stoffwechseltage Bad Mergentheim. Schriftenreihe der Diabetes Akademie Bad Mergentheim Bd 13, S 120–131

12. Faber O, Binder C (1977) C-peptide response to glucagon: a test for the residual B-cell function in diabetes mellitus. Diabetes 26: 605–610

13. Schober E, Schernthaner G, Frisch H, Fink M (1984) Beta-cell function recovery is not the only factor responsible for remission in type I diabetics: Evaluation of C-peptide secretion in diabetic children after first metabolic recompensation and at partial remission phase. J Endocrinol Invest 7: 507–512

14. Mühlhauser I, Jörgens V, Berger M, Voss HE, Gürtler W, Scholz V, Hornke L, Kunz A, Graninger W, Schernthaner G (1983) Bicentric evaluation of a diabetes teaching and treatment programme for type I (insulin-dependent) diabetic patients: Improvement of metabolic control and other parameters of diabetes care for up to 22 months. Diabetologia 25: 470–476

15. Schernthaner G, Treiber G, Sachs G, Kunz A, Binder M, Nakrour A (1985) Basal-Bolus insulin therapy device with Ultratard HM injected at bedtime and Actrapid HM substituted with insulin-pen (Novopen). In: Proceedings of the 3rd International Hvidore Symposium, Copenhagen, pp 73–79

16. Schernthaner G, Bruck S, Kunz A (1989) Strategien der modernen Insulintherapie im Jahre 1989. Therapiewoche Österreich 4: 18-29

17. Kofoed-Enevoldsen A, Borch-Johnsen K, Kreiner S, Nerup J, Deckert T (1987) Declining invidence of persistent proteinuria in type I (insulin-dependent) diabetic patients in Denmark. Diabetes 36: 205–209

18. Stephenson JM, Schernthaner G (1989) Dawn phenomenon and somogyi effect in insulin-dependent diabetes mellitus: Clinical relevance and intraindividual comparison during conventional and basal-bolus insulin therapies. Diabetes Care 12: 245–251

19. Andreani D, Kolb H, Pozzilli P (1989) Immunotherapy of type I diabetes. Wiley & Sons, pp 1–251

20. Drash AL, Laporte R, Becker DJ, Singh B, Fishbein H, Goldstein D (1980) The natural history of diabetes mellitus in children: Insulin requirement during the initial two years. International Study Group on diabetes in Children and Adolescents Bulletin 4: 4–7

21. Knip M, Sakkinen A, Huttunen NP, Kaar ML, Lankela S, Mustonen A, Akerblom HK (1982) Postinitial remission in diabetic children – an analysis of 178 cases. Acta Paediatr Scand 71: 901–908

22. Feutren G, Papoz L, Assan R, Vialettes B, Karsenty G, Vexiau P, DuRostu H, Rodier M, Sirmai J, Lallemand A, Bach JF (1986) Cyclosporin increases the rate and length of remission in insulin-dependent diabetes of recent onset. Lancet II: 119–124

23. The Canadian/European Randomized Control Trial Group (1988) Cyclosporininduced remission of IDDM after early intervention: association of 1 year of cyclosporin treatment with enhanced insulin secretion. Diabetes 37: 1574–1582

24. Madsbad S, Krarup T, Faber OK, Binder C, Regeur L (1982) The transient effect of strict glycaemic control on B cell function in newly diagnosed type I (insulin-dependent) diabetic patients. Diabetologia 22: 16–20
25. Cobb WE, Molitch M, Reichlin S (1980) Levamisol in insulin-dependent diabetes mellitus. N Engl J Med 303: 1065–1066
26. Secci A, Pontiroli AE, Falqui L, Pastore MR, Scorza R, Carenini A, Meroni PL, Pozza G (1986) Prednisone, indomethacin or theophylline administration and the remission phase in recent onset Type I insulin-dependent diabetic patients. Transplant Proc 18: 1540–1542
27. Moncada E, Subira ML, Barberia JJ, Sanchez-Ibarrola A, Salvador J, Toni F, Oleaga A, Cano I (1987) Effect of thymic hormone and azathioprine administration on remission rate and insular function of 35 recent diagnosed type I (insulin-dependent) diabetic patients. A one year follow-up study. Diabetologia 30: 559 A
28. Ludvigsson J, Heding L, Lieden G, Marner B, Lernmark A (1983) Plasmapheresis in the initial treatment of insulin-dependent diabetes mellitus in children. Br Med J 286: 176–178
29. Marner B, Lernmark A, Ludvigsson J, MacKay P, Matsuba I, Nerup J, Rabinovitch A (1985) Islet cell antibodies in insulin-dependent (type I) diabetic children treated with plasmapheresis. Diabetes Res 2: 231–236
30. Rabinovitch A, MacKay P, Ludvigsson J, Lernmark A (1984) A prospective analysis of islet-cell cytotoxic antibodies in insulin-dependent diabetic children. Transient effects of plasmapheresis. Diabetes 33: 224–228
31. Leslie RD, Pyke DA, Denman AM (1985) Immunosuppressive therapy in diabetes. Lancet I: 516
32. Eisenbarth GS, Srikanta S, Jackson R, Rabinowe SL, Dolinar R, Aoki T, Morris MA (1985) Anti-thymocyte globulin and prednisone immunotherapy of recent onset type I diabetes mellitus. Diab Res 2: 271–276
33. Silverstein J, Riley W, Barret D, MacLaren N, Rosenbloom A (1983) Immunosuppressive therapy for newly diagnosed insulin-dependent diabetes mellitus with antithymocyte globulin and prednisone. Pediatr Res 71: 295
34. Rand KH, Rosenbloom AL, MacLaren NK, Silverstein JH, Riley WJ, Butterworth BE, Yoon JW, Rubenstein AH, Merigan TC (1981) Human leukocyte interferon treatment of two children with insulin dependent diabetes. Diabetologia 21: 116–119
35. Koivisto VA, Aro A, Cantell K, Haatja M, Huttunen J, Karonen SL, Mustajoki P, Pelkonen R, Seppala P (1984) Remission in newly diagnosed type I (insulin dependent) diabetes: influence of interferon as an adjunct to insulin therapy. Diabetologia 27: 193–197
36. Stiehm ER, Ashida E, Sik Kim K, Winston DW, Haas A, Gale RP (1987) Intravenous immunoglobulins as therapeutic agents. Ann Int med 107: 367–382
37. Heinze E, Thon A, Vetter U, Gaedicke G, Zuppinger K (1985) Gamma-Globulin therapy in 6 newly diagnosed diabetic children. Acta Pediatr Scand 74: 605–606
38. Usadel KH, Teuber J, Schmeidl R, Schwedes U, Bicker U, Herz M (1986) Management of type I diabetes with ciamexone. Lancet II: 567
39. Usadel KH (1989) Immunotherapy of type I diabetes with ciamexone a multicenter double-blind trial. 1st International Symposium on Immunotherapy of type I diabetes, Rome, Italy
40. Lazarus SS, Shapiro SH, (1973) Influence of nicotinamide and pyridine nucleotides on streptozotocin and alloxan induced pancreatic B-cell cytotoxicity. Diabetes 22: 499–506
41. Vague PH, Vialettes B, Lassemann-Vague V, Vallo JJ (1987) Nicotinamide may extend remission phase in insulin-dependent diabetes. Lancet I: 619
42. Pozzilli P, Visalli N, Ghirlanda G, Manna R, Papa G, Procaccinni E, Andreani D (1988) Nicotinamide therapy in patients with newly-diagnosed type I (insulin-dependent) diabetes. Diabetologia 31: 533A
43. Harrison LC, Colman PG, Dean B, Baxter R, Martin FIR (1985) Increase in remission rate in newly diagnosed type I diabetic subjects treated with azathioprine. Diabetes 34: 1306–1308
44. Cook JJ, Hudson I, Harrison LC, Dean B, Colman PG, Werther GA, Warne GL, Court JM (1989) A double-blind controlled trial of azathioprine in children with newly diagnosed type I diabetes. Diabetes (in press)

45. Silverstein J, MacLaren N, Riley W, Spillar R, Radjenovic D, Johnson S (1988) Immunosuppression with azathioprine and prednisone in recent onset IDDM. N Engl J Med 319: 599–604

46. Majon JL, Arkison P, Dawson KG, Dupré J, Jenner MR, Mehta A, Momah CI, Paul TL, Stiller CR (1989) Methylprednisolone combined with cyclosporine in remission induction in Typ I diabetes. Autoimmunity (in press)

47. Stiller CR, Dupre J, Gent M, Jenner MR, Keown PA, Laupacis A, Martell R, Rodger NW, v. Graffenried B, Wolfe BMJ (1984) Effects of cyclosporine immunosuppression in insulin-dependent diabetes mellitus of recent onset. Science 223: 1362–1367

48. Assan R, Bach JF, DuRostu H, Feutren G, Karsenty G, Lallemand L, Papoz L, Rodier M, Sirmai J, Vexiau P, Vialettes B (1985) Metabolic and immunological effect of cyclosporine in recently diagnosed type I diabetes mellitus. Lancet I: 67–71

49. Schernthaner G, Aschauer-Treiber G, Gaube S, Klösch-Kasparek D, Müller C, Zielinski C (1988) Ergebnisse der Cyclosporin-A-Terhapie in der Frühphase des Tpy I-Diabetes mellitus. Wiener Klinische Wochenschrift 100: 454–459

50. Schernthaner G, Gaube S, Klauser R, Müller C, Prager R, Zielinski CC (1987) Insulin action and insulin secretion following arginine, glucagon or i.v. glucose administration in type I-diabetic patients during cyclosporin-A induced total remission. International Research Symposium "The Immunology of Diabetes", Woods Hole, MA, USA. American Diabetes Association 38

51. Müller C, Zielinski CC, Kalinowski M, Wolf H, Mannhalter JW, Aschauer-Treiber G, Klösch-Kasparek D, Eibl MM, Schernthaner G (1989) Effects of Cyclosporin A upon humoral and cellular immune parameters in insulin-dependent diabetes mellitus type I: A long-term follow-up study. J Endocrinol 121: 177–183

52. Dupré J, Stiller CR, Gent M, Donner A, von Graffenried B, Heinrichs D, Jenner M, Keown P, Mahon J, Martell R, Momah CI, Murphy G, Rodger NW, Wolfe BM (1988) Clinical Trials of Cyclosporin in IDDM. Diabetes Care [Suppl 1] 11: 37–44

53. Müller C, Schernthaner G, Kovarik J, Kalinowska W, Zielinski C (1987) Natural killer cell activity and antibody dependent cellular cytotoxicity in patients under various immunosuppressive regimens. J Clin Immunol Immunopathol 44: 12–19

54. Sibley RK, Sutherland DER, Goetz FC, Michael AF (1985) Recurrent diabetes mellitus in the pancreatic iso- and allograft period: a light and electron-microscopic and immunohistochemical analysis of four cases. Lab Invest 53: 132–144

55. Dupré J, Stiller CR, Gent M, Donner A, Mahon J, Jenner MR, Keown PA, Laupacis A, Martell R, Rodger NW, von Graffenried B (1988) Effects of immunosuppression with cyclosporine in insulin dependent diabetes mellitus of recent onset: the Canadian open study at 44 months. Transplant Proc 20: 184–192

56. Bougners PF, Carel JC, Castano L, Boitard C, Gardin JP, Landais P, Hors J, Mihatsch MJ, Paillard M, Chaussain JL, Bach JF (1988) Factors determining very early remission of type I diabetes in children treated with cyclosporin A. N Engl J Med 318: 663–671

57. Yki-Jarvinen H, Koivisto VA (1984) Insulin sensitivity in newly diagnosed type I diabetics after ketoacidosis and after three months of insulin therapy. J Clin Endocrinol Metab 59: 317–378

58. Shah SC, Malone JI, Simpson NE (1989) A randomized trial of intensive insulin therapy in newly diagnosed insulin-dependent diabetes mellitus. N Engl J Med 320: 550–554

59. Mordes JP, Rossini AA (1987) Keys to understanding autoimmune diabetes mellitus: the minimal models of insulin-dependent diabetes mellitus. Baillière s Clin Immunol Allergy 1: 29–52

60. Gottlieb PA, Rossini AA, Mordes JP (1988) Approaches to prevention and treatment of IDDM in animal models. Diabetes Care 11: 29–36

61. Oschilewski U, Kiesel U, Kolb H (1985) Administration of silica prevents diabetes in BB rats. Diabetes 34: 197–199

62. Charlton B, Bacelj A, Mandel TE (1988) Administration of silica particels or anti-Lyt2 antibody prevents β-cell destruction in NOD mice given cyclophosphamide. Diabetes 37: 930–935

63. Koike T, Hoh Y, Ishi T, Ito I, Takabayashi K, Maruyama N, Tomioka H, Yashida S (1987) Preventive effect of monoclonal anti-L3T4 antibody on development of diabetes in NOD mice. Diabetes 36: 539–541
64. Kantwerk G, Cobbold S, Waldmann H, Kolb H (1987) L3T4 and Lyt2 T cells are both involved in the generation of low-dose streptozotozin-induced diabetes in mice. Clin Exp Immunol 70: 585–592
65. Kiesel U, Kolb H (1983) Suppressive effect of antibodies to immune response gene products on the development of low-dose streptozotozin-induced diabetes. Diabetes 32: 869–871
66. Kelley VE, Gaulton GN, Hattori M, Ikegami H, Eisenbarth G, Strom TB (1988) Anti-interleukin 2 receptor antibody suppresses murine diabetic insulitis and lupus nephritis. J Immunol 140: 59–61
67. Hahn JH, Lucke S, Klöting I, Volk HD, Baehr KV, Diamantstein T (1987) Curing BB rats of freshly manifested diabetes by short-term treatment and a combination of a monoclonal anti-interleukin 2 receptor antibody and a subtherapeutic dose of cyclosporin A. Eur J Immunol 17: 1075–1078

Insulin Antibodies:
A Brief Review and Personal Contribution

D. ANDREANI

Zusammenfassung

Viele Jahre der Forschung haben die Identifikation der Faktoren ermöglicht, die die Antigenität von Insulin bestimmen und kontrollieren. Aufgrund zahlreicher Studien gewannen wir die Überzeugung, daß freies Insulin und Insulinantikörper, wahrscheinlich durch Immunkomplexbildung ein Dysäquilibrium erreichen, das die Gewebsaffinität des Hormones reguliert. Ab einem gewissen Punkt unserer Untersuchungen wunderten wir uns und waren nahezu überzeugt, daß Immunkomplexe, mit oder ohne Insulin (Antigen), auf irgendeine Weise mit dem Auftreten früher diabetischer Sekundärkomplikationen, der „malignen Mikroangiopathie" und einigen Komplikationen bei schwangeren Diabetikerinnen und ihren Kindern verbunden sein müssen. Später konnte gezeigt werden, daß die Immunogenität von Insulin nicht nur durch Speziesunterschiede, sondern auch durch Verunreinigungen selbst in kleinen Mengen verursacht sein kann und das Hormon stärker immunogen werden läßt. In der Folge erwies sich gereinigtes Schweineinsulin am wenigsten immunogen. Trotzdem wurden einige Fälle von Insulinallergie auch bei Verwendung dieser neuen Insuline berichtet. Einen weiteren Schritt auf dem Weg der Insulinreinigung und zur sicheren Anwendung von Insulinpräparaten stellt die Synthese von humanem Insulin durch gentechnologisches Rekombinationsverfahren mit Hilfe von Baktereien oder durch einen semi-synthetischen Prozeß mit chemischer Modifikation von Schweineinsulin dar. Aber auch unter Humaninsulintherapie wurden noch einige Fälle von Insulinallergie beobachtet. Vor wenigen Jahren wurde das spontane Auftreten von Insulinautoantikörpern bei Erstmanifestation eines Typ I-Diabetes mellitus, sogar den Verwandten dieser Patienten und auch anderen Personen mit einem erhöhten Risiko für Typ I-Diabetes beschrieben. In Analogie zu anderen Autoimmunkrankheiten könnte man den Schluß ziehen, daß das autologe Hormon die Bildung von Autoantikörpern hervorruft, die für die Pathogenese dieser Krankheit von Bedeutung sein mögen. Diesen neuen Antikörpern zusammen mit komplementfixierenden Inselzellantikörpern und Inselzelloberflächenantikörpern wird die Rolle von Markern zugeschrieben. Obwohl nicht absolut spezifisch, haben Anti-Insulinautoantikörper eine prädiktive Bedeutung für Personen mit erhöhtem Risiko für Typ I-Diabetes. Zuletzt soll noch erwähnt werden, daß in den vergangenen Monaten über die Fähigkeit von Anti-Insulinautoantikörpern, die Insulinsekretion zu stimulieren und eine Hypoglykämie auszulösen berichtet wurde.

The first Journal to which we submitted the paper rejected it after many months with a comment by a referee to the effect that everyone knows that insulin does not make antibodies.
Perhaps of further interest is that although the paper was accepted (in 1956) by the next Journal, namely J. Clin. Invest., similar reservations on the interpretation of findings were expressed and we were not permitted to use the term insulin antibody in the title of the paper.

Rosalyn Yalow

Introduction

Though insulin immunogenicity had been previously suspected on a number of occasions we owe the precise approach to the subject to Berson and Yalow whose important findings more than 30 years ago opened the door to a great flux of research and publications [1].

It would be impossible to give a complete and satisfactory overview of the information accumulated to date after the discovery that insulin was antigenic and was able to raise antibodies in the human body. Therefore, I will limit myself to underlining a few data from the literature which seem to me relevant and to discussing some points which have emerged from the research performed by my group over this period of time.

First of all, it is worthwhile recapitulating the conditions which are nowadays believed to be connected with the effects of insulin antibodies. The picture seems clear, but discussion is still going on to determine the real impact of insulin antibodies in certain conditions and the modalities of their intervention. Among other questions it is important to take into consideration the question why insulin antibodies may have opposite effects, as illustrated by biological and clinical conditions where insulin antibodies are involved:

1. Allergic reactions, local and systemic; anaphylactic shock
2. Lipodystrophy (hypertrophic and atrophic)
3. Reduced free insulin; insulin resistance
4. Blunted insulin peak after injection and worse glucose control
5. Buffer effect in insulin action
6. Late and/or unexpected hypoglycemia
7. Immune complexes disease
8. Fetal pathological conditions (hypoglycemia, respiratory distress syndrome, etc.)
9. Damage to β-cells
10. Stimulation of β-cells
11. Interference with insulin receptors

Over the course of the years it has been possible to identify the following factors which determine and control the antigenicity of insulin [2, 3, 5]:

1. Primary structure of the hormone (species differences, abnormal insulin molecule)
2. pH of insulin medium (acid insulin less tolerated)
3. Crystallization and polymerization
4. Presence of impurities such as proinsulin, glucagon, enteric hormones
5. Frequent withdrawal of insulin in treatment
6. Subcutaneous and/or intradermal deposition of insulin with access to macrophages
7. Addition of retarding substances; protamine, surfen, etc.
8. Intercurrent infectious disease

Most factors are related to the insulin itself, but also depend on the subject receiving the treatment.

As to the reactivity of insulin-treated subjects, age, sex, and genetic background are claimed to be of great relevance [4, 2], although this is disputed by other authors [6]. There is no doubt that some subjects react strongly to insulin and may produce high titers of antibodies, as happens in animal experiments.

My group has been studying insulin antibodies since 1960 [7] and therefore when the book by Federlin on the *Immunopathology of insulin* appeared in 1971 [8] we greeted it with enthusiasm. I found the book extremely illuminating and it has always had a special place in my library. In our own clinical observations and research we were impressed by the consequences of insulin immunogenicity and patients with different types of allergies, insulin resistance, and high antibody levels were followed with particular interest.

Lipodystrophy, whose origins were obscure at the beginning, was also thought to be in some way related to insulin immunogenicity [9]. This point has been clarified by Reeves et al. [10].

After a good number of studies we became convinced that free insulin and insulin antibodies, possibly forming immune complexes, reach an unstable equilibrium according to which the access of the hormone to tissues is regulated (Fig. 1). At a certain point in our investigations we wondered whether, and were almost convinced, that immune complexes, either associated with insulin or independent, might be in some way related to the early complications of diabetes and to "malignant microangiopathy" (Fig. 2) [11–13]. The picture became more complex when antibodies were also shown to interfere with insulin receptors [14].

We have also been led to believe that insulin antibodies are responsible for some complications in pregnant diabetic women and in their babies [15]. These include gestosis, hypoglycemia in the newborn infant, macrosomia, respiratory distress syndrome, hypoglycemia and hypocalcemia. It is very likely that insulin, in addition to poor metabolic control, may interfere with the course of pregnancy and normal fetal development.

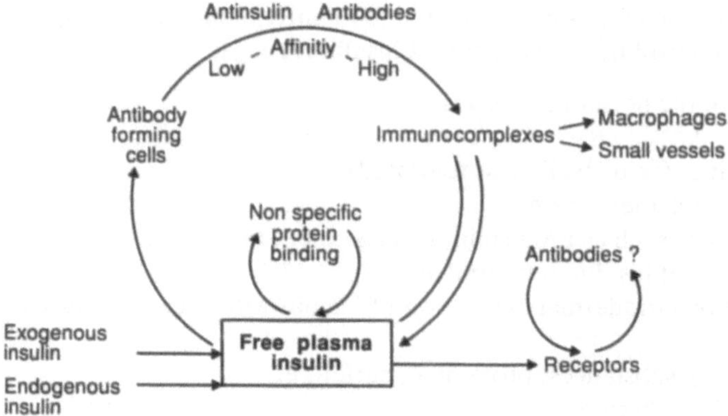

Fig. 1. Balance between free insulin and insulin antibodies. Exogenous and endogenous (when present) insulin contributes to the insulin pool, which is influenced by antibodies and receptors. Nonspecific protein binding and interference of antibodies on receptors are supposed. Immune complexes formed may have an impact on macrophages and small vessels

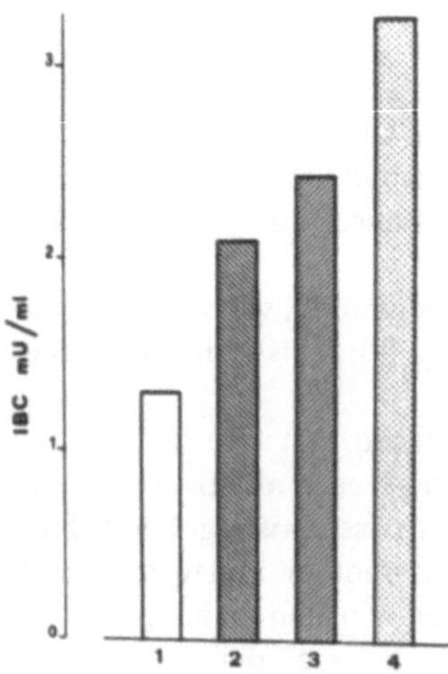

Fig. 2. IgG insulin antibody levels in long-standing insulin-treated diabetics without and with microangiopathy. *1*, 33 patients without microangiopathy. *2*, 45 patients with background retinopathy. *3*, 30 patients with proliferative retinopathy. *4*, 18 patients with malignant microangiopathy. *IBC*, Insulin binding capacity

Highly Purified Insulins

In the history of insulin antibodies, the remarkable contribution of Dr. Schlichtkrull [16] must be acknowledged; working with Novo Industri Copenhagen, he and his team were able to demonstrate that the immunogenicity of insulin was not only due to species differences but also to impurities which, even in small amounts, were capable of rendering the hormone more immunogenic. As a result of the research performed by Schlichtkrull et al. [17], as well as by Chance and others [18], it was clearly demonstrated that highly purified porcine insulins were the least immunogenic insulins. These investigations led to the production of "mono-component" and "monopeak" insulins.

When purified insulins became available their use confirmed that animal insulins deprived of impurities had a very low immunogenicity, and that the use of the highly purified monocomponent porcine insulins enabled most cases of allergy, resistance, and lipodystrophy to be avoided [19, 20].

It is of great relevance to note that today these inconveniences have become very rare and physicians can use insulin with no anxiety as far allergic reactions are concerned.

After more than 2 years of experimentation with monocomponent insulins, we were able to make the following observations [9]:

1. Highly purified insulins were capable of dramatically improving the clinical symptoms of immunological reactivity to exogenous insulin.
2. The use of purified insulin was accompanied by lower levels of circulating insulin antibodies. This phenomenon was most prominent in patients with the highest pretreatment levels.
3. During treatment with the new insulins a substantial decrease in insulin requirement was registered. Correspondingly, slight hypoglycemic crises were observed from time to time. However, it is worth noting that this finding has been confirmed by some authors, but not by others [2, 21].

Nonetheless, some cases of allergy have been reported even using the new insulins [22–24].

During long-term studies we observed that after 1 year antibody levels reached a lower level where they became stabilized for more than 4 years. Insulin requirements also reached a level which could be maintained for 3–4 years; in such cases, however, insulin requirement tended to increase again with the duration of treatment [25].

Human Insulin

Another step in the process of insulin purification and in the safe use of insulin preparations is represented by the synthesis of human insulin by a recombinant technique using bacteria, or a semisynthetic process involving the chemical modification of porcine insulin. The industrial production of human insulin has now made it possible for a large proportion of insulin-dependent diabetic subjects to take advantage of these purified, homologous insulins. But even with human insulin, some cases of allergy were still observed [26].

The experience of my group with human insulin has been on the whole favorable, insofar as we have observed a very low production of insulin antibodies, even less than with purified porcine insulins [27] (Fig. 3). Our experience indicates

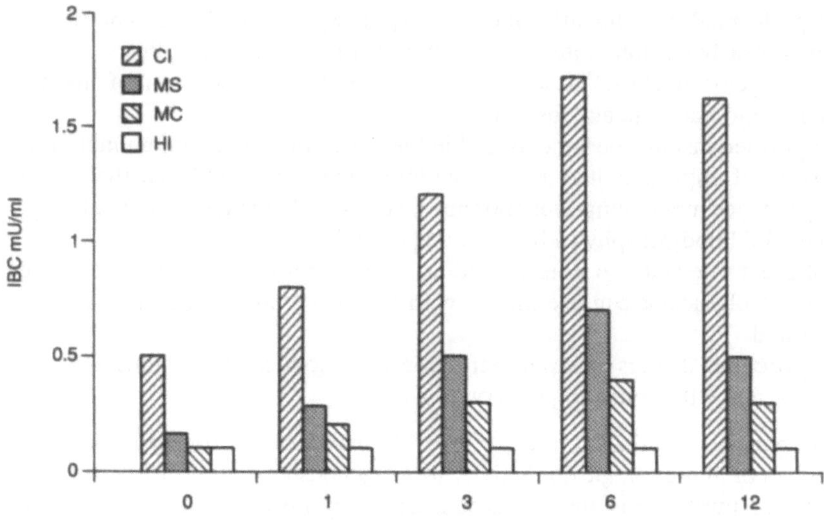

Fig. 3. IgG insulin antibody levels in newly diagnosed diabetics from the beginning of treatment with different insulins. *CI*, 20 patients treated with conventional insulins. *MS*, 15 patients treated with monospecies porcine insulin, *MC*, 25 patients treated with monocomponent porcine insulin. *HI*, 15 subjects treated with human monocomponent insulin. *IBC*, Insulin binding capacity

that if allergic phenomena appear, they are of minor relevance (e.g., some red spots at the place of injection). In our studies there was a slight difference between newly diagnosed subjects starting treatment ex novo and subjects already treated with other types of insulins including porcine monocomponent insulins, who were subsequently shifted to the human hormone. The latter showed a slight reduction in insulin antibody levels, but these levels rose again to the earlier values as treatment continued. It seems likely, therefore, that once the immune reaction has been elicited even the use of homologous purified insulin is not capable of making antibodies disappear. At the same time, there was no drop in the insulin requirement [28].

I must add that in our experience on few occasions when a patient was transfered from human insulin produced by one firm to human insulin produced by another firm the allergic reaction was no longer observed. It may be that the degree of purity is not always the same, or that polymerization or some other physicochemical change takes place in some preparations.

Insulin Autoantibodies

Reports have recently been published concerning the spontaneous appearance of insulin autoantibodies in newly diagnosed diabetic patients [29] and even in the relatives of type I diabetics and in other subjects at risk for insulin-dependent diabetes [30–32].

Data on insulin autoantibodies have provided the best demonstration that insulin can behave as an antigen in the same body in which it is produced. This represents a final and interesting step in our knowledge of insulin immunogenicity. Insulin is not only antigenic when it comes from a different species or when, even having being made as homologous, it is injected exogenously, but also when it is produced in the same organism and thus behaves like a autoantigen.

In parallel with other autoimmune diseases, in insulin-dependent diabetes one may speculate that the autologous hormone elicits the formation of autoantibodies which may be relevant to the pathogenesis of the illness. But, of course, the interpretation of the autoimmune process is very complex and would deserve a much longer discussion.

Anti-insulin autoantibodies (a-IAAb) have been revealed at diagnosis in a large number of patients. Together with CF-ICA and ICSA, these new antibodies have been accorded the role of markers [31, 33, 34]. It is interesting to note that by combining and adding the figures obtained by a-IAAb determination with those of CF-ICA and ICSA, a very high percentage of newly diagnosed diabetic patients show a humoral marker of β-cell aggression. It seems therefore that the antigens freed by the immunoaggreesion on the β-cells are many and of different kinds. This finding brings type I diabetes into line with other endocrine autoimmune syndromes, such as some thyroid diseases. In this respect, I must add that a-IAAb have been found in patients with other endocrine autoimmune diseases who show no signs of clinical diabetes [35–37]. One point of great interest, which was highlighted by Eisenbarth's group in close association with our group, is that, although not absolutely specific, a-IAAb also have a predictive value in subjects at risk of developing type I diabetes. In fact, subjects at risk have shown a remarkable increase in a-IAAb levels shortly before the clinical appearance of the disease, and together with ICA and reduced response to i.v. glucose they may be indicators of the development of clinical diabetes.

A final point which I would like to raise is that over the last few months anti-insulin antibodies have been reported as being capable of stimulating insulin secretion and producing hypoglycemia [38]. This finding parallels what is observed in thyroid disease, to the point that the condition which derives from these stimulating anti-insulin antibodies has been imaginatively called "Graves' disease of islets" [39].

Anti-insulin antibodies accompanying hypoglycemia were described in the past in the insulin autoimmune syndrome [40] and in acanthosis nigricans and hirsutism in which insulin antibodies are active on insulin receptors. But in this condition the insulin antibodies are probably of a different kind.

If these observations are confirmed they will provide a complete picture of the immune phenomena concerning insulin and will contribute to our knowledge of autoimmune syndromes in diseases of the endocrine glands. But the story does not end here. Many factors are still missing or need to be confirmed. The missing bricks still need to be found and installed in their right place before the whole house is built.

References

1. Yalow RS, Bauman A, Rothschild MA, Berson SA et al. (1956) Insulin 131I metabolism in human subjects. Demonstration of insulin binding globulin in insulin treated subjects. J Clin Invest 35: 170–190
2. Reeves WG (1981) Antibody production during insulin therapy. Pattern of response and clinical sequels. In: Keck K, Erb P (eds) Basic and clinical aspects of immunity to insulin. De Gruyter, Berlin, p 219–235
3. Arquilla ER, Valdes I, Thompson R, Michelski RF, Thomas K (1981) Differences in insulin antibodies induced with varying antigenic forms. In: Keck K, Erb P (eds) Basic and clinical aspects of immunity to insulin. De Gruyter, Berlin, pp 163–189
4. Schernthaner G, Mayr WR (1981) Insulin antibody formation following conventional or monocomponent insulin treatment is influenced by genes of the HLA-DR locus. In: Keck K, Erb P (eds) Basic and clinical aspects of immunity to insulin. De Gruyter, Berlin pp 263–274
5. Federlin K, Velovsky HG, Maser E (1981) Clinical aspects of immunity to insulin. In: Keck K, Erb P (eds) Basic and clinical aspects of immunity to insulin. De Gruyter, Berlin, pp 203–215
6. Asplin CA, Dornan TL, Raghu PK, Hansen JA, Plamer JP (1984) The antibody response to insulin therapy. Diabetes 33: 966–69
7. Andreani D, Negri M, Sereno L, Grevo V, Cramarossa L (1960) Osservazione sul turnover e sul livello plasmatico dell'insulina. Folia Endocrinol 32: 1146
8. Federlin K (1971) Immunopathology of insulin. Springer, Berlin Heidelberg New York
9. Andreani D, Iavicoli M, Tamburrano G, Menzinger G (1974) Comparative trials with monocomponent (MC) and monospecies (MS) pork insulin in the treatment of diabetes mellitus. Influence of antibody levels on insulin requirement and some complications. Horm Metab Res 6: 447–454
10. Reeves WG, Alley BR, Tattersall RB (1980) Insulin induced lipodystrophy: evidence for an immune pathogenesis. Br Med J 1: 1500–1503
11. Irvine WJ, Di Mario U, Guy K, Iavicoli M, Pozzilli P, Lumbroso B, Andreani D (1980) Immune complexes and diabetic microangiopathy. In: Irvine WJ, Immunology of diabetes, Teviot, Edinburgh, pp 325–336
12. Andreani D (1980) Malignant microangiopathy. Diabetologia 18: 255–256
13. Di Mario U, Ventriglia L, Iavicoli M, Guy K, Andreani D (1983) The correlation between insulin antibodies and immune complexes in diabetics with and without microangiopathy. Clin Exp Immunol 52: 575–580
14. De Pirro R, Fusco A, Spallone V, Magnatta R, Lauro R (1980) Insulin antibodies prevent insulin-receptor interactions. Diabetologia 19: 118–122
15. Fallucca F, Di Mario U, Gargiulo P, Iavicoli M, Galfo C, Musacchio N, Pachi A, Andreani D (1985) Humoral immunity in diabetic pregnancy; interrelation with maternal/neonatal complication and maternal metabolic control. Diabete Metab 11: 386–396
16. Schlichtkrull J, Brague J, Eze H, Hallund D, Heding LG, Jorgens K, Markussen J, Stahenke P, Sundby F, Volund A (1970) Proinsulin and related proteins. Diabetologia 6: 63
17. Schlichtkrull J, Brauge J, Christiansen AH, Heding J, Hallund O, Jorgensen KA (1972) Clinical aspects of insulin antigenicity. Diabetes [Suppl 2] 21: 649
18. Chance RE, Root MA, Galloway JA (1976) The immunogenicity of insulin preparation. Acta Endocrinol (Copenh) [Suppl] 205: 185–198
19. Andreani D, Iavicoli M, Colletti A, Menzinger G (1972) Esperienze sul trattamento del diabete con le insuline monocomponenti e monospecie. Folia Endocrinol 25: 516
20. Waldhäusl WK, Fresch H, Haydl RH (1974) Elevated insulin binding capacity incidence and treatment by MC insulin. In: Bastenie PA, Gepts W (eds) Immunity and autoimmuntiy in diabetes mellitus. Excerpta Medica, Amsterdam, pp 54–62
21. Peacock I, Taylor a, Tattersall RB, Douglas CA, Reeves WG (1983) Effects of new insulins on insulin and C peptide antibodies, insulin dose and diabetic control. Lancet I: 149–151
22. Leslie D (1977) Generalized allergic reaction to monocomponent insulin. Br Med J 2: 735

23. Simmonds JP, Russell FI, Cowley AJ, Servell HH, Heamshawn V (1980) Generalize allergy to porcine and bovine monocomponent insulin. Br Med J 2:355
24. Carini C, Brostoff J, Kurtz AB (1982) An anaphylactic reaction to highly purified pork insulin. Diabetologia 22: 324–326
25. Andreani D, Menzinger G, Di Mario U, Scarsella M, Iavicoli M (1977) Clinical use of monocomponent insulin preparations. XIV International Congress of Therapeutics, Montpellier. Expansion Scientifique Française, Paris, pp 9–25
26. Fineberg SE, Galloway JA, Fineberg NJ, Rathburn MJ, Hufferd SH (1983) Immunogenicity of recombinant DNA human insulin. Diabetologia 25: 465–469
27. Iavicoli M, Andreani D (1984) Formation of IgG specific for insulins: clinical consequences. In: Andreani D, Di Mario U, Federlin K, Heding LG (eds) Immunology in diabetes. Kimpton, London, pp 221–230
28. Di Mario U, Arduini P, Tiberti C, Lombardi G, Pietravalle P, Andreani D (1986) Immunogenicity of biosynthetic insulin. Diabetes Res Clin Pract 2: 317–324
29. Palmer JP, Asplin CM, Clemens P, Lyen K, Tatpati O, Raghu PK, Paguette IL (1983) Insulin antibodies in IDD before insulin treatment. Science 222: 1337–39
30. Wilkin T, Hotkins PJ, Armitage M, Rodier M, Casey C, Diaz JL, Ryke DA, Leslie RDG (1985) Value of insulin autoantibodies as serum markers for insulin-dependent DM. Lancet I: 480–487
31. Vardi P, Dib SA, Tuttleman M, Connelly JE, Grinbergs M, Radizabeh A, Riley WJ, McLaren NK, Eisenbarth GS, Soeldner S (1987) A competitive insulin autoantibodies assay. Prospective evaluation of subjects at high risk for type I diabetes mellitus. Diabetes 36: 1286–1291
32. Becker T, Helmke K, Sessewiss K, Sauer HR, Federlin K (1988) Islet cell antibodies (ICA), Insulin autoantibodies (IAA): prevalence and correlation to metabolic testing in type I diabetics and their I relatives. Diabetologia 3: 468A
33. Dean BM, Becker F, McNally JM, Schwartz G, Gale EAM, Bottazzo GF (1986) Insulin autoantibodies in the prediabetic period: correlation with ICA and development of diabetes. Diabetologia 29: 339–342
34. Ludvigsson J, Binder C, Mandrup-Poulsen T (1988) Insulin autoantibodies are associated with islet cell antibodies. Diabetologia 31: 647–651
35. Betterle C, Presotto F, Pedrini B, Moro L, Slack RS, Zanette F, Zanchetta R (1987) Islet cell and insulin autoantibodies in organ-specific autoimmune patients. Diabetologia 30: 724–726
36. Armitage M, Scott-Morgan L, Tuck A, Wilkin TJ (1988) Insulin autoantibodies are as frequent in poliendocrine autoimmune disease as in insulin dependent diabetes mellitus. Diabetic Med [Suppl] 5: 16
37. Di Mario U, Perfetti R, Anastasi E, Contreas G, Amendola MA, Masala C (1989) Autoantibodies to insulin do appear in non-diabetic patients with autoimmun disorders: comparison with anti-immunoglobulin antibodies and other autoimmune pheonema (in press)
38. Wilkin TJ, Hammonds P, Mirza I, Bone A, Webster K, Armitage M (1988) Graves' disease of the islet: a new antibody that stimulates the beta cell to secrete insulin. Diabetic Med [suppl] 5: 8
39. Wilkin TJ, Hammonds P, Mirza IH, Bone AJ, Webster K (1988) Islet cell stimulating antibodies: a new cause of hypoglycemia. Diabetologia 31: 560A
40. Hirata Y (1987) Autoimmune insulin syndrome up to date. In: Andreani D, Marks V, Lefebvre P (eds) Hypoglycemia. Raven, New York, pp 105–118

Discussion I

Chairman: K. F. WEINGES

E. F. Pfeiffer:
One comment on Andreani's report about Rosalyn Yalow: She referred the story at the funeral of Sol Berson, when she was giving the eulogy for him. She projected all the letters from editors who had rejected the paper on the insulin antibodies. Only to tell it to your associates at home when you return, right when they are up in the moment in which they did not get accepted their paper directly. She persisted, and finally they passed the paper through, but with comments to the effect that they were not permitted to put "antibodies" in the title. And then afterwards they were awarded the Nobel prize. So I think if one of your associates has a paper rejected at least 20 times, then he is very near to the Nobel prize.

Dynamische Aspekte
der Insulinsubstitution

Physiologische Grundlagen der Insulinsubstitution

W. Waldhäusl

Summary

Insulin replacement in an insulin deficient state has been a routine treatment since more than 60 years, but the strategy applied remains a conventional pharmacological one for the majority of patients. Attempts to mimic more closely physiological insulin release when designing strategies of insulin replacement were delayed by the success of conventional insulin treatment in reducing the incidence of diabetic ketoacidosis and coma. However, the rising prevalence of diabetes associated complications forced a reappraisal of the available forms of insulin therapy. From this it was concluded that algorithms for more appropriate insulin replacement must be derived from normal endogenous insulin release. Such a strategy perceives basal (= fasting) and prandial insulin requirement as separate and independent entities and requires the patient to correct immediately blood glucose values beyond given target levels. Such functional insulin treatment permits up to 50 % of type I diabetic patients to consistently renormalize their HbA_{1c} levels, and helps pregnant type I diabetic patients to maintain near-euglycemia throughout pregnancy. It is the aim of this overview to discuss physiological knowledge of insulin release and carbohydrate metabolism pertinent to the design of a rational strategy for functional insulin treatment.

Einleitung

Ziel jeder Insulinersatztherapie ist die weitgehende Anpassung der Metabolik des Diabetikers an normale Verhältnisse. Dies gilt insbesondere für den Patienten mit Typ I-Diabetes und absolutem Insulinmangel, wobei letzterer vor der Verfügbarkeit von Insulin Ursache von schwerster Katabolie und Kachexie war. Heute bewahrt ein ausreichender Ersatz des Insulindefizites mit mindestens 1–2 Insulininjektionen je Tag den Patienten vor Ketoazidose, Katabolie und einem frühen Tod, nicht jedoch vor den Spätkomplikationen der Erkrankung. Diese auch als „konventionell" bezeichnete Form der Insulintherapie verlangt zur Vermeidung insulinbedingter Hypoglykämien eine, an bestimmte Zeiten gebundene Nahrungsaufnahme definierter Zusammensetzung, was höchster Disziplin seitens des Patienten bedarf. Das Fehlen jeglicher Flexibilität bezüglich Insulindosierung und Nahrungszufuhr verhindert bei dieser Vorgangsweise bei der Mehrzahl der Patienten die Annäherung an normale metabolische Verhältnisse. Die Ursache für das partielle Versagen der konventionellen Insulintherapie muß in der Art der damit verbundenen unphysiologischen Insulinzufuhr gelegen sein, die in keinem Fall in der Lage ist, natürliche Verhältnisse der Insulininkretion nachzuahmen. Grundvoraussetzung für eine patientenorientierte Lösung des Problems sind daher ausreichende Kenntnisse über den normalen Ablauf von Insulinsekretion und -wirkung und die Übertragung dieses Wissens durch den Arzt bzw. den Diabetesberater in verständlicher und praktikabler Form auf den insulinpflichtigen Diabetiker [1]. Ziel der vorliegenden und notwendigerweise unvollständigen Zusammenfassung ist eine Besprechung der physiologischen Grundlagen der Insulinersatztherapie und der Möglichkeiten einer praktischen Umsetzung des vorhandenen Wissens.

Physiologische Grundlagen

Die Planung einer rationellen Insulintherapie basiert somit auf dem Wissen um die Dynamik der Insulinsekretion beim Gesunden, um das Verhalten der hepatischen Glukoseproduktion und der Glukoseutilisation durch periphere Gewebe, wie auch um die Beeinflußbarkeit der Insulinsekretion durch endogene und exogene Faktoren.

Insulinsekretion

Wesentlich für das Verständnis der Zusammenhänge ist zunächst die Feststellung, daß Insulin nicht nur zu den Mahlzeiten (= „prandiales Insulin"), sondern auch im Fastenzustand (= „basales Insulin") sezerniert wird. Die Freisetzung erfolgt pulsatil in enger Wechselwirkung mit den anderen in den Langerhans'schen Inseln produzierten Hormonen Glukagon, Somatostatin und pankreatisches Polypeptid sowie in Dosisabhängigkeit von der jeweiligen Substratzufuhr. Die Relation zwischen dem basal und prandial freigesetzten Insulin beträgt beim Erwachsenen bei gewichtserhaltender Ernährung etwa 1 : 1. Als Substrate für die Stimulation der Insulinsekretion dienen vor allem Glukose und Aminosäuren, wobei zu beachten ist, daß auf isokalorischer Basis die Insulinsekretion durch Glukose etwa 3- bis 4-fach stärker stimuliert wird als durch ein gleichwertiges Eiweißsubstrat. Die Hauptaufgabe des freigesetzten Insulins ist eine anabole. Sie dient der Speicherung von Glukose und verzweigtkettigen Aminosäuren sowie der Proteinsynthese und der Energiebereitstellung durch Glukoseoxydation.

Die Komplexität der endokrinen Antwort auf die Zufuhr eines Substrates wird besonders gut nach oraler Glukosezufuhr erkennbar. So stimuliert Glukose nicht nur die splanchnische Abgabe von Insulin und C-Peptid sowie vorübergehend auch von pankreatischem Polypeptid [2], sondern hemmt parallel dazu auch die Glukagon- und Wachstumshormonsekretion [3]. Diese Veränderungen werden von einem frühen Anstieg von Noradrenalin im Plasma und später auch von einem solchen des Plasmaadrenalins begleitet [3]. Stimulierende Modulatoren der Insulinsekretion sind weiter eine erhöhte Aktivität des Nervus vagus sowie verschiedene gastrointestinale, pankreatische, adrenale und hypophysäre Hormone. Im Gegensatz dazu hemmen Insulin selbst [4] sowie pharmakologische Mengen von Proinsulin [5], Somatostatin [6, 7] und alpha-adrenerge Agonisten die Insulinsekretion. Insgesamt erlaubt diese Feinregulation bei gesunden Personen eine Konstanz der Blutglukosekonzentration zwischen 4.5 mmol/l nüchtern und 8.9 mmol/l 60 Minuten nach Einnahme einer sehr kohlenhydratreichen Mahlzeit [8].

Der mit einer Periodizität von 8–30 Minuten ablaufenden pulsatilen Freisetzung von Insulin, C-Peptid und Glukagon [9, 10] dürfte bei der Optimierung der jeweiligen Hormonwirkung besondere Bedeutung zukommen. So wurde *in vitro* gezeigt, daß pulsatile Insulinzufuhr in der Lage ist, bei gleichbleibender metabolischer Wirkung die glukagonstimulierte hepatische Glukoseproduktion auch nach Halbierung der Insulingesamtdosis noch im gleichen Ausmaß zu unterdrükken wie bei Verabreichung einer doppelt so großen kontinuierlich zugeführten Insulinmenge [11]. In analoger Weise wurde auch eine größere Wirksamkeit einer pulsatilen gegenüber einer kontinuierlichen Insulinzufuhr auf die Suppression von hepatischer Glukoseproduktion und peripherer Glukoseutilisation bei Typ I-Diabetikern nachgewiesen [12].

Insulin wird nach seiner Freisetzung aus den Langerhans'schen Inseln zu etwa 50% durch die Leber extrahiert [2, 13], wobei zu beachten ist, daß die fraktionelle hepatische Insulinextraktion nach Glukosezufuhr vorübergehend absinkt [2, 14]. Die Aufgabe des durch die Leber zurückgehaltenen Insulins dürfte es vor allem sein, die glukagonbedingte Glykogenolyse nach Kohlenhydratzufuhr zu drosseln [15] und damit hepatisch gespeichertes Glykogen für die Abdeckung des Bedarf bei Fehlen einer exogenen Glukosezufuhr bereitzustellen.

Quantitativ kann beim Gesunden mit einer Insulinsekretion von 14–17 mE/min [2, 16] oder etwa einer Einheit je Stunde gerechnet werden. Nach Zufuhr von Glukose steigt die Insulinsekretion dosisabhängig etwa um 0.9 E je 150 min nach Einnahme von 10 g Glukose an [2, 16, 17]. Derartige Berechnungen sind durch die Erfassung der Abgabe von C-Peptid aus dem Splanchnikusgebiet mittels Lebervenenkathetertechnik möglich, da Insulin und C-Peptid in äquimolaren Mengen aus den Betazellen freigesetzt werden und C-Peptid durch die Leber nicht retiniert wird. Ähnliche Befunde wurden auch nach kinetischer Analyse der Insulinsekretion von anderen Untersuchern beobachtet [14]. Aus diesen Untersuchungen läßt sich unter Berücksichtigung der mehr als 210 min dauernden Substratresorption aus dem Darm eine Insulinfreisetzung von etwa 1.35 E/12 g Glukose, entsprechend einer Broteinheit, ableiten [2, 16, 18].

Hepatische Glukoseproduktion

Die Aufrechterhaltung einer normalen Blutglukosekonzentration bedarf einer gesicherten hepatischen Glukoseproduktion, die im postabsorptiven Zustand etwa 2 mg/kg min beträgt [16, 19] und durch orale Glukosezufuhr um etwa 50% unterdrückt wird [19], was zu einer Einsparung an Leberglykogen führt. Das parallel dazu eintretende postprandiale Ansteigen der Glukoseabgabe aus dem Splanchnikusgebiet ist somit überwiegend exogener Natur, da die aus dem Darm resorbierte Glukose lediglich zu 10–30% von der Leber aufgenommen wird [2, 19, 20], wie mittels radioaktiver Tracer-Technik nachgewiesen werden konnte [19, 20].

Periphere Glukoseutilisation

Der Verbrauch an Glukose durch extrahepatische Gewebe entspricht im Nüchternzustand der hepatischen Glukoseproduktion von etwa 2 mg/kg min. Dieses Gleichgewicht ist von großer Wichtigkeit für die Aufrechterhaltung der Euglykämie. Postprandial werden 70–80% [21, 22] der oral eingenommenen Glukose für extrahepatische periphere Gewebe zur Verfügung gestellt, wobei die begleitende verstärkte Insulinsekretion durch Unterdrückung der hepatischen Glukagonwirkung für eine Unterbindung der hepatischen Glykogenolyse sorgt. Dieser Effekt wird umso stärker, je größer die zugeführte Glukosemenge ist.

Zu beachten ist zudem, daß jede körperliche Anstrengung die Glukoseutilisation durch die Muskulatur verstärkt und daß dieser Effekt beim Gesunden im Fastenzustand durch eine vermehrte hepatische Glukoseproduktion ausgeglichen wird [23]. So findet sich bei hypoglykämischen Episoden nach körperlicher Anstrengung eine verstärkte hepatische Glykogenolyse [24], die auf eine erhöhte Freisetzung von Glukagon, Adrenalin und/oder Noradrenalin [25, 26] zurückgeführt werden kann. Euglykämie wird aber auch während einer länger dauernden körperlichen Anstrengung durch eine erhöhte hepatische Glukoseproduktion gewährleistet. Die Quelle für diese durch die Leber freigesetzte Glukose wird durch Glukoneogenese aus C3-Verbindungen, wie Laktat, Pyruvat und Alanin seitens der arbeitenden Muskulatur zur Verfügung gestellt. Die synergistische Wechselwirkung von körperlicher Belastung und Insulin auf die muskuläre Glukoseaufnahme ist zeitabhängig [27] und hält nach Beendigung der körperlichen Tätigkeit weiter an [28], was bei Typ I-Diabetikern auch nach der Beendigung der körperlichen Belastung zu hypoglykämischen Episoden führen kann [29].

Modulation der Insulinwirkung

Besondere Bedeutung für die Modulation der Insulinwirkung kommt den gegenregulatorischen („diabetogenen") Hormonen wie Katecholaminen [30], Kortisol [31], Wachstumshormon [32] und Glukagon [31] zu. Sie alle erhöhen die hepatische Glukoseproduktion wie auch die Insulinresistenz der peripheren Gewebe.

Die stärkste Wirkung in diesem Sinn besitzen Adrenalin und Kortisol, so wie dies bei Gesunden [33] und Typ I-Diabetikern [34] nachgewiesen werden konnte. So finden sich bei schweren diabetischen Ketoazidosen deutlich überhöhte Werte der erwähnten Hormone im Plasma, was die unter diesen Bedingungen zu beobachtende Insulinunterempfindlichkeit erklärt [35]. Ein Befund der schon von Cori und Cori [36] *in vitro* erhoben wurde. Die überragende klinische Bedeutung der erwähnten Streßhormonwirkungen wurde bereits von Houssay und Penhos [37] erkannt, die nachwiesen, daß Adrenalektomie und Hypophysektomie die hyperglykämische Wirkung einer Pankreatektomie beim Hund aufheben können.

Osmolalität

Neben den Streßhormonen muß auch einer erhöhten Osmolalität, so wie sie bei schweren metabolischen Entgleisungen vorkommt, eine die Insulinresistenz begünstigende Wirkung zuerkannt werden. Dies gilt sowohl für Diabetiker [35] als auch für Gesunde nach intravenöser Zufuhr von Mannitol [38] und für Beobachtungen *in vitro* [39]. Das bedeutet umgekehrt, daß eine hypoosmolale Rehydratation bei Patienten mit schwerer Hyperglykämie und diabetischem Koma die Insulinempfindlichkeit der Gewebe wesentlich verbessert, was sowohl auf einen Abfall der Osmolalität, wie auch der Streßhormone zurückgeführt werden kann [35].

Dawn-Phänomen

Dieser Terminus beschreibt ein Ansteigen der Glykämie in den frühen Morgenstunden bei Diabetikern und möglicherweise auch der Insulinsekretion bei Gesunden [40]. Als Ursache des „Dawn-Phänomens" werden einerseits nächtliche hypoglykämische Episoden [41, 42] angesehen, so daß in diesem Fall von posthypoglykämischen Hyperglykämien („Somogyi-Effekt" [41]) gesprochen werden kann [43], während andererseits ein Insulinmangel in den frühen Morgenstunden als Erklärung herangezogen wird [41, 44]. Eine wesentliche Rolle für die Entstehung morgendlicher Hyperglykämien dürfte aber auch der reaktiven Ausschüttung gegenregulatorischer Hormone nach [41] oder unabhängig von nächtlichen Hypoglykämien [45–47] oder bei Insulinmangel zukommen [41, 44]. Weitere Ursachen einer morgendlichen Hyperglykämie bei Diabetikern sind in einer Gewebsunterempfindlichkeit gegenüber Insulin oder in der Größe des aktuellen hepatischen Glykogenpools und seiner Reaktion auf glykogenolytische Reize zu suchen. So konnte gezeigt werden, daß die Dauer einer vorangegangenen Fastenperiode sowohl morgens als auch abends wesentlichen Einfluß auf die periphere Glukoseutilisation besitzt, so daß die Insulinempfindlichkeit von Gesunden mit zunehmender Fastendauer abnimmt [1]. Zusätzlich wurde beobachtet, daß die hepatische Glukoseproduktion nach Setzen eines adäquaten Reizes durch intravenöse Verabreichung von Glukagon (6 ng/kg min) nach hyperkalorischer Ernährung wesentlich größer ist als nach einem Tag niedrig kalorischer Ernährung.

Aus diesen Befunden ist ableitbar, daß frühmorgendliche Hyperglykämien ein Sekundärphänomen im Sinne einer physiologischen Reaktion auf eine metabolische Abweichung darstellen. Dabei dürften der aktuellen Insulinempfindlichkeit des Patienten, der Größe seines hepatischen Glykogenpools sowie dessen Ansprechen auf gegenregulatorische Hormone besondere Bedeutung zukommen [41, 48, 49].

Die große Komplexität der Steuerung des Glukosehaushaltes bedeutet, daß ein Umsetzen von physiologischem Wissen in therapeutische Maßnahmen nur durch ein vereinfachendes Abstrahieren der wesentlichen Steuerungsfaktoren für praktisch-therapeutische Notwendigkeiten möglich werden kann.

Insulintherapie bei Typ I-Diabetes

Aus dem Gesagten wird ersichtlich, daß die Steuerung des Kohlenhydrathaushaltes nicht nur durch die Komponenten Insulin und Glukose, sondern auch durch eine Vielzahl anderer Faktoren in einem wohlgeordneten Zusammenspiel erfolgt. Wesentliche Bausteine dieses Systems sind die Menge (I) der hepatischen Glukoseproduktion und der durch den Darm angebotenen Glukose; (II) der durch das Splanchnikusgebiet und insbesondere durch die Leber postprandial retinierten Glukose sowie das Ausmaß der damit untrennbar verbundenen Veränderungen der hepatischen Glukoseproduktion aus Glykogenolyse und Glukoneogenese; (III) der durch periphere Gewebe aufgenommenen und oxydierten Glukose (= Glukoseutilisation); (IV) des während des Fastens und nach Nahrungszufuhr freigesetzten Insulins sowie dessen Abhängigkeit von den modulierenden Einflüssen der Streßhormone und der körperlichen Aktivität; und (V) die Möglichkeit der kontinuierlichen Blutglukosemessung durch die Betazelle.

Verfügbare Strategien der Insulintherapie stellen ein Kontinuum vom einfachen bis zum aufwendigen Behandlungssystem dar und können mit den Stichworten „konventionell", „intensiviert", „mehr physiologisch" und „funktionell" umschrieben werden. Als Hilfen für die Planung einer entsprechenden Therapie stehen physiologische Kenntnisse über den basalen und prandialen Zielbereich der Glykämie beim Gesunden und über die parallel dazu ablaufende Insulinsekretion, sowie quantitatives Wissen über die Veränderungen der Blutglukose nach körperlicher Belastung und Streßhormonexposition zur Verfügung. Zusätzliche technische Hilfsmittel sind die Messung von Glukose in Blut und Harn sowie der Azetonurie und die Korrektur von aberranten Blutglukosewerten durch Altinsulin an Hand von Erfahrungswerten. Die Güte der bei Typ I-Diabetes erzielbaren metabolischen Kontrolle hängt von der jeweiligen Strategie und damit von den eingesetzten Wissenskomponenten ab.

Ziel ist in jedem Fall die Vermeidung der akuten metabolischen Entgleisung, was mit jeder Form der Insulintherapie bei richtiger Durchführung erreicht werden kann und eine möglichst normnahe metabolische Kontrolle. Letzteres ist bei konventioneller Insulintherapie nur bei einem sehr geringen Prozentsatz der Patienten erreichbar [50], gelingt aber umso häufiger, je mehr sich die Form der Insulinzufuhr den physiologischen Verhältnissen annähert. In der Praxis wird letzteres vor allem durch Blutglukoseselbstmessungen in Verbindung mit prompten Blutglukosekorrekturen durch den Patienten erreicht.

Konventionelle Insulintherapie

Die Vielfalt der zu beachtenden Faktoren macht es notwendig, daß sich der Arzt darauf beschränkt, klinisch anwendbares Wissen für die symptomatische Behandlung von Insulinmangelzuständen, insbesondere bei Typ I-Diabetes, aus den Kenndaten des normalen Kohlenhydrathaushaltes (Tabelle 1) auszuwählen. Dies war in der Vergangenheit im Rahmen der konventionellen Insulintherapie nur in beschränktem Maße möglich, da nur das Angebot an Nahrung und Insulin normiert werden konnte, aber keine Möglichkeit einer Blutglukoseselbstmessung bestand. Eine genau einzuhaltende, unflexible Verordnung von Nahrungs- und Insulinzufuhr an Hand starrer Spielregeln, die der Patient präzis einzuhalten hatte, war das Ergebnis. Diese Vorgangsweise hat dazu geführt, daß die Häufigkeit des diabetischen Komas rasch abgenommen hat und die Blutglukosewerte mehrheitlich um 11.7 mmol/l (211 mg/dl) eingestellt werden konnten. Das Auftreten diabetischer Spätkomplikationen mußte hingegen in Kauf genommen werden [50, 51].

Heute verwendet die konventionelle Insulintherapie eine Mischung von kurzwirkendem Normalinsulin mit einem Intermediärinsulin [52]. Ausgebildete Typ I-Diabetiker sind dabei in der Lage, die Insulindosis wechselnem Bedarf anzupassen, z. B. durch Verminderung der Altinsulinkomponente innerhalb der zu verabreichenden Mischung vor einer sportlichen Betätigung oder bei Reduktion einer zuzuführenden Nahrungsmenge. Die einmal tägliche Injektion eines Langzeitinsulins ist in diesem Zusammenhang obsolet, kann aber gelegentlich zur Basalinsulinisierung von insulinpflichtigen Typ II-Diabetikern eingesetzt werden.

Tabelle 1. Ausgewählte Kenndaten des normalen Kohlenhydrathaushaltes [17]

Hepatische Glukoseproduktion (HGP, mg/kg min)
- Neugeborene: 4.2 − 5.4
- Erwachsene: 2.3 ± 0.1
- Suppression/oGTT: 55 ± 5.0 %

Basaler peripherer Glukoseverbrauch = Basale HGP

Hepatische Glukoseextraktion: 10–25 %

Insulinproduktionsrate
- Basal: 0.7–1.0 E/h
- Prandial: 1.35 E/12 g Glukose (BE)
- Quotient Basal/Prandial/24 h: ca. 1.0

In diesem Fall dient die meist spät abends gegebene Langzeitinsulindosis dem Absenken der basalen hepatischen Glukoseproduktion [53].

Die bei konventioneller Insulintherapie induzierte weitgehend starre Hyperinsulinämie verlangt eine gleichmäßige, pünktliche Aufnahme von Kohlenhydraten, um näherungsweise eine Konstanz des Blutglukosespiegels zu gewährleisten. Die Abstimmung der Nahrungszufuhr erfolgt insulinbezogen in Form von 5–7 Mahlzeiten. Wesentlich ist dabei die Feststellung, daß der Zeitpunkt der Insulininjektion jenen der nachfolgenden Nahrungsaufnahme fixiert, da anderenfalls mit schweren Hypoglykämien zu rechnen ist. Die qualitative Zusammensetzung und der Kaloriengehalt der Nahrung entspricht hinsichtlich des relativen Anteils an Kohlenhydraten (45–60 %), Fett (20–40 %)und Protein (15 %) jenem von gesunden Personen.

Eine derartige konventionelle Insulintherapie erlaubt selbst unter den günstigen Bedingungen einer klinischen Diabetesambulanz nur bei knapp 20 % aller Typ I-Diabetiker eine Normalisierung des HbA_{1c} und damit teilweise auch des Kohlenhydrathaushaltes [50]. Dieses Ergebnis reduziert sich im ländlichen Raum auf 4 % [51]. Das bedeutet, daß die Mehrzahl der konventionell mit Insulin behandelten Patienten während ihrer gesamten Lebenszeit stets den Gefahren einer chronischen Glukoseintoxikation ausgesetzt bleibt.

Intensivierte Insulintherapie

Erste Hinweise darauf, daß der unbefriedigende Erfolg der konventionellen Insulintherapie weiter verbessert werden kann, wurden mit dem zu Forschungszwecken entwickelten künstlichen Pankreas gewonnen [54, 55]. Das auf diese Weise, wie auch durch physiologische Untersuchungen [1] abgesicherte Wissen, daß Insulin nicht nur prandial sondern auch im Hungerzustand erforderlich ist, führte zur Intensivierung der konventionellen Insulintherapie. Dazu kam, daß die Einführung der Blutglukoseselbstmessung nunmehr auch unsystematische Korrekturen aberranter Blutglukosewerte durch Altinsulin ermöglichte. Die dafür notwendige Strategie wurde dem Patienten in strukturierten Ausbildungsprogrammen vermittelt [52, 56].

Dementsprechend könnte der Begriff der „intensivierten konventionellen Insulintherapie" all jene Therapieformen umfassen, die bei fixer Nahrungs- und Insulinzufuhr über den Aufwand der einfachen konventionellen Insulintherapie hinausgehen und zusätzlich Maßnahmen zur Verbesserung der Blutglukosekontrolle, einsetzen. Dazu gehören die gelegentliche bis häufige Selbstmessung von Blut- und/oder Harnglukose durch den Patienten mit allfälliger unsystematischer Korrektur von Hypo- und Hyperglykämien sowie eine gelegentliche, jedoch unsystematische Insulindosisanpassung. Letztere vermittelt dem ausgebildeten Patienten eine größere Sicherheit bei der Durchführung der Insulintherapie.

Funktionelle Insulintherapie

Der Versuch einer funktionellen Insulintherapie mit dem Ziel einer Nahe-Normoglykämie ist dann erfolgversprechend, wenn der Patient lernt, physiologisch zu agieren und das basale, den Fastenzustand abdeckende Insulin vom prandialen gedanklich und praktisch abzutrennen.

Diese Form der Insulinsubstitution wurde einerseits durch die klinische Anwendung von Insulininfusionspumpen empirisch vorbereitet [57, 58] und andererseits durch die systematische Übertragung physiologischer Kenndaten in die Therapie des insulinabhängigen Diabetes ermöglicht [1, 18, 56, 59, 60]. Der Ersatz des basalen Insulins kann dabei außer durch eine 2x täglich im Abstand von 12 Stunden vorzunehmende Injektion von Langzeitinsulin (= basale Insulinsubstitution) auch mit Insulininfusionsgeräten durchgeführt werden. Getrennt davon und nahrungsangepaßt ist zudem unmittelbar vor der Mahlzeit der prandiale Insulinbedarf mit Altinsulin abzudecken. Die bei funktioneller Insulintherapie unbedingt erforderliche Blutglukoseselbstmessung verschafft dem insulinabhängigen Diabetiker die Möglichkeit, allfällige Abweichungen der Blutglukosekonzentration von vorgegebenen Kenndaten anhand einfacher, in die Praxis umsetzbarer Algorithmen zu korrigieren (Tabelle 2). Die Richtwerte für die Korrektur zu hoher Blutglukoseabweichungen wurden erstmals von Schade und Mitarbeitern (56) empfohlen.

Der am Morgen im Rahmen der Basalversorgung meist vorhandene Insulinmehrbedarf von 2–6 Einheiten ist bei der Mehrzahl der Patienten mit rasch wirkendem Normalinsulin (= Altinsulin) abzudecken. Im Falle einer morgendlichen Hyperglykämie ist das abendliche Basalinsulin durch ein NPH-Insulin spät vor dem Schlafengehen zu ersetzen, wodurch die am frühen Morgen verfügbare Insulinmenge erhöht werden kann. Das mahlzeitenbezogene Insulin ist unter Bedachtnahme auf die zugeführte Kohlenhydratmenge zu dosieren (1.5 E Altinsulin je BE; ausschließliche Eiweißzufuhr bedarf etwa 0.5 E Altinsulin/100 kcal). Die erwähnten Empfehlungen gelten naturgemäß nur bei absolutem Insulinmangel und fehlender Insulinresistenz. Bei abnormer Insulinempfindlichkeit ist eine entsprechende Sekundäranpassung der erwähnten, näherungsweisen Kennwerte der Insulinsubstitution erforderlich. Die Vermittlung des Wissens erfolgt zweckmäßigerweise mit einer ausgefeilten Didaktik [60].

Die Vorgangsweise erlaubt bei entsprechend ausgebildeten und motivierten Patienten eine wesentliche Verbesserung der metabolischen Kontrolle, die sich bei mehr als zweijährigen funktionellem Insulinersatz bei ca. 48% der Erwachsenen (Abb. 1) und 20% der kindlichen [61] insulinabhängigen Diabetiker mit einem HbA_{1c} <6.3% bemerkbar macht.

Dem insulinabhängigen Patienten erlaubt diese Vorgangsweise auch unter ambulanten Bedingungen und im Berufsleben wesentlich häufiger eine anhaltende, „Beinahe-Normalisierung" der Blutglukose als dies bei konventioneller Insulinsubstitution möglich ist. Dies gilt auch für besondere Lebenssituationen wie Krankheit und Gravidität, die bei konventionellem, nicht aber bei funktionellem Insulinersatz große Schwierigkeiten bereiten können. So werden vor allem während der Gravidität von Typ I-Diabetikerinnen mit Hilfe der Strategie einer

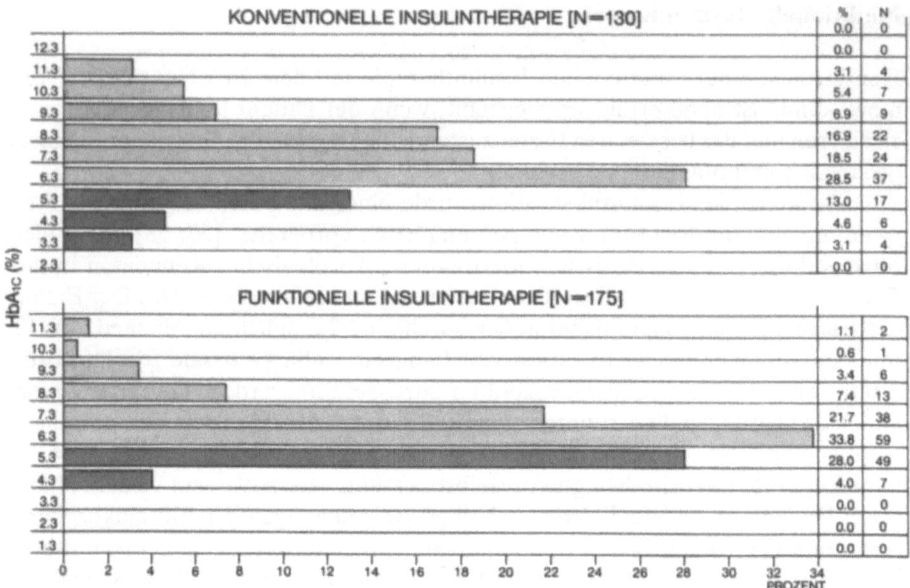

Abb. 1. Histogramm des HbA$_{1c}$ (normal <5.8%) bei Patienten mit Diabetes mellitus Typ I während konventioneller Insulintherapie (HbA$_{1c}$ <5.8%: 20.7%; <6.8%: 49.5%. N = 130) und nach mehr als zweijähriger funktioneller Insulintherapie (Mittelwert von mehr als vier Messungen. HbA$_{1c}$ <5.8%: 32%; <6.8%: 65.8%. N = 175). Krankengut der I. Med. Univ. Klinik, Wien

funktionellen Insulintherapie optimale Ergebnisse bezüglich der Kontrolle von HbA$_{1c}$ und Blutglukose erzielt [62]. Bei der Behandlung gravider Typ I-Diabetikerinnen ist zu beachten, daß der tägliche Insulinbedarf mit fortschreitender Gravidität zunimmt und mit der Geburt, sowie bei manchen Frauen auch einige Tage vorher, abnimmt (Abb. 2).

Der Vorteil der funktionellen Insulintherapie gravider Typ I-Diabetikerinnen liegt nicht nur im Erreichen einer sehr guten Stoffwechselkontrolle, sondern auch in der Möglichkeit einer fast ausschließlich ambulanten Betreuung der geschulten Patientin, was die früher übliche, lang dauernde Hospitalisierung zu vermeiden erlaubt [62].

Schlußfolgerung

Stellt man die Strategien von konventioneller und funktioneller Insulintherapie einander gegenüber, so besteht der wesentliche Unterschied darin, daß die nach wie vor überwiegend angewendete konventionelle Insulinersatztherapie die tägliche Insulindosis und Kohlenhydratzufuhr fixiert und nur unsystematische Kor-

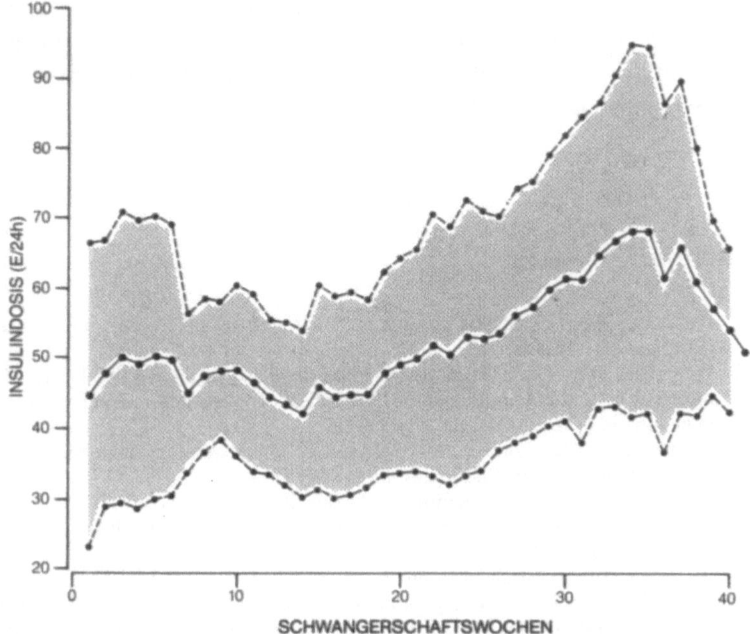

Abb. 2. Verhalten des täglichen Insulinbedarfes mit Fortschreiten der Gravidität bei Typ I-Diabetikerinnen (N = 18; $\bar{x} \pm$ SD. HbA$_{1c}$ bei Entbindung: 4.8% $\pm$ 0.5%). Krankengut der I. Med. Univ. Klinik, Wien

Tabelle 2. Primäre Richtwerte für die Durchführung einer funktionellen Insulintherapie bei Typ I-Diabetes [1, 17, 18, 56, 59, 60]

● Basal (B):	0.7–1.0 E/h
● Prandial (P):	ca. 1.5 E/BE
● Quotient B/P:	ca. 1.0
● Blutglukose-Korrektur:	ca. − 40 mg/dl je 1 E Altinsulin
	ca. + 40 mg/dl je BE Glukose
● Dynamische Bezugswerte:	0 60 120 min pp
	100 160 140 mg/dl

rekturen einer abnormen Glykämie anbietet. Dem gegenüber wird bei Ausschöpfung des physiologischen Wissens über die Steuerung des Kohlenhydrathaushaltes bei funktioneller Insulintherapie ein dynamischer Algorithmus eingesetzt (Tabelle 2) und der Patient zu einer systematischen Glykämiekontrolle verpflichtet, wie dies schon von Stolte [63] 1939 konzipiert worden ist. Die Möglichkeit der Selbstbemessung von Insulindosis und Nahrungsaufnahme ermöglicht dem Patienten einen Freiraum, der seine Motivation zur Mitarbeit erhält und es ihm ermöglicht, langfristig akzeptablere Werte der mittleren Blutglukose [1, 17] und des HbA_{1c} [64] zu erzielen. Wichtig bleibt dabei, daß stets der Arzt das anzustrebende Ziel bestimmt und damit darüber entscheidet, ob nun eine konventionelle oder funktionelle Insulinersatzstrategie, die nach Möglichkeit jedem Typ I-Diabetiker zugängig sein sollte, anzustreben ist.

Literatur

1. Waldhäusl WK (1986) The physiological basis of insulin treatment – clinical aspects. Diabetologia 29: 837–849
2. Waldhäusl WK, Gasic S, Bratusch-Marrain P, Nowotny P (1983) The 75-g oral glucose tolerance test: effect on splanchnic metabolism of substrates and pancreatic hormone release in healthy man. Diabetologia 25: 489–495
3. Kleinbaum J, Shamoon H (1982) Selective counterregulatory hormones responses after oral glucose in man. J Clin Endocrinol Metab 55: 787–790
4. Waldhäusl WK, Gasic S, Bratusch-Marrain P, Korn A, Nowotny P (1982) Feedback inhibition by biosynthetic human insulin of insulin release in healthy human subjects. Am J Physiol 243: E476–E482
5. Waldhäusl W, Bratusch-Marrain P, Gasic S, Komjati M, Heding L (1986) Inhibition by proinsulin of endogenous, C-peptide release in healthy man. Am J Physiol 251: E139–E145
6. Gerich JE (1981) Somatostatin Vol 1. In: Brownlee M (ed) Diabetes mellitus. Wiley, New York, pp 297–354
7. Waldhäusl W, Bratusch-Marrain P, Dudczak R, Deutsch E (1977) The diabetogenic action of somatostatin in healthy subjects and in maturity onset diabetics. J Clin Endcrinol Metab 44: 876–883
8. Fajans SS, Conn JW (1965) Prediabetes subclinical diabetes and latent clinical diabetes. In: Leibel BS, Wrenshall GH (eds). On the nature and treatment of diabetes. Excerpta Medica Foundation, Amsterdam, pp 641–656
9. Lang A, Matthews DR, Pero J, Turner RC (1979) Cyclic oscillations of basal plasma glucose and insulin concentrations in human beings. N Engl J Med 301: 1023–1027
10. Hansen BC, Jen KLC, Pek SB, Wolfe RA (1982) Rapid oscillations in plasma insulin, glucagon und glucose in obese and normal weight humans. J Clin Endocrinol Metab 54: 785–792
11. Komjati M, Bratusch-Marrain PR, Waldhäusl W (1986) Superior efficacy of pulsatile versus continuous hormone exposure on hepatic glucose production in vitro. Endocrinology 11: 312–319
12. Bratusch-Marrain PR, Komjati M, Waldhäusl W (1986) Efficacy of pulsatile versus continuous insulin administration on hepatic glucose production and glucose utilization in insulin dependent diabetic man. Diabetes 35: 922–926
13. Field JB (1973) Extraction of insulin by liver. Am Rev Med 24: 309–326
14. Eaton RP, Allen RC, Schade JS (1983) Hepatic removal of insulin in normal man: dose response to endogenous insulin secretion. J Clin Endocrinol Metab 56: 1294–1300
15. Unger RH, Raskin P, Srikant CB, Orci L (1977) Glucagon and the A-cells. Rec Progr Horm Res 33: 477–517
16. Waldhäusl W, Bratusch-Marrain P, Gasic S, Korn A, Nowotny P (1979) Insulin production rate following glucose ingestion estimated by splanchnic C-peptide output in normal man. Diabetologia 17: 221–227
17. Waldhäusl W, Bratusch-Marrain P (1987) Factors regulating the disposal of an oral glucose load in normal, diabetic and obese subjects. Diabetes/Metabolism Reviews 3: 79–109
18. Waldhäusl W, Bratusch-Marrain PR, Francesconi M, Nowotny P, Kiss A (1982) Insulin production rate in normal man as an estimate for calibration of continuous intravenous insulin infusion in insulin dependent diabetic patients. Diabetes Care 5: 18–24

19. Ferranini E, Björkman O, Reichard GH, Pil A, Olsson M, Wahren J, DeFronzo R (1985) The disposal of an oral glucose load in healthy subjects. Diabetes 34: 580–588
20. Radziuk J, McDonald TJ, Rubenstein D, Duprè J (1978) Initial splanchnic extraction of ingested glucose in normal man. Metabolism 27: 657–669
21. Katz LD, Glickman MG, Rapoport S, Ferranini E, DeFronzo RA (1983) Splanchnic and peripheral disposal of oral glucose in man. Diabetes 32: 675–679
22. Nickelson MJ, Butterfield WJH (1971) Peripheral glucose uptake during the oral glucose tolerance in normal and obese subjects and borderline and frank diabetes. Clin J Med 40: 261–273
23. Zinman B, Murray FT, Vranic M, Albisser AM, Leibel BS, McClean PA, Marliss EB (1977) Glucoregulation during moderate exercise in insulin treated diabetics. J Clin Endocrinol Metab 45: 641–652
24. Lawrence RD (1926) The effects of exercise on insulin action in diabetes. Br Med J 1: 648–652
25. Pequignot JM, Peyrin L, Peres G (1980) Catecholamines fuel interrelationship during exercise in fasting men. J Appl Physiol 48: 109–113
26. Hansen I, Firth R, Haymond M, Cryer P, Rizza R (1986) The role of autoregulation of the hepatic glucose production in man. Diabetes 35: 186–191
27. James DE, Burleigh KM, Kreagen EW (1985) Time dependence of insulin action in muscle and adipose tissue in the rat in vivo. Diabetes 34: 1049–1054
28. Bogardus C, Thuillez P, Ravussin E, Vasquez B, Namiriga M, Azhar S (1983) Effect of muscle glycogen depletion on in vivo insulin action in man. J Clin Invest 72: 1605–1610
29. Calles J, Cunningham JJ, Nelson L, Brown N, Nadel E, Sherwin RS, Felig P (1983) Glucose turnover during recovery from intensive exercise. Diabetes 32: 734–738
30. Deibert DC, DeFronzo RA (1980) Epinephrine induced insulin resistance in man – a Beta-receptor mediated phenomenon. J Clin Invest 65: 717–721
31. Shamoon H, Hendler R, Sherwin RS (1980) Altered responsiveness to cortisol, epinephrine and glucagon in insulin-infused juvenile onset diabetes. A mechanism for diabetic instability. Diabetes 29: 284–291
32. Bratusch-Marrain P, Gasic S, Waldhäusl WK, Nowotny P, Komjati M, Korn A (1987) The effect of growth hormone on splanchnic glucose and substrate metabolism following oral glucose loading in healthy man. Diabetes 33: 19–25
33. Waldhäusl WK, Gasic S, Bratusch-Marrain P, Komjati M, Korn A (1987) Effect of stress hormones on splanchnic substrate and insulin disposal following glucose ingestion in healthy man. Diabetes 36: 127–135
34. Bratusch-Marrain P, Waldhäusl W, Grubeck-Loebenstein B, Korn A, Vierhapper H, Nowotny P (1981) The role of diabetogenic hormones on carbohydrate and lipid metabolism following oral glucose loading in insulin dependent diabetics: effects of acute hormone adminstration. Diabetologia 21: 387–393
35. Waldhäusl W, Kleinberger G, Korn A, Dudczak R, Bratusch-Marrain P, Nowotny P (1979) Severe hyperglycemia: effects of rehydration on endocrine derangements and blood glucose concentration. Diabetes 28: 577–584
36. Cori CF, Cori GF (1928) The mechanism of epinephrine action II. The influence of epinephrine and insulin on the carbohydrate metabolism of rats in the postabsorptive state. J Biol Chem 19: 321–341
37. Houssay BA, Penhos JC (1956) Diabetogenic action of pituitary hormones on adrenalectomized hypophysectomized dogs. Endocrinology 59: 637–641
38. Bratusch-Marrain P, DeFronzo RA (1983) Impairment of insulin mediated glucose metabolism by hyperosmolality in man. Diabetes 32: 1028–1034
39. Komjati M (1982) Einfluß der Osmolalität auf Kohlenhydratstoffwechsel und Ketogenese in vivo. Thesis, TU Wien
40. Schmidt M, Hadji-Georgopoulos A, Rendell M, Margolis S, Kowarski A (1981) The dawn phenomenon, an early morning glucose rise: implications for diabetic intraday blood glucose variation. Diabetes Care 5: 579–585
41. Somogyi M (1938) Insulin as a cause of extreme hyperglycemia and instability. Bull St Louis Med Soc 32: 498–500

42. Boller R, Pilgerstorfer W (1938) Blutzuckerstudie über Protamin-Zink-Insulin. ZS Klin Med 134: 300–320
43. Joslin EP, Gray H, Root HF (1922) Insulin in hospital and home. J Metab Res 2: 651–699
44. Schmidt M, Hadji-Georgopoulos A, Rendell M, Magolis S, Kowarski D, Kowarski AA (1979) Fasting hyperglycemia and associated free insulin and cortisol changes in "Somogyi-like" patients. Diabetes Care 2: 457–464
45. Molnar GD, Fatourechi V, Ackerman E, Taylor WF, Rosevear JW, Gatewood LC, Service FJ, Moxness KE (1971) Growth hormone and glucose interrelationships in diabetes: studies of inadvertent hypoglycemic episodes during continuous blood glucose analysis. J Clin Endocrinol Metab 32: 426–437
46. Olefsky S, Shreeve DR, Sutcliffe CH (1974) Brittle diabetes. Q J Med 43: 113–125
47. Bolli G, Irving S, Gottesman IS, Campbell PJ, Haymond MW, Cryer PE, Gerich JE (1984) Glucose counterregulation and waning of insulin in the Somogyi phenomenon (posthypoglycemic hyperglycemia). N Engl J Med 311: 1214–1219
48. Mintz DH, Finster JL, Taylor AL, Fefer A (1968) Hormonal genesis of glucose intolerance following hypoglycemia. Am J Med 45: 187–197
49. Oakley NW, Jacobs HS, Turner RC, Williams J, Aquino CS, Nabarro JDN (1970) The effect of hypoglycemia on oral glucose tolerance in normal subjects and patients with pituitary and adrenal disorders. Clin Sci 39: 663–674
50. Waldhäusl W, Howorka K, Derfler K, Bratusch-Marrain PR, Holler C, Zyman H, Freyler H (1985) Failure and efficacy of insulin therapy in insulin dependent (Type I) diabetic patients. Acta diabetol lat 22: 279–294
51. Derfler K, Waldhäusl W, Zyman HJ, Howorka K, Holler C, Freyler H (1986) Diabetes Care in a rural area: clinical and metabolic evaluation. Diabetes Care 9: 509–517
52. Berger M, Jörgens V, et al (1983) Praxis der Insulintherapie. Springer, Berlin Heidelberg New York Tokyo (2. Auflage 1986)
53. Riddle MC (1985) New tactics for type 2 diabetes: regimes based on intermediate acting insulin taken at bedtime. Lancet I: 192–194
54. Waldhäusl W, Howorka K, Bratusch-Marrain P (1988) Konventionelle oder funktionelle Insulintherapie? Wien Klin Wschr 100: 430–435
55. Pfeiffer EF, Thum Ch, Clemens AH (1974) Die künstliche Betazelle. Naturwissenschaften 61: 455
56. Schade DS, Santiago JV, Skyler JS, Rizza RA (1983) Intensive insulin therapy, Excerpta Medica, Amsterdam
57. Hepp KD, Renner R, v Funke JH, Mehnert H, Haerten R, Kresse H (1975) Intravenous insulin therapy under conditions imitating physiological profiles. Diabetologia 11: 349
58. Tamborlane WV, Sherwin RS, Genel M, Felig P (1980) Outpatient treatment of juvenile onset diabetes with a preprogrammed pro table subcutaneous insulin infusion system. Am J Med 68: 190–196
59. Czerwenka-Howorka K, Bratusch-Marrain P, Waldhäusl W (1984) Algorithmen der normoglykämischen Insulinsubstitution der Typ I-Diabetes. Erste Langzeitergebnisse. Wien Klin Wochenschr 96: 558–559
60. Howorka K (1987) Funktionelle, nahe-normoglykämische Insulinsubstitution. Lehrinhalte, Praxis und Didaktik. Springer, Berlin Heidelberg New York Tokyo
61. Schober E, Borkenstein M, Frisch H (1987) Basis-Bolus-Therapie bei diabetischen Kindern und Jugendlichen unter Verwendung des Novo Pens. Wien Klin Wochenschr 99: 312–313
62. Feiks A, Howorka K, Nowotny C, Dadak C, Waldhäusl W (1987) Diabetes mellitus Typ I und Schwangerschaft: Ein interdisziplinäres Betreuungsprogramm. Wien Klin Wochenschr 99: 228–232
63. Stolte K, Wolff J (1939) Die Behandlung der kindlichen Zuckerkrankheit mit freigewählter Kost. Erg Inn Med Kinderheilkd 56: 154–193
64. Howorka K, Waldhäusl W (1986) Feasibility of long-term near-normoglycaemic insulin substitution (NIS) by multiple injections. In: Proceedings of the 2nd Assisi International Symposium on Advanced Models for the Therapy of Insulin-Dependent Diabetes, 20.–23. 4. 1986. Raven Press

Aktuelle Diätetik beim insulinspritzenden Patienten

H. MEHNERT

Summary

Principles of dietary therapy in diabetes mellitus include a qualitatively sufficient nutrition, a patient-adjusted energy supply, and a balanced food intake at regular intervals to stabilize metabolism and to reduce the risk of chronic diabetic late complications. Furthermore, the dietary regimen should be adjusted to individual eating customs. These principles of a diabetes-specific dietary regimen are internationally accepted and can be realized in several different ways. The caloric composition of the diabetes diet should be 50% carbohydrates, 35% fat, and 15% proteins. When calculating the caloric requirements of diabetic patients one must remember that the majority of diabetic patients, particularly type II diabetics, are obese and have to have caloric intake restrictions. Type I diabetic patients are usually not obese, nevertheless dietary patterns must be tailored to avoid these patients gaining weight. Hyper- or hypoglycemia can be avoided in different ways. It is most important to fit the caloric intake and medication to be individual's activity and exercise schedule. It is equally important to divide the food intake into many small meals, to avoid glucose as a sweetener, to consider the differences in digestion and resorption of carbohydrates, and to include fiber in the diet. Furthermore, it is crucial to remember the blood glucose-lowering effect of alcohol, particularly without simultaneous carbohydrate intake. The use of special diabetic foods is questionable. Most useful are nonglucose-type sweeteners, specifically prepared beverages, and canned food. An important principle of modern diabetes therapy is instruction of all patients to enable them to calculate their nutrition adequately. Beside insulin treatment, the diet therapy is the most efficient way to influence the long-term prospects of diabetic patients.

Ziele der Diabetesdiät (Tabelle 1)

Qualitativ vollwertige Ernährung

Selbstverständlich hat auch und gerade die Ernährung bei der Stoffwechselkrankheit Diabetes mellitus qualitativ vollwertig zu sein und die physiologischen Be-

Tabelle 1. Ziele der Diabetesdiät

1. Qualitativ vollwertige Ernährung
   (Deckung physiologischer Bedürfnisse,
   insbesondere infolge Wachstum, Gravidität, Arbeitsleistung)

2. Bedarfsgerechte Energiezufuhr
   (Erreichen und Erhalten des wünschenswerten Körpergewichts,
   insbesondere Gewichtsreduktion bei adipösen Diabetikern)

3. „Geregelte" Ernährung zur Stabilisierung des Stoffwechsels
   (Vermeidung von Hyper- und Hypoglykämien,
   Abstimmung der Faktoren Insulin, Arbeit, Nahrungsaufnahme)

4. Reduktion des Risikos chronischer Spätschäden
   (insbesondere Mikro- und Makroangiopathie, Neuropathie, Katarakt)

5. Berücksichtigung individueller Ernährungsgewohnheiten im Rahmen der Diätverordnung

dürfnisse zu decken. Die Aufteilung der Nährstoffe ist über Jahre und Jahrzehnte
Gegenstand lebhafter Diskussionen gewesen. In den letzten Jahren hat sich aber
immer mehr jener Standpunkt durchsetzen können, der auf eine eher kohlenhy-
dratreiche sowie fettarme und nicht allzu eiweißreiche Diät abzielt.

Gemäß internationalen Übereinkünften sollten die Kohlenhydrate mindestens
ca. 50% der Gesamtkalorien und das Fett höchstens 35% ausmachen. Der Ei-
weißgehalt, der früher bis zu 20% angegeben wurde, sollte nicht mehr als 15%
betragen und im übrigen besser als obere Grenze mit 0.8 g/kg Körpergewicht
angegeben werden.

Wegen der Katabolie der Stoffwechsellage bei instabilem oder schlecht eingestelltem Diabetes, aber auch wegen des Wachstums und der Gravidität sowie bei
vermehrter körperlicher Arbeit hatte man früher den Eiweißbedarf des Organismus insbesonders beim insulinspritzenden Patienten sehr hoch gesetzt. Wie erwähnt, ist man in jüngster Zeit damit zurückhaltender geworden, auch wenn man
annehmen muß, daß immer wieder ein Teil des Körpereiweißes in Phasen der
verstärkten Glukoneogenese gleichsam eingeschmolzen wird. Untersuchungen
von Brenner [3] und Bending [2] haben nämlich erkennen lassen, daß möglicherweise eine allzu eiweißreiche Kost sich als ungünstig im Hinblick auf die Entwicklung renaler diabetischer Gefäßschäden erweist.

Während der Phasen des Wachstums ist insbesondere die Energiezufuhr (s.u.)
erhöht. Hier muß man bedenken, daß wegen der mitunter exzessiven Kohlen-
hydratmengen bei der obigen Nährstoffrelation unter Umständen stärkere Fett-
zulagen nicht zu vermeiden sind. Das gleiche gilt für die vermehrte Arbeitsleistung. In der Gravidität liegt der Schwerpunkt weniger auf einer vermehrten
Energie- und damit Fettzufuhr, als in der Beachtung der Tatsache, daß überhaupt
genügend Kalorien (trotz Komplikationen wie Schwangerschaftserbrechen, Ge-
stose etc.) zugeführt werden. Ein Energie- und Nährstoffmangel, der durch solche

Komplikationen auftreten kann, bedarf unter Umständen der Korrektur durch parenterale Ernährung.

Bedarfsgerechte Energiezufuhr

Wenn man eine „kaloriengerechte" Diät verordnet, dann erfüllt man die Forderung nach einer bedarfsgerechten Energiezufuhr mit Erreichen und Erhalten des wünschenswerten Körpergewichts [27]. Selbstverständlich ist die Reduzierung des Körpergewichts das Hauptanliegen bei mehr als 90 % aller Typ II-Diabetiker [18], während die Typ I-Diabetiker häufig Normalgewicht haben. Andererseits muß man aber bedenken, daß es eben nicht nur um das Erreichen, sondern auch um das Erhalten des wünschenswerten Körpergewichts geht und daß Typ I-Diabetiker in dieser Hinsicht, d. h. im Hinblick auf eine etwaige stärkere Gewichtszunahme, mindestens genauso gefährdet sind wie normalgewichtige stoffwechselgesunde Personen im jugendlichen Alter. Man darf sogar behaupten, daß insulinspritzende Diabetiker wegen der häufigen Nahrungszufuhr zur Vermeidung von Hypoglykämien und auch wegen des Insulins selbst als potentiellem Faktor für die Mastfettsucht gefährdeter sind, übergewichtig zu werden als stoffwechselgesunde Personen. Aus diesem Grunde bedarf es also auch bei Typ I-Diabetikern der rechtzeitigen und richtigen Schulung im Hinblick auf die bedarfsgerechte Energiezufuhr.

„Geregelte" Ernährung zur Stabilisierung des Stoffwechsels

Die verschiedenen Wege zu einer geregelten Ernährung, die Hyper- und Hypoglykämien vermeiden kann, werden später besprochen. Natürlich steht die Abstimmung der Faktoren Insulin, Arbeit und Nahrungsaufnahme im Vordergrund der Bemühungen, ist aber nicht der alleinige Weg zu diesem Therapieziel.

Nachdem man in den letzten Jahren zunehmend die Bedeutung einer normnahen Blutzuckereinstellung für die Prognose des Diabetes erkannt hat [10, 23], besteht kein Zweifel mehr daran, daß alle Maßnahmen, die den Stoffwechsel in diesem Sinne stabilisieren können, in den Therapieplan eingebaut werden sollen. Keinesfalls dürfen diese Maßnahmen aber mit dem Therapieziel der bedarfsgerechten Energiezufuhr kollidieren, wie es bei alleiniger Berücksichtigung der unterschiedlichen Digestion und Resorption von Kohlenhydraten der Fall ist und auf Austauschtabellen, die sich nur nach diesem Gesichtspunkt richten, zutrifft [21].

Reduktion des Risikos chronischer Spätschäden

In einer Verlautbarung des Ernährungsausschusses der British Diabetic Association [6] wird als Therapieziel zu Recht auf die Beeinflussung von Gefäßschäden hingewiesen. Wie bereits oben erwähnt, hilft hierfür sicherlich eine eher kohlen-

hydratreiche und fettarme Kost mit der in besonderer Weise modifizierten Fettzufuhr (s.u.). Wichtig ist der Hinweis, daß Diabetiker – so nach den Zahlen der
von Janka durchgeführten Schwabinger Studie [11] – zu 50 % an Hypertonie leiden
und daß deswegen eine Kochsalzrestriktion ins Auge gefaßt werden muß. Die
englischen Autoren weisen darauf hin, daß eine Kostform mit einem niedrigen
Kohlenhydratanteil, dafür aber mit mehr Eiweiß (Käse, Räucherwaren, Fleisch),
wesentlich mehr Kochsalz enthält und auch aus diesem Grunde für das Gros der
Diabetiker unerwünscht ist.

Berücksichtigung individueller Ernährungsgewohnheiten im Rahmen der Diätversorgung

Die Berücksichtigung individueller Ernährungsgewohnheiten bei der Diätverordnung ist ein wichtiges Ziel der Ernährungsbehandlung. Eine gute Mitarbeit (Compliance) des Patienten wird sich sicherlich nur dann erreichen lassen, wenn der
Patient entsprechend motiviert wird. Petzoldt [22] weist zu Recht darauf hin, daß
Verhaltensweisen, Gewohnheiten, Vorlieben oder äußere Bedingungen die erfolgreiche Durchführung der Diabetesdiät beeinträchtigen können. Es muß deswegen neben der Beachtung wichtiger ernährungsphysiologischer Grundsätze
auch auf die individuelle Situation des Diabetikers eingegangen werden. „Diät
für den Diabetiker muß flexibel sein, sie muß wie ein 'Maßanzug' angepaßt
werden" (Petzoldt).

Wege der Diabetesdiät (Tabelle 2)

Aufteilung der Nährstoffe

Bei den Zielen der Diabetesdiät wurde die Aufteilung der Nährstoffe mit 50 %
Kohlenhydraten, 35 % Fett und 15 % Eiweiß bereits angegeben. Die Verteilung
der Fette zu je einem Drittel auf solche mit gesättigten Fettsäuren, einfach ungesättigten und hoch ungesättigten Fettsäuren ist wünschenswert.

Deckung des Energiebedarfs

Das alles in allem wichtigste Gebot in der Diabetesdiät ist, wie gesagt, die Forderung, daß diese Kostform kaloriengerecht, d. h. zumeist kalorienknapp, zu sein
hat. Je nach Lebensalter, Körpergewicht, Geschlecht und beruflicher Tätigkeit
des Patienten wird die zuzubilligende Kalorienmenge etwa zwischen 20 und 45
Kilokalorien/kg Sollgewicht des Patienten liegen. Natürlich ist die Gewichtsreduktion – wie oben erwähnt – bei den meisten Typ II-Diabetikern die Therapie
der Wahl. Kaloriengerechte Ernährung bedeutet aber auch, daß Typ I-Diabetiker,

Tabelle 2. Wege der Diabetesdiät

1. Aufteilung der Nährstoffe
2. Deckung des Energiebedarfs
3. Vermeidung von Hyper- und Hypoglykämien (Adjustierung der medikamentösen Therapie und der körperlichen Arbeit an die Diät, Verabreichung vieler kleiner Mahlzeiten, Vermeidung von Zuckern vom Glukose-Typ, Beachtung der unterschiedlichen Digestion und Resorption von Kohlenhydraten, Einsatz von Ballaststoffen, Berücksichtigung der blutzuckersenkenden Wirkung von Alkohol)
4. Einsatz von diätetischen Lebensmitteln
5. Vermittlung des diätetischen Wissens an den Patienten
6. Berechnung der Kost und Einhaltung der Diät durch den Patienten

die jetzt noch normalgewichtig sind, nicht übergewichtig werden. Deswegen ist die bedarfsgerechte Kalorienmenge der nach Broteinheiten, Gramm Fett und ggf. Gramm Eiweiß zu berechnenden Diät auch für den Typ I-Diabetiker wichtig.

Vermeidung von Hyper- und Hypoglykämien

Eine Fülle von Maßnahmen steht zur Verfügung, um die so wichtige Stabilisierung des Stoffwechsels im Sinne der Vermeidung von Hyper- und Hypoglykämien zu erreichen.

Adjustierung der medikamentösen Therapie und der körperlichen Arbeit an die Diät

Sicherlich die wichtigste Maßnahme zur Stoffwechselstabilisierung ist in der Anpassung von Medikamenten und körperlicher Tätigkeit an die Nahrungsaufnahme zu sehen. Eine noch so gut zusammengestellte Diät wird dann nicht zur Stoffwechselstabilisierung beitragen, wenn beispielsweise die gewählte Insulintherapie falsch durchgeführt wird. Der häufigste Fehler liegt in der zu seltenen Applikation von zu lang wirkenden Insulinen, die ihrerseits nicht in der Lage sind, die Stoffwechselschwankungen gerade bei Typ I-Diabetikern zu beherrschen. Die ideale Adjustierung des Insulins an die Nahrungszufuhr besteht darin, daß viele kleine Mahlzeiten durch viele kleine Insulininjektionen abgedeckt werden und für die Nacht ein länger wirkendes Insulin verabreicht wird. Bei körperlicher Arbeit, insbesondere bei Leistungssport, soll der Diabetiker dem physiologischen Bedürfnis nach vermehrtem Energiebedarf Rechnung tragen und einige Broteinheiten – je nach Intensität und Dauer des ausgeübten Sportes – zusätzlich zu sich nehmen. Wegen des erheblich insulineinsparenden, blutzuckersenkenden Effekts der Muskelarbeit wird er aber in den meisten Fällen auch gleichzeitig die Insulindosis zu reduzieren haben. Das Gebot, daß der Diabetiker sich mit der Nahrungszufuhr dem Wirkungsablauf des gespritzten Insulins anpassen soll, läßt sich lockern oder ganz aufheben, je mehr der Patient auf die Nahrungszufuhr mit einer akuten Insulinzufuhr reagieren kann. Zwar wird man auch bei intensivierter konventioneller Therapie mit 4–5 Insulininjektionen und auch bei der Insulinpumpentherapie (basale Insulinrate plus kleine abgerufene Alt-Insulinmengen) noch bei einigen Diätprinzipien, wie sie vorher und im folgenden skizziert werden, bleiben müssen. Aber z. B. der Zeitpunkt der eingenommenen Mahlzeiten kann sicher eher differieren als bei einer starren Behandlung mit nur einer oder mit zwei Insulininjektionen. Der extrem seltene Idealfall ist natürlich beim erfolgreich transplantierten Diabetiker zu erreichen, dessen neue Bauchspeicheldrüse die Funktion der Insulinproduktion voll übernommen hat und wie beim Gesunden zeit- und bedarfsgerecht das Hormon in die Blutbahn absondert. Nur solche Diabetiker brauchen keine eigentliche Diabetesdiät zu halten, sondern „nur" eine vernünftige Ernährung beachten, um nicht übergewichtig zu werden und um andere Risikofaktoren zu vermeiden (Abb. 1).

Verabreichung vieler kleiner Mahlzeiten

Ein wichtiger Grundsatz der Diabetesdiät ist das Gebot vieler kleiner anstelle weniger großer Mahlzeiten. Man soll die Patienten auffordern, nicht weniger als 6–7 Mahlzeiten täglich einzuhalten. Der Sinn dieser häufigen Mahlzeiten ist leicht

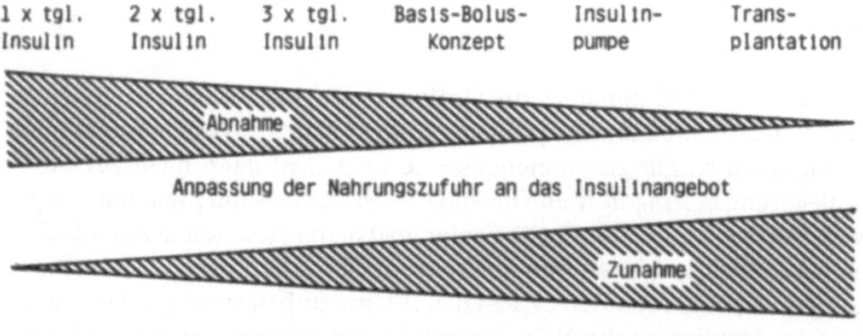

NB. Je intensivierter die Insulintherapie durchgeführt wird, desto weniger ist eine Anpassung der Nahrungszufuhr an das Insulinangebot erforderlich; vielmehr richtet sich dann das Insulinangebot nach dem gewünschten Zeitpunkt und nach dem Ausmaß der Nahrungszufuhr.

Abb. 1. Anpassung der Nahrungszufuhr an das Insulinangebot (und umgekehrt): Abhängigkeit vom jeweiligen Therapieregime beim insulinspritzenden Diabetiker

verständlich. Patienten, die noch über eine gewisse körpereigene Insulinproduktion verfügen, sollen ihre Bauchspeicheldrüse schonen, indem sie die erlaubten Nahrungsmittelmengen dem Organismus in kleinen Portionen zuführen und somit die Insulinproduktion nicht überfordern. Diabetiker, die Insulin spritzen, haben ihre Nahrungszufuhr in der Regel der Wirkungsweise des Insulins anzupassen (Ausnahmen s.o.). Sie müssen häufig etwas essen, damit parallel zu dem langsam in die Blutbahn aufgenommenen Fremdinsulin auch ausreichende Nahrungsmittelmengen zur Verfügung stehen. Wenige große Mahlzeiten führen bei solchen Patienten infolge zu geringer Wirkung des Fremdinsulins zu Blutzuckerspitzen, während das Auslassen der Mahlzeiten das Gegenteil, nämlich die ebenfalls gefährlichen Unterzuckerreaktionen, hervorrufen kann.

Die erforderliche individuelle Betrachtungsweise für die Notwendigkeit vieler kleiner oder weniger großer Mahlzeiten erhellt jedoch aus der Tatsache, daß Pumpenträger unter den Insulinpatienten – und das sind praktisch nur Typ I-Diabetiker – bei entsprechender Kooperation durchaus nur wenige große Mahlzeiten zu sich nehmen können (s.o.), also gerade das Prinzip nicht zu beachten brauchen, das als so zwingend für alle Typ I-Diabetiker beschrieben wurde.

Vermeidung von Zuckern vom Glukosetyp

Weder in quantitativer noch in qualitativer Hinsicht darf der Diabetiker „alles" essen. Dies gilt sowohl für den Typ I- als auch für den Typ II-Diabetes. Zucker von Glukosetyp (Glukose, Maltose, Saccharose) sollten von allen Diabetikern gemieden werden. Im Hinblick auf die Freigabe von Zucker in der Diabetesdiät hat Gries zu Recht von den „Risiken eines Dammbruchs" gesprochen, die dann im Hinblick auf die Überschreitung aller Diätgebote bestehen. Im übrigen gibt es unter den diätetischen Lebensmitteln genügend Möglichkeiten, dem Süßungsbedürfnis des Patienten zu entsprechen (s.u.).

Beachtung der unterschiedlichen Digestion und Resorption von Kohlenhydraten

Nicht nur die chemischen Eigenschaften bestimmen die Aufschließbarkeit der in einem Nahrungsmittel enthaltenen Kohlenhydrate, sondern auch die Verarbeitung und Zubereitung durch Mahlen, Kochen und Backen [22]. Ebenso wichtig ist aber – wie schon oben erwähnt – die Kombination von Kohlenhydraten und Fetten oder Ballaststoffen in einem Nahrungsgemisch oder in einer Mahlzeit im Hinblick auf die nach der Digestion erfolgende Resorption der Glukose. Wie erwähnt, bedingen Fette ebenso wie Ballaststoffe eine Beeinflussung der Magenentleerung und eine Verzögerung der Kohlenhydratresorption. Es unterliegt keinem Zweifel, daß jenen Kohlenhydraten und jenen Nahrungsgemischen, die zu einer verlangsamten Resorption von Glukose führen, im Prinzip der Vorzug zu geben ist. Zwei Einschränkungen sind dabei aber zu machen: Einmal darf man nicht – wie oben skizziert – das Prinzip der fettarmen Diät zugunsten des resorptionsverzögernden Effekts der Fettbeigabe vernachlässigen, und zum anderen darf man die Möglichkeiten, mit einem „glykämischen Index" zu arbeiten, nicht überschätzen. Wir stimmen Coulston [5] zu, daß ein glykämischer Index, basierend auf der Untersuchung isoliert verabreichter Kohlenhydrate, von minimalem klinischen Nutzen ist und die Diätetik nicht bereichern kann. Diese strikte Aussage soll aber keineswegs besagen, daß die unterschiedliche Digestion und Resorption der Kohlenhydrate unbeachtet bleiben sollte. Im Gegenteil: Man sollte versuchen, nur bestimmte Nahrungsmittelgruppen gegeneinander auszutauschen, wie sie in den Kohlenhydrataustauschtabellen der Deutschen Diabetes Gesellschaft geordnet sind. Dies gilt auch trotz des Einwandes, daß starke Schwankungen hinsichtlich der Aufschließbarkeit und Resorption innerhalb der Gruppen bestehen [22]. Im Moment steht aber kein besserer Weg zur Verfügung. Im übrigen sollte man in erster Linie grundsätzliche Fehler vermeiden, wie z. B. die alleinige Gabe von Kohlenhydraten (womöglich in Form von rasch resorbierbaren Fruchtsäften) zum ersten Frühstück, in dessen Gefolge der Diabetiker sowieso den höchsten Blutzuckerwert aufweist. Gerade hier ist also die Verabreichung von Brot aus grob geschrotetem Korn oder einem entsprechenden Müsli mit Fett bzw. Milch durchaus erwünscht, um die postprandialen Hyperglykämien abzuschwächen.

Einsatz von Ballaststoffen

Der Einsatz von Ballaststoffen [12, 14, 15, 25] ist im Hinblick auf die Vermeidung von Hyperglykämien sicherlich sinnvoll. Es konnte gezeigt werden, daß nicht resorbierbare Nahrungsbestandteile (dietary fiber) den postprandialen Blutzuckerwert, den HbA_I-Wert und die Urinzuckerausscheidung bei Diabetikern verringern. Kombinationen von Kostformen mit hohen Kohlenhydrat- und Ballaststoffgehalten verbessern die Diabeteseinstellung und senken die Blutlipide.

Berücksichtigung der blutzuckersenkenden Wirkung von Alkohol

Alkohol – besonders in höheren Konzentrationen und bei Fehlen gleichzeitiger Kohlenhydratzufuhr – wirkt blutzuckersenkend.

Es wird empfohlen, am ehesten einen Austausch von Alkohol gegen Fettkalorien herbeizuführen, damit nicht der Alkohol bei reduzierter Kohlenhydratzufuhr zu Hypoglykämien führt [22]. Dieses Problem ist von unterschiedlicher Relevanz und besonders bei jüngeren, insulinspritzenden Langzeitdiabetikern gefürchtet. Gerade diese Patienten verlieren oft die Eigenschaft, Hypoglykämien rechtzeitig zu bemerken und können durch die Alkoholhypoglykämie ohne ausreichende Kohlenhydratzufuhr schwerste Schäden, ja sogar den Tod erleiden.

Einsatz von diätetischen Lebensmiteln

Gewisse Zucker oder Zuckeralkohole werden nicht nur bedeutend langsamer als Glukose, Saccharose und Maltose resorbiert, sondern weisen auch noch einen weitgehend vom Insulin unabhängigen Stoffwechsel auf.

Aber auch im Hinblick auf Hypoglykämien sind diese Zuckeraustauschstoffe von Nutzen, da sie bei Bedarf – also bei einer drohenden Hypoglykämie – sinnvollerweise in die Glukoneogenese einbezogen werden [24]. Es ist also nicht erforderlich, daß insulinspritzende Diabetiker bei Austausch eines anderen Kohlenhydrats gegen Fruktose oder Sorbit weniger Insulin spritzen. Wichtig ist vielmehr, daß der Diabetiker die Zuckeraustauschstoffe voll in die Kohlenhydratberechnung einbezieht. Dies wurde durch eine Änderung der Diätverordnung berücksichtigt, wonach auch Zuckeraustauschstoffe nach Broteinheiten berechnet werden müssen [17].

Die besonders langsame Resorption der Zuckeralkohole Sorbit und Xylit wäre an sich ein Vorteil. Leider geht die Resorption aber so langsam vor sich, daß man z. B. schon bei Verabreichung von täglich 40 g Sorbit mit Durchfällen rechnen müßte. Aufgrund älterer und neuerer Untersuchungen besteht kein Zweifel, daß die Zuckeraustauschstoffe, insbesondere die am meisten gebrauchte und am besten verträgliche Fruktose, sich vorteilhaft gegenüber Zuckern vom Glukosetyp – also z. B. Saccharose – unterscheidet [s. 18]. Untersuchungen von Haslbeck et al. [7] konnten dies sogar für den Einsatz der Zucker in gemischten Mahlzeiten, bei denen also die Zuckerresorption sowieso schon verzögert wird, zeigen (Abb. 2).

Neben Zuckeraustauschstoffen sind Süßstoffe (Saccharin, Cyclamat, Aspartame, Acesulfam) wichtig, um dem Süßungsbedürfnis des Diabetikers entgegenzukommen. Gerade bei übergewichtigen Patienten sind diese fast kalorienfreien Süßstoffe von großem Vorteil und können praktisch unbegrenzt eingesetzt werden.

Ein Schwerpunkt in der Herstellung diätetischer Lebensmittel für Diabetiker liegt bei Getränken und in der Konservennahrung.

Vermittlung des diätetischen Wissens an den Patienten

Die Einhaltung der verordneten Diabetesdiät ist ganz wesentlich von Zeit und Mühen bestimmt, die die behandelnden Ärzte und Diätassistentinnen darauf verwenden [22]. Je mehr Mühe man sich mit der Diätberatung für Diabetiker gibt, desto größere therapeutische Erfolge kann man auch bei Typ I-Diabetikern erzielen. Dies erweist sich besonders an der Reduzierung von Medikamenten bei Patienten, die den Diätanweisungen Folge geleistet haben. Die Diätberatung der Patienten steht am Beginn der Behandlung und muß durch ergänzenden Unterricht immer wieder erweitert werden.

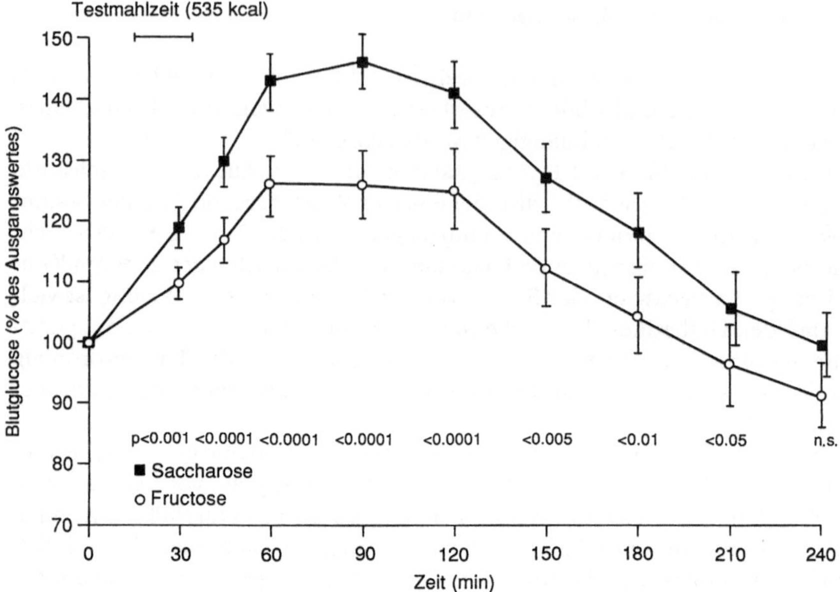

Abb. 2. Verhalten der Blutglucose (in Prozent des Ausgangswertes) bei 30 Patienten mit Typ II-Diabetes nach Zufuhr von Saccharose bzw. Fruktose in einer Testmahlzeit. (Zusammensetzung: 30 g Fruktose bzw. Saccharose, 32.5 g Stärke, 20 g Fett und 23 g Eiweiß). $\bar{x}$ ± Sem, Wilcoxon-Test (Paarvergleich)

Berechnung der Kost und Einhaltung der Diät durch den Patienten

Angesichts der großen Fortschritte, die in den vergangenen Jahren auf dem Gebiet der Diabetestherapie gemacht wurden, mag es verwunderlich erscheinen, daß seitens der Diabetologen immer wieder die Forderung nach einer Verbesserung der Diabetesdiät erhoben wird [4, 8, 9, 16]. Unter Verbesserung ist dabei aber nicht eine qualitative oder quantitative Änderung der Kostform anzusehen, deren Grundsätze nunmehr im wesentlichen geklärt sind, sondern vielmehr eine Intensivierung der Diätberatung und eine Förderung der Kooperation der Patienten. Der Engpaß in der Diätetik ist für Ärzte und Diätassistentinnen nicht im mangelnden Wissen um die erwünschte Art oder Menge der Diätkost zu suchen, sondern vielmehr in der Schwierigkeit, dieses Wissen dem Patienten zu übermitteln und ihn zur dauernden Mitarbeit zu bewegen. Gerade auch bei insulinspritzenden Patienten sollte man sich vor Augen halten, welche schwerwiegenden Folgen eine Ignorierung diätetischer Maßnahmen mit sich bringt: bei insulinspritzenden Typ II-Diabetikern bedingt sie die Konservierung des Übergewichts und beim Typ I-Diabetiker die Provozierung einer sich allmählich entwickelnden Adipositas. Bei beiden Diabetestypen führt darüber hinaus die fehlende Adjustierung von Nahrungsmittelangebot, Nahrungsmittelqualität, Muskelarbeit und Insulininjektion zu der langfristig schädlichen Hyperglykämie und kurzfristig zu der womöglich akut bedrohlichen Hypoglykämie.

Literatur

1. Bantle JP, Laine DC, Castle GW, Thomas JV, Hoogwert BJ, Goetz FC (1983) Postprandial glucose and insulin response in meals containing different carbohydrates in normal and diabetic subjects. New Engl J Med 309: 7

2. Bending JJ, Dodds R, Keen H, Viberti GL (1986) Lowering protein intake and the progression of diabetic renal failure. Diabetologia 29: 516

3. Bremer BM, Meyer TW, Hostetter TH (1982) Dietary protein intake and the progressive nature of kidney disease. The role of hemodynamically mediated glomerular injury in the pathogenesis of progressive glomerular injury in the pathogenesis of progressive glomerular sklerosis in aging, renal ablation, and intrinsic renal disease. New Engl J Med 307: 652

4. Buchenau H (1963) Diätberatung – Erfahrungen, Wünsche und Ziele. Der Diabetiker 13: 28

5. Coulston AM, Hollenbeck CB, Liu CD, Williams QA, Starick AH, Mazzaferri AL, Reaven AM (1984) Effect of source of dietary carbohydrate on plasma glucose, insulin, and gastrin inhibitory polypeptide responses to test meals in subjects with noninsulin-dependent diabetes mellitus. Am J Clin Nutr 40: 963

6. Dietary recommendations for diabetics for the 1980s – a policy statement by the British Diabetic Association (1982) Human Nutrition, Applied Nutrition 36A: 378

7. Haslbeck M, Rett K, Ladik T, Lotz N (1988) Einfluß von Kohlenhydraten in gemischter Kost auf den Blutzucker bei Typ II-Diabetes. In „Diätetische Lebensmittel in Praxis und Wissenschaft". Schriftenreihe des Bundesverbands der Diätetischen Lebensmittelindustrie 71: 34

8. Jahnke K (1971) Diätbehandlung des Diabetes mellitus. In: Pfeiffer EF (Hrsg), Handbuch des Diabetes mellitus. Lehmann, München

9. Jahnke K, Garbe R (1960) Bedeutung und Methodik von Ernährungs-Anamnesen. Nutr et Dieta 2: 115

10. Janka HU, Haupt E, Standl E (1984) Gefäßkrankheiten bei Diabetes mellitus. In: Mehnert H, Schöffling K (Hrsg) Diabetologie in Klinik und Praxis. Thieme, Stuttgart New York S 405 ff

11. Janka HU, Standl E, Bloss A, Oberparleiter F, Mehnert H (1978) Zur Epidemiologie der Hypertonie bei Diabetikern. Dtsch med Wochenschr 103: 1549

12. Jenkins DJA, Taylor RH, Wolever TMS (1982) The diabetic diet, dietary carbohydrate and differences in digestibility. Diabetologia 23: 477

13. Jenkins DJA, Wolever MS, Jenkins AL, Thorne MJ, Lee R, Kalmusky J, Reichert R, Wong GS (1983) The glycemic index of foods tested in diabetic patients: a new basis for carbohydrate exchange favouring the use of legumes. Diabetologia 24: 257

14. Laube H, Svedberg J (1981) Untersuchungen zur blutzuckersenkenden Wirkung von Guar bei Diabetes mellitus. Akt Endokrin 2: 102

15. Matzkies F, Webs B (1982) Ballastreiche Kostformen zur Behandlung des Diabetes mellitus. Akt Ernähr 7: 205

16. Mehnert H (1961) Zur diätetischen Behandlung des Diabetes mellitus. Dtsch med Wochenschr 86: 1469

17. Mehnert H (1976) Die Berechnung der Kohlenhydrate nach Broteinheiten. Dtsch med Wochenschr 101: 296

18. Mehnert H (1984) Diätetische Behandlung. In: Mehnert H, Schöffling K (1984) Diabetologie in Klinik und Praxis. Thieme, Stuttgart New York

19. Mehnert H (1985) Stoffwechselkrankheiten. Thieme, Stuttgart New York, S 157

20. Mehnert H, Standl E (1987) Ärztlicher Rat für Diabetiker. Thieme, Stuttgart New York

21. Otto H, Bleyer G, Pemartz M, Sabine G, Schauberger G, Spaethe R (1973) Kohlenhydrataustausch nach biologischer Äquivalenz. In: Otto H, Spaethe A (Hrsg) Diät bei Diabetes mellitus. Huber, Bern

22. Petzoldt R (1986) Diättherapie des Diabetes mellitus. In: Huth R, Kluthe R (Hrsg) Lehrbuch der Ernährungstherapie. Thieme, Stuttgart New York, S 142 ff

23. Pirart J (1978) Diabetes mellitus and its degenerative complications: A prospective study of 4400 patients observed between 1947 and 1973. Diabetes Care 1 168: 252
24. Rett K, Wicklmayr M, Schwiegelshohn B, Mickan C, Dietze G, Mehnert H (1986) Beeinflußbarkeit einer insulin-induzierten Hypoglykämie durch Fructose und Sorbit. Dtsch med Wochenschr 111: 780
25. Rottka H (1980) Der Verzehr von Pflanzenfaserballaststoffen in der Bundesrepublik Deutschland. In: Rottka H (1980) Pflanzenfaser-Ballaststoffe in der menschlichen Ernährung. Thieme, Stuttgart New York
26. Sauer H (1982) Gezielte Stoffwechselbeeinflussung: Erhöhung des Anteils der Kohlenhydrate. Akt Ernähr 7: 184
27. Wolfram G (1980) Was ist Idealgewicht? Ernährungs-Umschau 27: 351

Aktuelle Probleme der Therapie des Typ II-Diabetes mellitus mit Sulfonylharnstoffen

K. Schöffling

Summary

The β-cytotropic effects of sulfonylureas involve increased production of intracellularly stored insulin, lowering of the threshold for glucose-induced insulin secretion, and enhancement of glucose-induced insulin secretion. Extrapancreatic effects of sulfonylureas are often discussed. However, the peripheral therapeutic concentrations of sulfonylureas in vivo make this mechanism of action unlikely. Insulin therapy should therefore only be combined with sulfonylureas in C-peptide-positive patients.

Glibenclamide, the most potent sulfonylurea, is usually the drug of choice. Side effects occur in about $1\% - 2\%$, the most common and dangerous one being hypoglycemia at an incidence of about 0.24 per 100 patient-years. Another problem associated with sulfonylurea therapy is the secondary failure of these drugs. The mean annual secondary failure rate is about 8%. However, differentiation between true drug failure and dietary failure is difficult and they are probably often a combined phenomenon.

Treatment with sulfonylureas cannot replace adequate dietary measures. It must be stressed that sulfonylureas should not be misused as a therapy of convenience. Patients with diabetes mellitus have an increased mortality. Whether treatment with sulfonylureas will influence the mortality in patients with noninsulin-dependent diabetes mellitus, however remains, unanswered.

Einleitung

Vor wenigen Jahren haben wir weltweit den sechzigsten Geburtstag des Insulins in Vorträgen und Symposien gefeiert. Bei der Vorbereitung dieses Referates habe ich nun auch zurückgerechnet und festgestellt, daß es auch schon vor 45 Jahren war, als Janbon und Mitarbeiter in Montpellier die starke blutzuckersenkende Wirkung eines Sulfonamids, des IPDT, beobachteten [10]. Bevor wir das halbe Jahrhundert der Sulfonylharnstofftherapie auch noch feiern, ist es sicher angebracht, diese Behandlungsform der Zuckerkrankheit kritisch unter die Lupe zu nehmen und bei der Anwendung jeweils über den Nutzen, aber auch über die

Gefahren und Probleme nachdenken und entsprechend handeln. Wie Ihnen nur zu gut bekannt ist, entartete die Behandlung schon sehr früh zu einer „Therapie der Bequemlichkeit" [20], oft wurde und wird der Indikationsbereich und die zeitlich begrenzte Anwendbarkeit außeracht gelassen, und nicht selten wird die Gefahr von Hypoglykämien, insbesondere bei älteren Patienten unterschätzt. Eine Neubesinnung unter besonderer Beachtung dieser drei Probleme der oralen Therapie erscheint mir daher geboten.

Die Wirksamkeit der Sulfonylharnstoffe beim Typ II-Diabetes ist inzwischen millionenfach erwiesen und bedarf keiner weiteren Diskussion. Die Milligramm-substanzen werden heute bevorzugt, da sie eine höhere Spezifität und eine größere Potenz haben. Glibenclamid ist das wirksamste Präparat [20].

Wo ist nun gegenwärtig der Platz der Sulfonylharnstoffe in unserem Plan zur Behandlung der Typ II-Patienten? Zunächst ist es grundsätzlich geboten, Patienten mit Adipositas von denen ohne Fettsucht, leider die wesentlich kleinere Gruppe, abzugrenzen. Die Europäische Konsensusgruppe [1] spaltet diese beiden Untergruppen (Abb. 1) klar auch im Behandlungsplan von einander ab. Sie finden die Therapieform „Sulfonylurea" in dem Entscheidungsbaum unserer Gruppe an unterschiedlichen Plätzen.

Nebenwirkungen

Nebenwirkungen allergischer und toxischer Art werden bei Anwendung der neueren Substanzen nur noch bei ca. 1–2% der Behandelten beobachtet, während diese früher bei den Grammsubstanzen doch häufiger gesehen wurden [20].

Die Nützlichkeit und Risikoarmut der Behandlung des Typ II-Diabetes mit Sulfonylharnstoffen wurde 1970 durch die Ergebnisse der UGDP-Studie [12] in Zweifel gezogen, nachdem man glaubte festgestellt zu haben, daß eine statistisch signifikante Differenz der Plazebo- und der Tolbutamid-Gruppe im Bezug auf die kardiovaskuläre Mortalität besteht. Damalige eigene Untersuchungen [18] und viele andere Arbeiten haben die Resultate der UGDP-Studie nicht bestätigt. Nachdem diese Untersuchungen zunächst umstritten blieben und Planung, Ausführung und Interpretation von uns und vielen anderen einer Kritik unterzogen wurden, wurde 1978/79 von Mitgliedern der UGDP-Studie selbst die klinische Relevanz der Ergebnisse völlig in Abrede gestellt. Kilo und Williamson [11] zeigten in ihrer Auswertung damals die große Zahl von Fehlern, die dieser Studie anhaften und kommen nach ausführlicher Darstellung aller Irrtümer und Fehlinterpretationen zu dem Schluß, daß die aus der Studie primär gezogenen Schlußfolgerungen „falsch und in gefahrvoller Weise irreführend" sind.

Ein weiteres Übel dieser UGDP-Studie ist die Tatsache, daß seit dieser Untersuchung bis zum heutigen Tage Therapieerfolge und Mißerfolge mit Hilfe von Mortalitätsstatistiken gemessen werden. Auf diese Problematik komme ich am Schluß des Referates noch einmal kurz zurück.

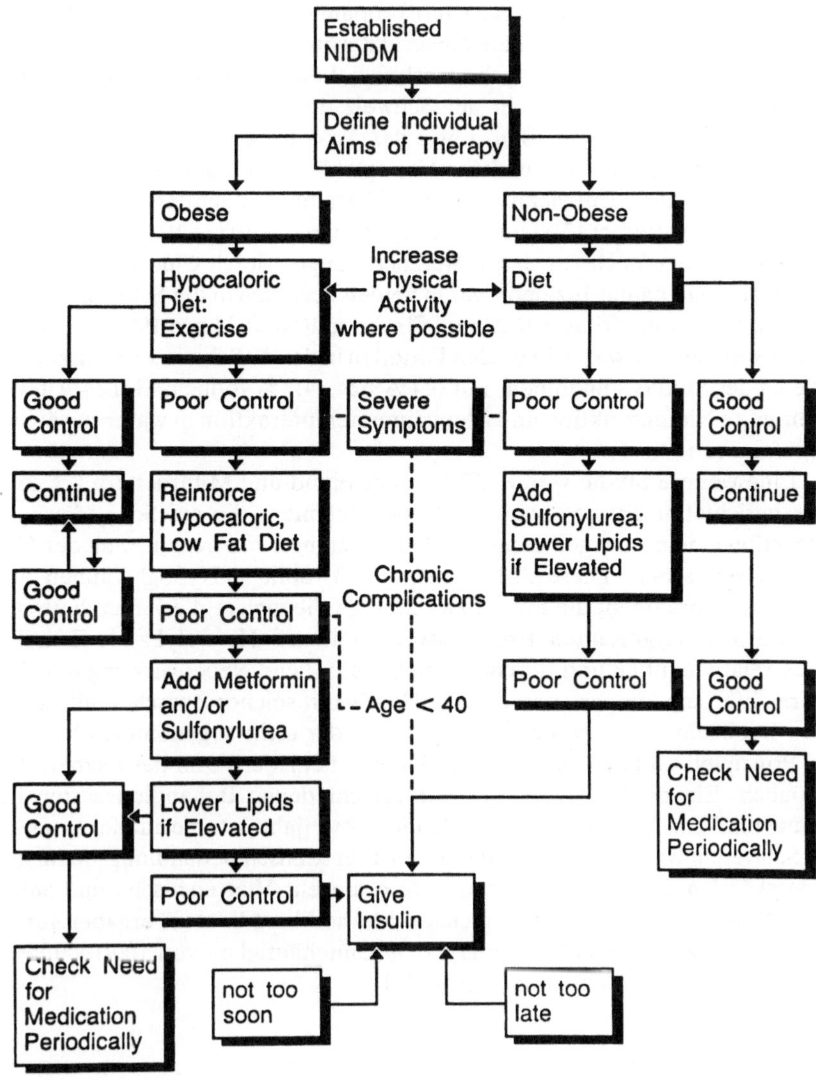

Abb. 1. Therapieplan der Consensuskonferenz beim Typ II-Diabetes

Hypoglykämien

Eine problematische und gefährliche Nebenwirkung, die eigentlich Ausdruck der Wirkung dieser potenten Substanzen ist, sind die Hypoglykämien. Sie wurden vor 30 Jahren in der Bundesrepublik Deutschland glücklicherweise sehr selten mit Carbutamid und Tolbutamid, den damals eingesetzten Präparaten, beobachtet. Ich war daher, sicher ebenso wie viele andere, 1973 überrascht, als Seltzer [15] über 473 schwere Hypoglykämien aus den Staaten berichtete. Fast alle Beobachtungen bezogen sich auf Chlorpropamid, das zwar auch in Deutschland entwickelt, aber praktisch kaum eingesetzt worden war. Eine ähnliche Studie über den Zeitraum 1960–1969 erschien schon 1 Jahr zuvor von W. Berger aus Basel [4], wobei wiederum auch in der Schweiz das Chlorpropamid mit der langen Halbwertszeit von 40 Stunden, sowie das Acetohexamid, das in Deutschland nie eine Bedeutung hatte, die meisten Hypoglykämien verursacht hatte.

Heute ist nach Entwicklung von Milligramm-Präparaten die Situation eine andere und W. Berger [5] sieht für den Zeitraum von 1975–1984 die Glibenclamid-Hypoglykämien noch vor den Unterzuckerungen durch Chlorpropamid. Die relative Hypoglykämie-Inzidenz war in beiden Perioden in der Schweiz vergleichbar und betrug für die frühere 0.22 und für die spätere 0.24 pro 1000 Patientenjahre. Die Zwischenfälle waren in beiden Perioden in den 50 Schweizer Krankenhäusern, die an der Studie teilnahmen, mit 6.4% bzw. 4.3% tödlich. Hohes Alter, eingeschränkte Nierenfunktion und Medikamenteninteraktionen waren zusätzliche Risikofaktoren.

Eine weitere Studie wurde 1983 von Asplund und Mitarbeitern [2] vorgelegt. Sie berichteten über 57 schwere Hypoglykämien, die am Schwedischen Drug Reaction Committee gemeldet worden waren und von denen 10 an der Hypoglykämie verstarben. Diese Arbeit zeigt, daß tödliche Hypoglykämien auch bei Patienten vorkamen, die nur 5 bzw. 2.5 mg Glibenclamid erhalten hatten.

Die hier dargestellten Ergebnisse zeigen, daß Hypoglykämie-Zwischenfälle eine relativ häufige und durchaus auch gefährliche Nebenwirkung der Sulfonylharnstoffe sein können, und daß die Häufigkeit solcher Zwischenfälle gegenüber den Beobachtungen aus den 60er Jahren leider nicht abgenommen hat.

Prinzipiell sind natürlich Hypoglykämien bei jeder Form der Diabetestherapie möglich. Ein direkter Vergleich der verschiedenen Behandlungsarten liegt bis heute im Weltschrifttum nicht vor. In einer Zweijahresstudie auf der Insel Gotland in Schweden wurden 4.2/1000 Patienten/Jahr klinisch behandlungsbedürftige Hypoglykämien durch Sulfonylharnstoffe ermittelt. Vier englische und amerikanische Studien, die sich in etwa gleicher Methodik bedienten, ergaben für insulinbehandelte Zuckerkranke eine Hypoglykämiehäufigkeit von 100/1000 Patienten/Jahr, also eine deutlich größere Zahl [7].

Sekundärversagen

Ein wichtiges und oft wenig beachtetes Problem der Sulfonylharnstofftherapie ist das nicht rechtzeitige Erkennen des Übergangs in das Sekundärversagen. Wir haben auf dieses Phänomen schon 1961 [19] hingewiesen und damals auf dem Genfer IDF-Kongress unsere Beobachtungen aus den ersten 5 Jahren mitgeteilt, die im folgenden Jahr aus der Joslin-Clinic bestätigt wurden [6]. Damals ergab sich bei 1218 Diabetikern und 244 Sekundärversagern eine mittlere, jährliche Versagerquote von 8%. Wir hielten daher 1961 eine zeitliche Begrenzung der Anwendbarkeit der Sulfonylharnstoffe für wahrscheinlich.

Wir haben diese Studie 1977 mit Haupt [9] wiederholt und in den 10 Jahren von 1968–1977 bei 306 von 914 NIDDM-Patienten mit Sulfonylharnstoffen ein Sekundärversagen festgestellt (Abb. 2).

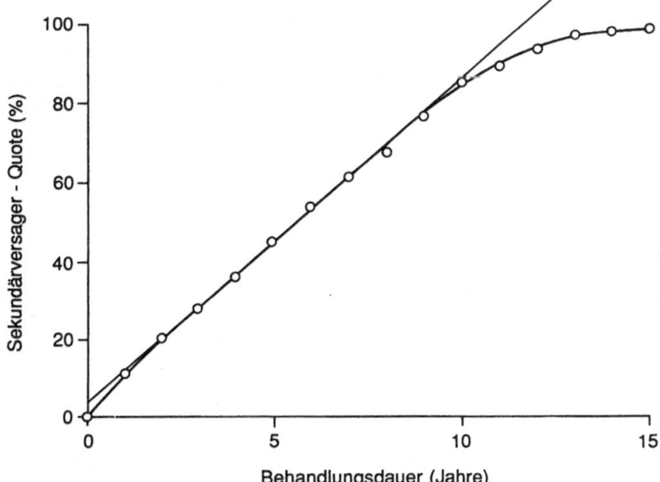

Abb. 2. Abhängigkeit der Sekundärversagerquote von der Behandlungsdauer [9]

Die Berechnung der kumulativen Häufigkeit des Sekundärversagens der Studie von 1977 zeigt, daß die schon in den ersten Jahren aufgestellte Hypothese richtig war, und daß Sulfonylharnstoffe bei der Mehrzahl der Kranken nur zeitlich begrenzt Anwendung finden können.

Exzessiver Gebrauch von Sulfanylharnstoffen

Der größte Fehler der Sulfonylharnstofftherapie, den ich abschließend als das 3. Problem besprechen möchte, ist die falsche Anwendung der Sulfonylharnstoffe. Sie werden immer wieder als „Tabletten der Bequemlichkeit" [16] mißbraucht, indem sie nicht nur gegeben bzw. genommen werden, wenn die alleinige Ernährungstherapie zur Erzielung einer guten Dauerstoffwechsellage, d. h. in der Regel Euglykämie, nicht mehr ausreicht, sondern indem sie anstelle der diätetischen Behandlung Anwendung finden. Diese Tatsache ergibt sich nicht nur aus täglichen Erfahrungen und aus dem erfolgreichen Bemühen um Ersatz der Tabletten durch die richtige Ernährungstherapie, sie ließ sich auch statistisch beweisen. Unsere Untersuchungen aus dem Jahre 1976 [17] zeigen, daß in keinem anderen Land so häufig eine Diabetes-Pharmokotherapie (Insulin plus Sulfonylharnstoffe plus Biguanide) erfolgte wie in der Bundesrepublik (Tabelle 1). Die Zahl der Diabetiker, die nach diesen Untersuchungen damals Pharmaka erhalten hatten, war größer als die Zahl der Zuckerkranken, die bei der Münchner Früherfassungsaktion ein paar Jahre [13] zuvor als manifeste Zuckerkranke entdeckt worden waren.

Tabelle 1. Pharmakotherapie des Diabetes mellitus 1976 (17)

Reihenfolge	Land	Einwohnerzahl	‰ der Einwohner mit Diabetes-Pharmakotherapie
1	Deutschland	60 650 000	22.1
2	Schweden	8 127 000	17.2
3	Frankreich	51 280 000	11.7
4	USA	207 010 000	11.1
5	Großbritannien	55 570 000	7.6
6	Italien	53 857 000	7.5
7	Spanien	34 490 000	5.2
8	Japan	106 900 000	3.2

Gleiche Zahlen konnten 1981 Berger und Standl [3] aus den IMS-Unterlagen ermitteln, wobei Berger 1986 in Davidsons Lehrbuch noch feststellte, daß auch in der DDR mit einem exzessiven Gebrauch der Sulfonylharnstoffe zu rechnen ist.

Diese Feststellung wurde auf der EASD-Konferenz mit exakten Zahlen belegt. Dort wurden Fünfjahres-Ergebnisse der sogenannten DIS-Studie (Diabetes-Interventions-Studie) von Hanefeld und Julius [8] vorgelegt. In dieser Studie wurden in den Jahren 1977 – 1980 insgesamt 1139 neu manifeste, initial diätetisch führbare Typ II-Diabetiker aus 16 Beratungsstellen der DDR aufgenommen. Mittels Randomisierung wurden sie 3 Gruppen zugeteilt: Basis-Intervention plus Clofibrinsäure bzw. Basis-Intervention plus Placebo (Doppelblindprinzip) und Kontrollgruppen mit der in den Beratungsstellen üblichen Diabetestherapie. Die Basis-Intervention bestand aus intensivierten Diätberatungen, großen Bemühungen um eine Gewichtsreduktion und Hypertonieführung sowie Hinweisen zum körperlichen Training. Nach dem DIS-Manual sollte bei den Interventionspatienten erst bei Überschreitung eines postprandialen Blutzuckerwertes von 13.9 mM/l = 250 mg/dl und eine Glukosurie von mehr als 20 g eine antidiabetische Pharmakotherapie begonnen werden. In der Kontrollgruppe gab es keine gesonderten Vorschriften, es wurden also die allgemeinen üblichen Kriterien benutzt.

Nach 5 Jahren Follow-up war in beiden Interventionsgruppen noch 2/3 der Kranken diätetisch sehr gut zu führen, während dies bei weniger als der Hälfte der Patienten der Kontrollgruppe möglich war. Trotz des viel häufigeren Einsatzes der Sulfonylharnstoffe in der Kontrollgruppe, kam es bei ihr im Verlaufe der 5 Jahre zu einer signifikanten Verschlechterung des mittleren Jahresblutzuckers. Diese Ergebnisse belegen eindeutig den guten Effekt der nicht-medikamentösen Diabetes-Therapie in den beiden Interventionsgruppen und zeigen eindeutig den Mißerfolg der sogenannten „üblichen Therapieform" beim Typ II-Diabetes.

Exakte Zahlen über den wirklichen Einsatz von oralen Antidiabetika und nicht sogenannte Verkaufszahlen kenne ich nur aus der DDR, da dort nur die staatlichen Ambulanzen Insulin und Tabletten an Zuckerkranke ausgeben können. Wie sich in der DDR die Situation 1985 darstellte, zeigt die nächste Darstellung (Tabelle 2), fast die Hälfte der Zuckerkranken nimmt Tabletten und, wie sie aus der DIS-Studie entnehmen konnten, wäre sie nur bei einem Viertel erforderlich gewesen.

Tabelle 2. Diabetestherapie in der DDR 1985 (8)

Insuline		14,8 %
Orale Antidiabetica		44,4 %
– *Glibenclamid*	*33,3 %*	
– *Tolbutamid*	*8,2 %*	
– *Buformin*	*0,8 %*	
– *SH + Buformin*	*2,1 %*	
Diät		40,9 %

Zusammenfassung

Abschließend muß ich mich noch einmal auf Grund der vielen Interpretationen der UGDP-Studie der Schlüsselfrage zuwenden: „Hat unsere gesamte Therapie mit der richtigen Ernährung, mit der Bewegungstherapie, dem Insulin, den Sulfonylharnstoffen und auch den Biguaniden einen Einfluß auf die Mortalität und auf die Lebenserwartung gehabt?" Ich kann Ihnen ebensowenig wie irgend jemand sonst auf der Welt auf diese Frage eine befriedigende Antwort geben. In der Darstellung von Panzram [4] (Tabelle 3) hat er den nur möglichen bescheidenen Vergleich erstellt, der zeigt, daß wir bei unseren Patienten mit Typ II-Diabetes in den 20 Jahren wahrscheinlich keine Lebensverlängerung erreicht haben. Ältere Studien dürfen wir nicht heranziehen, denn in ihnen wurde noch nicht einmal der Versuch unternommen, die beiden Diabetestypen zu trennen, die wir damals zudem alle anders benannt haben und bei denen der chemische und subklinische Diabetes, d. h. die heutige „gestörte Glukosetoleranz", nicht ausgeklammert worden war. So ist auch die Antwort auf die Frage nach dem Nutzen oder dem Schaden der Sulfonylharnstoffe mit Hilfe von Mortalitätsstatistiken zumindest heute noch nicht möglich und es war ein übler Fehler, daß die UGDP-Studie sich dieser statistischen Methode bediente.

Tabelle 3. Altersbezogene Reduktion der Lebenserwartung (14)

Age (years)	Marks and Krall 1971 [32]	Goodkin 1975 [25]	Panzram and Zabel-Langhennig 1981 [27]
10/ <15	(17)	27	–
15–19	16–17	23	–
20–29	12–14	16	–
30–39	10–11	11	–
40–49	8– 9	10	7–8
50–59	6– 7	6	5–6
60–69 (70)	4– 5	5	3–4
70+	–	–	3

Diesen realistischen negativen Erkenntnissen können wir aber unsere eigenen Erfahrungen aus den letzten 40 Jahren über das Leben unserer Zuckerkranken – zu unserem eigenen Trost und zu dem unserer Patienten – gegenüberstellen. Seit Ende des 2. Weltkrieges hat sich die Diagnostik und Therapie ständig verbessert und wir alle waren daran nicht unbeteiligt.

Die akute schwere Stoffwechselentgleisung, das Coma diabeticum ist selbst in einer Universitätsklinik zur Rarität geworden, und das Kind der diabetischen Mutter hat eine wesentlich größere Chance normal und gesund geboren zu werden. Die um vieles größer und besser gewordene Lebensqualität des Diabetikers hat viele Väter, einer von ihnen ist der Sulfonylharnstoff. Wichtig ist es daher auch, daß wir nicht nur an den Nutzen der Sulfonylharnstoffe denken, sondern daß wir ihre Risiken und Probleme in der gleichen Weise vor Augen haben und uns so auch in der Zukunft diese Therapieform erhalten.

Literatur

1. Alberti KGMM, Gries FA (1988) Management of Non-Insulin-dependent Diabetes mellitus in Europe- A Consensus View. Diabetic Med 5: 275
2. Asplund K, Wiholm BE, Lithner F (1983) Glibenclamide– associated hypoglycaemia: a report on 57 cases. Diabetologia 24: 412
3. Berger M, Standl E (1981) Sulfonylharnstoffe in der Diabetestherapie. Dtsch Med Wochenschr 106: 1443
4. Berger W (1971) 88 schwere Hypoglykämiezwischenfälle unter der Behandlung mit Sulfonylharnstoffen. Schweiz Med Wochenschr 101: 1013
5. Berger W, Caduff F, Pasquet M, Rump A (1986) Die relative Häufigkeit der schweren Sulfonylharnstoff-Hypoglykämie in den letzten 25 Jahren in der Schweiz. Schweiz Med Wochenschr 116: 145
6. Camerini-Davalos R, Marble A (1962) Incidence and causes of secondary failure in treatment with Tolbutamide. J Amer Med Assoc 181: 1
7. Ferner RE, Neil HAW (1988) Sulfonylureas and hypoglycaemia. Brit Med J 296: 949
8. Hanefeld M, Schulze J, Fischer S, Julius U, Schimke H, Haller H (1985) The Diabetes Intervention study. In: James RW, Pometta D (ed) Dyspoproteinemias and diabetes. Karger, Basel
9. Haupt E, Laube F, Loy H, Schöffling K (1977) Neue Untersuchungen zum Sekundärversagen der Therapie mit blutglucosesenkenden Sulfonamidderivaten. Med Klin 72: 1529
10. Janbon N, Chaptal C, Vedel A, Schaap I (1942) Accidents hypoglycemiques graves par un sulfonamidothiodiazol. Montpellier Med 85: 441
11. Kilo C, Miller IP, Williamson IR (1979) The achilles heel of the University Group Diabetes Program. J Am Med Assoc 243: 450
12. Klimt CR, Knatterud GL, Meinert CL, Prout TE (1970) A study of the effects of hypoglyemic agents on vascular complications in patients with adult-onset diabetes. Diabetes [Suppl 2] 19: 747
13. Mehnert H, Sewering H, Reichenstein W, Vogt H (1968) Früherfassung von Diabetikern in München 1967/68 Dtsch Med Wochenschr 93: 2044
14. Panzram G (1987) Mortality and survival in Typ 2 (non-insulin-dependent) diabetes mellitus. Diabetologia 30: 123
15. Seltzer H S (1972) Drug-Induced hypoglycaemia: a review based on 473 cases. Diabetes 21: 955
16. Schöffling K (1962) Orale Antidiabetika. Dtsch Z Verd-Stoffwechselk 21: 269
17. Schöffling K (1976) Die vier Säulen der Diabetes-Therapie. Langerhansvorlesung (12. Jahrestagung der Deutschen Diabetes-Gesellschaft, Braunlage)

18. Schöffling K (1979) Möglichkeiten und Risiken der Behandlung des Zuckerkranken mit oralen Antidiabetika. Therapiewoche 29: 5024
19. Schöffling K, Ditschuneit H, Pfeiffer EF (1961) Die zeitliche Begrenzung der Anwendbarkeit von Sulfonylharnstoffen in der Behandlung des Altersdiabetes. 4th Congress Intern Diab Fed, Genf
20. Schöffling K, Mehnert H, Haupt E (1984) Behandlung mit Sulfonylharnstoffen. In: Mehnert H, Schöffling K Diabetologie in Klinik und Praxis (Hrsg) Thieme, Stuttgart New York

Applikation von Normal- und Verzögerungsinsulin per injectionem – vorwiegend unter pharmakokinetischen Aspekten

H. Sauer

Summary

First of all this paper discusses some present clinically relevant data on the pharmacokinetics of in particular, retarded forms of insulin. The influence of galenic preparations are then discussed in detail with regard to species specificity, inconstancy of absorption, and the dependency of the absorption rate on the dose of insulin.

Because of the distinct trend to human NPH insulin the list of available insulins is less complex than one might conclude from the total of 25 preparations for routine therapy. The high number of combined preparations appears unnecessary and perhaps with respect to intensive insulin therapy not even desirable. This should not influence the decision to start with so-called „free" individual mixtures and should also not affect dose adaptation.

Einleitung

Die Veränderungen in der „Insulinlandschaft", wie sie sich in den letzten 10 Jahren bei etwa gleichbleibender Zahl von Präparaten insgesamt ergeben haben, lassen sich wie folgt zusammenfassen:

Der Anteil an Humaninsulin liegt z. Zt. bei etwa 80 % (in den USA bei 20 %, in England bei 80 %), Schweineinsulin und vor allem Rinderinsulin haben einen dementsprechenden Rückgang zu verzeichnen. Unter den Verzögerungsinsulinen hat sich der NPH-Typ mit heute etwa 75–80 % Marktanteil gegenüber ungefähr 15 % vor 10 Jahren durchgesetzt. Der Hauptgrund ist die gute Eignung für die heutige Insulintherapie sowie der Umstand, daß die überwiegende Zahl der Human-Verzögerungsinsuline auf NPH-Basis hergestellt werden. Die Zahl der Kombinationspräparate mit Normalinsulin hat stark zugenommen, von 5 im Jahre 1982 auf heute 15, davon 12 auf NPH-Insulin-Basis (Tabelle 1).

Die Insulinkonzentration der Routinepräparate beträgt 40 E/ml (U 40) bei weltweiter Tendenz zu U 100. In der Bundesrepublik werden U 100-Präparate für

die sog. Pen und für Insulinpumpen sowie von einem Hersteller für insulinresi-
stente Patienten geliefert.

Trotz der großen Zahl von Präparaten und der Fortschritte in Richtung zur
intensivierten Behandlung mit Selbstkontrolle und Dosisanpassung bleiben die
alten Probleme des konventionellen Regimes, d. h. der Injektionstherapie – ob
mit Spritzen oder Pen im Rahmen des sog. Basis-Bolus-Konzeptes – praktisch
unverändert bestehen. Das Fehlen einer Autoregulation der Insulinversorgung
wie beim Gesunden sowie die unphysiologische Pharmakokinetik der Insulinpräparate, insbesondere die Schwierigkeiten, eine konstante Basal- und eine prompte
Prandial-Versorgung zu erzielen, erschweren nach wie vor die Bemühungen um
eine Nahezu-Normoglykämie. Angesichts dieser Umstände hat die Pharmakokinetik der diversen Präparate in den letzten Jahren, v. a. die Insulinabsorption im
subkutanen Gewebe, zunehmende Aufmerksamkeit gefunden. Die in zahlreichen
Studien erhobenen Befunde haben die Kenntnisse über den Wirkungsablauf der
einzelnen Präparate einschl. ihrer Mischungen mit Normalinsulin erweitert und
damit die Grundlage für eine differenziertere Therapie geschaffen. Zur Orientie-
rung über die Absorptionsverhältnisse bzw. zur Ermittlung der Pharmakokinetik
stehen außer der Blutzuckerbestimmung die seit 1948 durchgeführten Absorp-
tionsmessungen von injiziertem markierten Insulin zur Verfügung sowie die Be-
stimmungen der Plasmainsulinkurve post inj. und die Clamp-Technik [5, 6, 7, 15,
30, 51–55].

Absorptionsraten und Insulinfreisetzung. Die Absorptionsraten sind abhängig von
den Eigenschaften des betreffenden Präparates, vor allem von ihrem pyhsikalisch-
chemischen Zustand sowie von den am Injektionsort herrschenden Verhältnissen
einschl. der darauf einwirkenden Faktoren.

Bei den Normalinsulinen handelt es sich um neutrale Lösungen. Das Prinzip
der heute gängigen Verzögerungsinsuline basiert im wesentlichen auf der Suspension von Kristallen oder auch amorphen Partikeln wie bei Nr. 25–28 und Nr.
35 (Tabelle 1). Die Kristallisation erfolgt bei den NPH- (Neutrales Protamin
Hagedorn) Insulinen mit Protamin in einem phosphathaltigen Puffer mit Zusatz
von Phenol bzw. m-Kresol. Die Bildung der Kristalle bzw. amorphen Partikel
erfolgt dagegen bei den Insulin-Zink-Suspensionen in einem Acetatpuffer mit
überschüssigem Zinkgehalt. Nur die Surfen-Insuline liegen als saure Lösung vor,
aus denen erst im neutralen Gewebs-pH amorphe Insulin-Surfenpartikel ausfallen.

Für die Absorptionsraten ist von Bedeutung, daß Insulin am Injektionsort nicht
in Form eines rasch resorbierbaren, biologisch aktiven Monomers sondern vor
allem Hexamer mit stärkerer Tendenz zur Aggregation und langsamerer Absorption vorliegt. Studien in den letzten Jahren haben gezeigt, daß offenbar bestimmte
biologisch aktive Insulinanaloga anders als tierisches oder Humaninsulin nicht
polymerisiert werden, sondern in monomerem Zustand im Injektionsbereich ver-
bleiben [55].

Mit einer therapeutisch relevanten Insulindegradation durch Proteasen im subkutanen Gewebe muß nicht gerechnet werden außer in speziellen seltenen Fällen
von Insulinresistenz und möglicherweise beim Brittle-Diabetes [51, 57].

Tabelle 1. Insulinpräparate (lediglich U 40) zur Injektion – nicht für „Pen". S = Schweineinsulin, R = Rinderinsulin, H = Humaninsulin, SHI = semisynthetisches Humaninsulin, BHI = biosynthetisches Humaninsulin, IZS = Insulin-Zink-Suspension, NPH = Neutrales Protamin-Insulin Hagedorn, NI = Normalinsulin

Insulinsorte		Spezies	Wirkungsdauer (ca. in h)	Hersteller
Normal- (Alt-) Insuline				
1. H Insulin Hoechst		H (SHI)	5–6	Hoechst
2. Huminsulin Normal		H (BHI)	5–6	Lilly
3. Insulin Actrapid HM(ge)		H (BHI)	7–6	Novo
4. Insulin Hoechst		R	5–6	Hoechst
5. Insulin S Hoechst		S	5–6	Hoechst
6. Insulin Velasulin Nordisk		S	5–6	Nordisk
7. Insulin Velasulin human		H (SHI)	5–6	Nordisk

Verzögerungsinsuline (sämtlich IMI, auch in Kombination mit Normalinsulin)
NI-Anteil in %

Insulinsorte	NI-Anteil	Spezies	Wirkungsdauer (ca. in h)	Hersteller
NPH-Insuline (NI-Anteil)				
8. Basal-H-Insulin Hoechst		H (SHI)	20	Hoechst
9. Depot-H15-Insulin Hoechst	15	H (SHI)	20	Hoechst
10. Depot-H-Insulin Hoechst	25	H (SHI)	16	Hoechst
11. Komb-H-Insulin Hoechst	50	H (SHI)	12–16	Hoechst
12. Huminsulin Basal NPH		H (BHI)	20	Lilly
13. Huminsulin Profil I	10	H (BHI)	18	Lilly
14. Huminsulin Profil II	20	H (BHI)	16	Lilly
15. Huminsulin Profil III	30	H (BHI)	16	Lilly
16. Huminsulin Profil IV	40	H (BHI)	12–16	Lilly
17. Insulin Insulatard Nordisk		S	20	Nordisk
18. Insulin Mixtard 30/70 Nordisk	30	S	16	Nordisk
19. Insulin Mixtard 50/50 Nordisk	50	S	12–16	Nordisk
20. Insulin Insulatard human		H (SHI)	20	Nordisk
21. Insulin Mixtard 30/70 human	30	H (SHI)	16	Nordisk
22. Insulin Mixtard 50/50 human	50	H (SHI)	12–16	Nordisk
23. Insulin Protaphan HM(ge)		H (BHI)	20	Novo
24. Insulin Actraphane HM(ge) 40 IE	30	H (BHI)	16	Novo
Insulin-Zink-Suspension (IZS)				
25. Insulin Monotard HM(ge) (70 % Krist. + 30 % amorph)		H (BHI)	20	Novo
26. Insulin Novo Lente (70 % Krist, Nr. 27 + 30 % amorph, Nr. 35)		RS	24–28	Novo
27. Insulin Novo Ultralente		R	28	Novo
28. Insulin Ultratard HM(ge) 40 IE/ml		H (BHI)	24	Novo
Surfen-Insuline				
29. Depot-Insulin Hoechst		R	12–16	Hoechst
30. Depot-Insulin S Hoechst		S	12–16	Hoechst
31. Komb-Insulin	(33)	R	12	Hoechst
32. Komb-Insulin S	(33)	S	12	Hoechst

Tabelle 1 (Fortsetzung)

Nur noch selten verwendete Präparate			
33. Depot-Insulin Horm (Insulin-Zink-Protaminat)	R	20	Hormon-chemie
34. Insulin Novo Rapitard (75% Ins.-Kristall-Susp. + 25% Nr. 3)	RS	20	Novo
35. Insulin Novo Semilente (IZS, amorph)	S	12–16	Novo

Speziesbedingte Absorptionsunterschiede von klinischer Relevanz sind nur für die Insulin-Zink-Suspensionen, jedoch nicht für die NPH-Insuline von Bedeutung. Die langsamere Absorption [21, 35] insbesondere der kristallinen Insulin-Zink-Suspension vom Rind (in Tabelle 1 Nr. 27, z. T. auch Nr. 26) beruht auf seiner stärkeren Aggregationstendenz. Die nur minimal raschere Absorption von Humaninsulin im Vergleich zu Schweineinsulin ist auf seine stärkere Hydrophilie zurückzuführen, die es dem Threonin in der B 30-Position verdankt. Für die therapeutische Praxis ist dies jedoch ohne Bedeutung, so daß bei Human- und Schweineinsulin, sofern die Galenik übereinstimmt, wie z. B. bei Nr. 17 und 20 und mit einem etwa gleichen Wirkungsablauf gerechnet werden kann [24, 37, 38, 45].

Abgesehen von der Möglichkeit, daß der Wirkungsablauf durch stärkere Antikörperbildung modifiziert wird, ist es eher unwahrscheinlich, daß im Gegensatz zu den Insulin-Zink-Suspensionen durch speziesbedingte Präparate-Eigenschaften per se die Absorption von NPH-Insulinen nennenswert verändert wird. Ein mit dem Human- oder Schweineinsulin galenisch identisches und auch hochgereinigtes NPH-Insulin vom Rind steht hierzulande allerdings nicht zur Verfügung. Im übrigen wurde kürzlich nachgewiesen, daß bezüglich der Antikörperbildung und auch klinisch manifester Immunreaktionen zwischen einem hochgereinigten Schweineinsulin- und einem Rinder-Schweine-Präparat nur geringe Unterschiede bestehen [2].

Auf die Beeinflussung der Absorption und des Blutzuckerverlaufs durch humorale Antikörper wird nicht näher eingegangen. Eine stärker erhöhte Antikörperkonzentration – nicht die unter Human- oder hochgereinigtem Schweineinsulin zu findenden minimalen Titer – verzögern den Wirkungseintritt, verlängern die Wirkung und können in der Spätphase durch Dissoziation des Insulin-Antikörperkomplexes zu unvorhergesehenen Hypoglykämien führen [15, 32, 51, 54].

Weitere Faktoren von seiten des Präparates (s. auch Tabelle 2): Höheres Injektionsvolumen verzögert die Absorption, außerdem führt eine höhere Konzentration zur Verlangsamung. Von Interesse ist in diesem Zusammenhang die weltweite Tendenz zu U-100 (100 E/ml) Insulinen. Da sich die beiden Faktoren in etwa neutralisieren, ist mit einer nennenswerten Änderung der Insulinabsorption nicht zu rechnen, es sei denn, daß hochkonzentrierte Sonderanfertigungen, wie z. B. mit 500 E/ml, vorliegen.

Lange vernachlässigt und nicht ausreichend bekannt war die Abhängigkeit der Absorptionsrate von der Dosis. Höhere Dosierungen verlangsamen, niedrigere

Tabelle 2. Einflüsse auf die Insulin-Absorption (in Anlehnung an M. Berger, 1985)

Einwirkungen	Verhalten der Absorption	Bemerkungen
intraindividuelle Inkonstanz	VK 25 % – trotz gleichen Areals [5, 6, 30]	relativ konstant bei minimalem Injektionsvolumen
interindividuelle Inkonstanz	VK 50 % [5, 6, 30]	
Injektionsareal	Abdomen > Oberarm > Oberschenkel, Gesäß	Injektion nach „Etagenprinzip"
Temperatur	Beschleunigung bei Wärme, langsamer bei Kälte	ausgeprägt v.a. für NI
Muskeltätigkeit	Zunahme im Bereich der aktiven Muskulatur [27]	für NI untersucht
Massage	Zunahme [31]	
Nikotin	doch keine Abnahme [9a]	
Lipohypertrophie	verzögert (49)	
Injektion in induriertes Gewebe	unübersichtlich, wahrscheinlich verlangsamt	keine konkreten Daten wegen fehlender Studien, außer (43)

beschleunigen die Absorption mit entsprechender Auswirkung auf den Zeitpunkt des Wirkungsmaximums sowie auf die Gesamtwirkdauer [20, 29]. So wurde für NPH-Insulin nachgewiesen, daß eine Verdreifachung der Dosis nur mit einer Verdopplung der prozentualen Absorptionsrate einhergeht [30]. W. Berger ermittelte aufgrund einer Auswertung pharmakokinetischer Daten aus verschiedenen Studien, daß z.B. bei NPH-Insulin eine Reduzierung der Dosis von 24 auf 12 E zu einer Verkürzung der maximalen Insulin-Wirkungszeit um 2.5 Std. führt; für Normalinsulin lag der Wert bei einer Stunde, wenn statt 12 nur 6 E injiziert wurden (W. Berger, persönliche Mitteilung).

Bei sämtlichen Insulinpräparaten muß mit z.T. erheblichen Schwankungen der Absorption nicht nur von Patient zu Patient, sondern auch beim gleichen Patienten gerechnet werden [5, 6, 30, 55]. Der intraindividuelle Variationskoeffizient wurde bei Injektion in das gleiche Areal mit 25 % ermittelt; interindividuell lag er sogar bei 50 % [5, 6]. Die intraindividuelle Inkonstanz der Absorption ist eine der wesentlichen Ursachen für die Labilität vor allem bei fehlender Eigeninsulinproduktion wie beim Typ I-Diabetes. – Der Variationskoeffizient ist offensichtlich dosisabhängig und nimmt mit höheren Dosen zu. So ist umgekehrt der günstige Einfluß der kontinuierlichen subkutanen Insulinzufuhr durch die Pumpe (CSII) beim instabilen Diabetes u.a. darauf zurückzuführen, daß die Absorption des in minimalen Mengen kontinuierlich infundierten Insulins gleichmäßiger verläuft als die der größeren Volumina nach Injektion. Die z.T. ausgeprägten interindividuellen Differenzen erschweren im übrigen die Vorhersage über den Wirkungsablauf eines Insulinpräparates im Einzelfall.

Lauritzen et al zeigten, daß Phasen mit stark erhöhtem freien Insulin im Plasma mit Hypoglykämien korreliert waren und umgekehrt niedrige Insulinkonzentrationen mit hohem Blutzucker [29, 30]. Die Situation wird generell dadurch kompliziert und die Analyse der Blutzuckerschwankungen oft dadurch erschwert, daß auch andere von der jeweiligen Diabetessituation ausgehende Faktoren, wie Wechsel der Insulinempfindlichkeit, wie z.B. beim Dawn-Phänomen, Bindung an Insulinantikörper oder verstärkte Hypoglykämieneigung wegen Defektes der Gegenregulation mit dem Faktor der Absorption interferieren. Ziel et al. [50] fanden, daß die Schwankungen der Insulinwirkung von Tag zu Tag und damit auch des Blutzuckers in stärkerem Maße durch Veränderungen der Gewebsempfindlichkeit als durch die jeweilige Absorptionsrate beeinflußt werden. – Trotz einer so komplexen Situation darf nicht versäumt werden, banale exogene Einflüsse zu eruieren, wie beispielsweise unzweckmäßige Wahl des Injektionsortes, falsche Technik oder ungeeigneter Spritz-Eß-Abstand, und dementsprechende Korrekturen vorzunehmen.

Insulinmischungen. Die Bemühungen um eine bessere Diabeteseinstellung haben dazu geführt, daß das Normalinsulin als Einzelinjektion oder in einer Mischung mit Verzögerungsinsulin zunehmende Bedeutung erlangt hat. Kombinationspräparate mit ihrem fixierten Normalinsulin-Anteil sind wohl zur Beseitigung postprandialer Hyperglykämien geeignet, nicht aber für die Dosisadaptation an den Blutzuckerverlauf und an die Lebensumstände. Dafür kommen allein die sog. „freien", vom Patienten selbst herzustellenden Mischungen in Betracht. Für jede Art von Mischung ist aber von Bedeutung, ob und wie weit das dem Verzögerungspräparat zugesetzte Normalinsulin den gewünschten stärkeren Initialeffekt beibehält. Seit langem ist bekannt und durch neuere Studien bestätigt, daß bei der Mischung mit NPH-Insulin kein Wirkungsverlust eintritt [9, 17, 28, 33]. Anders ist die Situation bei den Insulin-Zink-Suspensionen, bei denen anhand von Blutzucker- und Plasmainsulin-Kurven sowie von Clamp-Studien ein geringerer Initialeffekt mit einer Abschwächung der Wirkung insgesamt beschrieben wurde [9, 11, 12, 17]. Nur Berger et al. [s. 51] fanden beim Schweineinsulin keine Wirkungsverminderung, sofern sogleich nach der Mischung injiziert wurde. Die Abschwächung des Initialeffektes ist auf den hohen Zinkgehalt der Insulin-Zink-Suspension zurückzuführen, der andererseits jedoch für die Stabilisierung der Suspension notwendig ist. Bei Verwendung der reinen kristallinen Suspensionen [Nr. 27, 28] soll wegen des höheren Zinkgehaltes sogar auf eine Mischung verzichtet und Normalinsulin getrennt injiziert werden. Insulin-Zink-Suspensionen sind deshalb auch nicht in Form von Kombinationspräparaten mit Normalinsulin im Handel. – Für den Normalinsulin-Zusatz zu Surfen-Präparaten [Nr. 31, 32] wurde eine Verstärkung des Initialeffektes eindeutig nachgewiesen; systematische Studien im Vergleich zu getrennter Injektion liegen jedoch nicht vor.

Unter den *Lokalfaktoren* [51] sind vor allem spezielle Verhältnisse am Injektionsort von Bedeutung. Die Absorption wird zu einem wesentlichen Teil durch die Gewebsart und die Durchblutung [51, 58] bestimmt. Seit langem ist die raschere Absorption im Bereich der Bauchhaut im Vergleich zum Oberarm, bes. zum Oberschenkel und Gesäß, bekannt [5, 6, 27, 51], ebenso die verlangsamte Absorption im Bereich einer Lipohypertrophie [49] und bei adipösen Patienten [6a]. Das gleiche ist für narbig veränderte Gewebspartien anzunehmen, obgleich nur eine dementsprechende Studie vorliegt [43]. Oft ist es allerdings schwierig, besonders bei instabilem Diabetes, die durch solche Lokalfaktoren bedingten Absorptionsunterschiede anhand der Blutzuckerprofile nachzuweisen. Die Schwankungen, die als Folge der primär inkonstanten Absorption auftreten, können so ausgeprägt sein, daß sie die durch Lokalität bedingten Unterschiede überdecken.

Die Absorptionsdifferenzen in den verschiedenen Injektionsarealen waren Anlaß, von dem früheren Rotationsverfahren abzurücken und nach dem sog. „Etagenprinzip" vorzugehen. Nichts hat sich jedoch an der Notwendigkeit geändert, die Injektionsstellen durch möglichst häufigen Wechsel im Bereich der einzelnen Areale zu schonen.

Eine unbeabsichtigte intramuskuläre Injektion führt zu beschleunigter Absorption. Damit muß bei geringer Dicke des subkutanen Fettgewebes gerechnet werden, wenn der Einstich senkrecht erfolgt [13, 41], was besonders bei Verwendung kurzer, 12 bis 13 mm langer, Nadeln und von Insulininjektoren, den sog. Pens, vorkommt. – Der ausgeprägte Einfluß von Wärme und Kälte auf die Insulinabsorption als Folge der veränderten Hautdurchblutung ist ebenfalls eindeutig dokumentiert, z.T. mit bis zu 30 bis 40%iger Zunahme unter Wärmeapplikation [51] – Massage führt nach Verabfolgung von Verzögerungsinsulin nur dann zu rascherer Absorption und niedrigem Blutzucker, wenn man der in der Praxis kaum realisierbaren Prozedur folgt und sie 30 Minuten nach der Injektion beginnen und für mindestens 30 Minuten durchführen läßt [31]. Dieser Effekt kommt offenbar nicht über die Durchblutung zustande, sondern durch eine druckbedingte stärkere Dispersion des Insulins in größere subkutane Areale.

Trotz optimaler Bedingungen im Injektionsareal ist der Anstieg des Plasmainsulins auch nach Injektion von Normalinsulin weniger prompt, der Blutzucker im Falle einer Nahrungsaufnahme dementsprechend höher als beim Stoffwechselgesunden. Die Möglichkeiten, derartige Blutzuckersteigerungen zu reduzieren, sind vielfältig und bestehen in dem Versuch, die Absorption zu beschleunigen etwa durch Wahl eines geeigneten Injektionsareales, durch Verlängerung des Spritz-Ess-Abstandes, durch Anpassung der Menge und Art der Kohlenhydratzufuhr sowie durch körperliche Aktivität zu einem geeigneten Zeitpunkt. Weitere Möglichkeiten (s. Tabelle 2), die Absorption zu erhöhen, sind kaum praktikabel.

Günstiger ist die Situation, wenn die *Applikationsart* geändert wird wie unter CSII, oder evtl. bei Verwendung eines Jet-Injektors oder einer Sprinkler-Nadel. – In Zukunft werden möglicherweise biologisch aktive Insulinanaloga oder andere „Normalinsuline" zur Verfügung stehen, die rascher als das tierische oder Humaninsulin absorbiert werden [26, 46].

Basales Insulin. Besonders im Rahmen der konventionellen intensivierten Insulintherapie ist eine einigermaßen konstante Versorgung mit „basalem" Insulin ein aktuelles, jedoch noch unvollkommen gelöstes Problem. Die Bedeutung der Basalversorgung hat ihren Niederschlag auch in dem Begriff Basis-Bolus-Konzept gefunden, der beinahe zu einem Modewort geworden ist und oft recht freigiebig zur Klassifizierung von Insulinregimen verwendet wird.

Bei einem Basalinsulin muß es sich um ein Langzeitpräparat ohne ausgeprägtes Wirkungsmaximum handeln, so daß, abgesehen von den allen Insulinen eigenen Absorptionsschwankungen, eine gleichbleibende Wirkung über 24 Std. gewährleistet ist. Die kristalline Insulin-Zink-Suspension Ultralente kommt unter den heute verfügbaren Präparaten dieser Forderung am nächsten [s. 39, 53]. Sie wird aber wegen ihrer Herkunft vom Rind und der daraus resultierenden etwas höheren Immunogenität vielerorts abgelehnt, an anderen Stellen aber weiter verwendet, zumal durch die Hochreinigung die Häufigkeit und Schwere von Immunreaktionen auch der Rinderinsuline entscheidend reduziert werden konnte [2].

Das „human Ultralente" Nr. 28 wurde von Holman et al. [22] dem entsprechenden Rinderinsulin [Nr. 27], das jedoch hinsichtlich der Absorption und der nach Injektion resultierenden Plasmainsulinkurve eine deutlich längere Wirkung zeigte [35], in klinischen Studien diesbezüglich für gleichwertig befunden. – Über ein Insulinanaloges mit gleichbleibendem Langzeiteffekt und geringen Absorptionsschwankungen, das die Kriterien für ein Basalinsulin besser erfüllt als humanes oder tierisches Insulin, wurde kürzlich berichtet [25].

Bereits Ende der 70er Jahre hatten Turner und Mitarbeiter [41] ein Konzept für die Kombination von basaler und prandialer Insulinversorgung entwickelt, und zwar zunächst auf der Basis der kristallinen Rinderinsulin-Zink-Suspension, später mit etwa gleichen Ergebnissen mit dem entsprechenden Humanpräparat [Nr. 28]. Darüber hinaus wurden, ausgehend vom Nüchternblutzucker, Dosierungsregeln für das Basalinsulin und aufgrund der präprandialen Blutzucker mittags und abends sowie des Spätwertes für das Normalinsulin, gegeben, das ein- bis dreimal täglich je nach Schwere bzw. Typ des Diabetes appliziert wurde.

In diese Formel (Tabelle 3) geht, sofern es sich um die Basalinsulin-Dosierung handelt, auch das Körpergewicht ein. Diese aufgrund klinischer Erfahrungen ermittelten Dosisempfehlungen haben sich nach den genannten Autoren bewährt und vor allem während der Einstellungsphase nur selten zu Hypoglykämien geführt, während sich derartige Regime andererorts nur bei einem Teil der Patienten als geeignet erwiesen.

Die meisten Regime der intensivierten Therapie werden heute im Sinne eines Basis-Bolus-Konzeptes interpretiert. Diese Bezeichnung wird nicht selten auch dann verwendet, wenn die Voraussetzungen einer basalen Insulinversorgung nicht erfüllt sind, wie beispielsweise für ein Regime mit dreimal „prandialem" Normalinsulin und spät einem NPH-Präparat, v.a. in niedriger Dosis. Wegen dessen Wirkungsdauer von nur 15 – 20 Stunden und bes. bei niedriger Dosierung läßt der Effekt im Laufe des folgenden Tages am späten Nachmittag bzw. gegen Abend nach. Tagsüber lassen sich solche Phasen einer unzureichenden Insulinwirkung i.a. durch Normalinsulininjektion zu jeder Hauptmahlzeit überbrücken, jedoch nur, wenn der Mahlzeitenabstand nicht zu groß, z. B. mehr als 5 Stunden beträgt. Bei längerem Intervall, vor allem zwischen der Injektion mittags und vor dem Abendessen, steigt der Blutzucker nicht selten ab 16 bis 17 Uhr an, da nicht mehr genug NPH-Insulin vom Abend vorher und auch nicht genug Normalinsulin von der Mittagsinjektion zur Verfügung stehen. Wenn dessen Dosis wegen Hypoglykämieneigung 2 bis 3 Stunden später nicht erhöht werden kann, soll eine geringe Dosis NPH-Insulin dem mittags applizierten Normalinsulin beigemischt werden.

Unter Umständen muß auch das humane Langzeitpräparat wegen Hypogly-kämieneigung niedriger dosiert werden als es dem 24-Std.-Bedarf an basalem Insulin entspricht, so daß eine zweimalige Injektion notwendig ist. Die Langzeit-insuline haben deshalb auch im Sinne des Bolus-Basis-Konzeptes zu keinem Durchbruch geführt. Es ist daher nicht verwunderlich, wenn vielerorts die Inter-mediärpräparate bevorzugt werden, oft zweimal, selten sogar dreimal am Tage.

Es konnte nur auf einige pharmakokinetische Aspekte der Insulintherapie und die sich daraus ergebenden therapeutischen Konsequenzen eingegangen werden. Faktoren von seiten des Patienten bzw. aufgrund seiner Diabetessituation beein-flussen den Blutzucker bzw. die Einstellungsqualität oft in stärkerem Maße als die Pharmakokinetik des Insulins. Eine adäquate Stoffwechselführung voraus-gesetzt handelt es vor allem um Änderungen der Insulinempfindlichkeit, nicht selten im Zirkadianrhythmus, z.B. mit einem Dawn-Phänomen, um eine ver-stärkte Hypoglykämieneigung bzw. -gefährdung als Folge eines Defektes der Gegenregulation sowie um eine Veränderung der Hypoglykämiesymptomatik mit Verlust der „Warnsymptome".

Allgemeine Hinweise zur derzeitigen Präparatesituation

Die derzeit umfangreiche Liste mit 28 Verzögerungs-Präparaten ist nur auf den ersten Blick verwirrend. Die inzwischen erfolgte Konzentration auf den NPH-Typ und auf die Spezies Human erleichtert die Übersicht, wenn berücksichtigt wird, daß zwischen den verschiedenen Human-NPH-Präparaten keine signifikan-ten Unterschiede bestehen [42] und NPH-Insulin vom Schwein einen etwa glei-chen Wirkungsablauf wie Humaninsuline identischer Galenik zeigte [37, 38, 42].

Tabelle 3. Kalkulation der Insulin-Basaldosis mit Korrektur für Übergewicht

Für Idealgewicht bei etwa 175 cm/70 kg:

Dosis für mg/dl $\quad \dfrac{\text{NBZ} - 50}{10}$

$\quad\quad$ mmol/l $\quad (\text{NBZ} - 3) \times 2$

Beispiel für NBZ 200 mg/dl: $\quad \dfrac{200 - 50}{10} = 15\ \text{E}$

Korrektur für Übergewicht:

Nach NBZ kalkulierte Dosis $\times \left[2{,}5\ \dfrac{\text{Ist-Gewicht}}{\text{Ideal-Gewicht}} - 1{,}5 \right]$

Danach ergibt sich für

120% Idealgewicht: 1,5 × höhere Dosis
140% Idealgewicht: 2,0 × höhere Dosis
160% Idealgewicht: 2,5 × höhere Dosis

Die Palette der Kombinationspräparate mit 10%, 15%, 20%, 25%, 30%, 33% (auf Surfenbasis), 40% und 50% ist allerdings umfangreicher als notwendig. Sie darf jedoch nicht zu einer Überschätzung der in diesen unterschiedlichen Relationen vermuteten Möglichkeiten für die Einstellung führen, oder gar von der „freien" Mischung mit den besseren Adaptationschancen abhalten. Die Kombinationspräparate mit fixiertem Normalinsulin-Anteil sind v.a. beim Typ II-Diabetes indiziert. Freie, vom Patienten selbst herzustellende und variable Mischungen sind hier i.a. unnötig und oft unzumutbar. So führten, wie Roland et al. in einer ambulanten Studie bei Typ II-Patienten zeigten, individuelle Mischungen auf NPH-Basis mit einem Normalinsulin-Anteil zwischen 20 und 70% zu keiner signifikant besseren Einstellung als 2 Kombinationspräparationen mit 30% bzw. 50% Normalinsulin [40].

Unter den Insulin-Zink-Suspensionen ist eine Konzentration auf das Human-Intermediärinsulin Nr. 25 und auf das protrahiert wirkende Nr. 28 zu verzeichnen. Die Surfeninsuline vom Schwein und bes. vom Rind (Nr. 29–32) werden zunehmend durch Humaninsuline vor allem vom NPH-Typ ersetzt, unnötigerweise bei vielen Patienten, die keine Immunreaktion aufweisen und die nach dem Wechsel ebensogut oder ebensoschlecht, in einigen Fällen sogar schlechter eingestellt sind als vorher.

Humaninsulin wird inzwischen bei allen Ersteinstellungen verwendet, ohne Vorteil jedoch gegenüber hochgereinigten Schweineinsulinen des gleichen Verzögerungstyps (s. Tabelle 1), allerdings auch ohne Nachteil hinsichtlich der Kosten.

In den letzten Jahren wurde mit Schwerpunkt in der Bundesrepublik und der Schweiz von Patienten berichtet, bei denen nach Übergang von tierischem auf Humaninsulin im Falle einer Hypoglykämie eine Abschwächung oder ein Ausbleiben der sog. Warnsymptome, vor allem Schwitzen und Hunger, aufgetreten und dadurch die zeitige Erkennung der Hypoglykämie erschwert sei. Eine Verminderung der Hypoglykämiesymptomatik unter Humaninsulin im Vergleich zu Schweineinsulin ergab die Auswertung einer Schweizer Doppelblindstudie [4]. Zu ähnlichen Befunden kam eine Studie aus der Bundesrepublik [24]. Keine Unterschiede zwischen tierischem und Humaninsulin ließen jedoch mehrere gemeinsam ausgewertete Doppelblindstudien aus den USA [1] und eine weitere Studie [16] hierzulande erkennen. Bisher gibt es außerdem keine Beweise, daß Hypoglykämien nach Übergang auf Humaninsulin häufiger und in schwererer Form auftreten, sofern die Einstellungsqualität unverändert und der Verzögerungstyp der gleiche blieb. Außer einer längeren Diabetesdauer führt insbesondere beim Typ I-Patienten eine sehr gute bzw. nahezu normoglykämische Einstellung als mindestens ebenso bedeutsamer Faktor zu einer Abschwächung der Hypoglykämiesymptomatik mit unawareness. In jedem Fall sind bei einem Wechsel des Insulinpräparates und nach Änderung des Insulin-Regimes erhöhte Aufmerksamkeit und sorgfältige Stoffwechselkontrolle wegen eventueller Hypoglykämiegefährdung erforderlich. In zwei kürzlichen Publikationen [14, 36] zur Frage der Hypoglykämie unter Humaninsulin wird als Ergebnis einer Bewertung der bisherigen Studien die Auffassung vertreten, daß eine „spezielle" humaninsulinbedingte unawareness nach Übergang von tierischem Insulin wenn überhaupt nur

Tabelle 4. Entwicklung der heute wichtigen Insuline und Stoffwechselführung. *MS* = Monospezies; *C* = Chromatographie; *SK* = Selbstkontrolle; *GHb* = Glykohämoglobin-Bestimmung

			1965		1970	1975	1980	1985
				MS	C		Human-Ins.	
Surfen		1940						→
NPH	seit	1948						→
IZS		1952						→
					BZ-SK	GHb	Insulin-Pumpe	„Pen"

bei wenigen, insbesondere bei Typ I-Patienten nach längerer Krankheitsdauer auftreten.

Welchen Einfluß hatten die „neuen" Insuline per se auf die therapeutischen Möglichkeiten in den letzten Jahren bis hin zu den Regimen der intensivierten Therapie? Zweifellos stehen mit der Entwicklung des Humaninsulins bessere Herstellungsverfahren zur Verfügung und vielleicht ist es außerdem zu einer Stimulierung der klinisch-wissenschaftlichen Forschung gekommen. Die entscheidenden Voraussetzungen für eine bessere Einstellungsqualität bis hin zu mehr Flexibilität auch im Hinblick auf die Lebensführung existieren jedoch bereits seit längerer Zeit, wie Tabelle 4 erkennen läßt. Dies gilt sowohl für geeignete, wenn auch noch keineswegs ideale Insulinpräparate mit minimaler Immunogenität und mit Mischungsstabilität bei Zusatz von Normalinsulin, für die mehrfache tägliche Injektion von Normalinsulin in unterschiedlichen Kombinationen mit Verzögerungspräparaten sowie in den erweiterten Modalitäten der Stoffwechselkontrolle und -führung einschl. der Adaptation. Hinzu kommt, daß die Möglichkeiten für eine Verbesserung der Diabeteseinstellung nun auch von Patienten und vor allem von Ärzten akzeptiert werden. Die Zukunft wird zeigen, ob es gelingt, Insulinpräparate bzw. -modifikationen mit noch günstigeren pharmakokinetischen Eigenschaften zu entwickeln. So könnten sich bestimmte Insulinanaloga eines Tages möglicherweise als „humaner" erweisen als Humaninsulin selbst oder auch das beinah „humane" Schweineinsulin.

Literatur

1. Anderson F, Galloway J, Spradlin T, Grimes J (1988) Lack of hypoglycemic unawareness with human insulin. Diabetes Res Clin Pract Suppl 1 Vol 5: 523
2. Asplin C, Raghu P, Clemons P et al. (1987) Randomized prospective trial of pure porcine and conventional bovine/porcine insulin. Diabetes Care 10: 337
3. Berger W, Althaus B (1986) Änderungen der Hypoglykämie-Frühsymptome bei Wechsel von tierischem Insulin auf Humaninsulin. Schweiz Ärztezeitung 67: 1130
4. Berger W, Honegger B, Keller U, Jaeggi E (1989) Warning symptoms of Hypoglycaemia during treatment with human an porcine insulin in Diabetes mellitus. Lancet I: 1041–1044

5. Binder C (1969) Absorption of injected insulin. A clinical-pharmacological study, Munksgaard, Copenhagen

6. Binder C, Lauritzen T, Faber O, Pramming S (1984) Insulin pharmacokinetics. Diabetes Care 7: 188–199

6a. Birtwell AJ, Burch A, Owens DR, Luzio S (1984) Subcutaneous insulin absorption in lean and overweight men. Diabetologia 27: 257A

7. Bottermann, P, Wahl K, Ermler R, Lebender A, Gyaram H (1985) Action Profiles and plasma concentrations of insulin after s.c. application of different insulin preparations. In: Beyer J, Albisser M, Schrezenmeir J, Lehmann L (eds). Computer systems of insulin adjustment in diabetes mellitus. Panscientia, Hedingen

8. Chantelau EA, Sonnenberg GE, Rajab A et al. (1985) Absorption of subcutaneously administered regular human and porcine insulin in different concentrations. Diabète Metab 11: 106

9. Colagiuri S, Villalobos S (1986) Assessing effect of mixing insulin by glucose-clamp technique in subjects with diabetes mellitus. Diabetes Care 9: 579–586

9a. Cüppers HJ, Könings P, Klingenbiel KJ, Mühlhauser I, Berger M (1984): Effekt von Zigarettenrauchen auf die Absorption von subkutan injiziertem Insulin. Aktuel Endokrinol Stoffw 5: 83

10. Federlin K (1988) Therapie mit Humaninsulin – tatsächlich ein Risiko für Patienten? Dtsch Ärztebl 85: C 1721–1722

11. Forlani G, Santacrose G, Ciavarella A et al. (1986) Effects of mixing short- and intermediate-acting insulins on absorption course and biologic effect of short-acting preparation. Diabetes Care 9: 587–590

12. Francis AJ, Hanning I, Alberti KGMM (1985) The Effect of Mixing Human Soluble and Human Crystalline Zinc-suspension Insulin: Plasma Insulin and Blood Glucose Profiles after Subcutaneous Injection. Diabetic Med 2: 177–180

13. Frid A, Gunnarsson R, Güntner P, Linde B (1988) Effects of Accidental Intramuscular Injection on Insulin Absorption in IDDM. Diabetes Care 1: 41–45

14. Gale EAM (1989) Hypoglycaemia and human insulin. Lancet II: 1264–1266

15. Galloway JA, Spradlin CT, Nelson RL et al. (1981) Factors influencing the absorption, serum insulin concentration and blood glucose responses after injections of regular insulin and various insulin mixtures. Diabetes Care 4: 366–376

16. Haupt E, Galle M, Oerter E (1989) Zum Verlust der Hypoglykämieempfindung von Typ I-Langzeitdiabetikern nach der Umstellung auf Humaninsulin. Erste Ergebnisse. Aktuel Endokrinol Stoffw 10: 95

17. Heine RJ, Bilo HJG, Fonk T et al. (1984) Absorption kinetics and action profiles of mixtures of regular and intermediate acting insulins. Diabetologia 27: 558–562

18. Hildebrandt P, Sestoft L, Nielsen SL (1983) The absorption of subcutaneously injected short-acting soluble insulin: Influence of injection technique and concentration. Diabetes Care 6: 459

19. Hildebrandt P, Birch K, Sestoft L, Vølund A (1984) Human monotard insulin: dose-dependent subcutaneous absorption. Diabetes Res 1: 183–185

20. Hildebrandt P, Birch K, Sestoft L, Vølund A (1984) Dose-dependent Subcutaneous Absorption of Porcine, Bovine and Human NPH Insulins. Acta Med Scand 215: 69–73

21. Hildebrandt P, Berger A, Volund A, Kuhl C (1985) The subcutaneous absorption of human and bovine ultralente insulin formulations. Diabetic Med 2: 355

22. Holman RR, Steemson J, Darling P, Reeves WG, Turner RC (1984) Human ultralente insulin. Brit med J 288: 665–668

23. Home PD, Mann NP, Hutchison A et al. (1984) A fifteen-month double-blind cross-over study of the efficacy and antigenicity of human and pork insulins. Diabetic Med 1: 93

24. Jakober B, Lingenfelser T, Glück H, Maassen M, Eggstein M (1989) Hypoglykämie bei Typ I-Diabetikern – Schweineinsulin versus Humaninsulin. Klin Wochenschr 67 (Suppl XVI): 201–202

25. Jørgensen ST, Vaag A, Langkjaer L, Hougaard PH, Markussen J (1989) NovoSol Basal: pharmacokinetics of a novel soluble acting insulin analogue. Br Med J 299: 415–419

26. Jörgensen S, Jörgensen KH, Jensen I, Hougaard P, Owens DR (1988) Mangnesium Insulin: a soluble Insulin with faster absorption in Man. Diab Res Clin Pract [Suppl 1] Vol 5: S478
27. Koivisto VA, Felig P (1980) Alterations in insulin absorption and blood glucose associated with varying insulin injection sites in diabetic patients. Ann Intern Med 92: 59–61
27a.Koivisto VA, Felig P (1978): Effects of leg exercise on insulin absorption in diabetic patients. New Engl Med 298: 79–83
28. Kølendorf K, Bojsen J, Deckert T (1983) Absorption an miscibility of regular porcine insulin after subcutaneous injection in insulin-treated diabetic patients. Diabetes Care 6: 6
29. Lauritzen T, Faber OK, Binder C (1979) Variation in ^{125}I-Insulin Absorption and Blood Glucose Concentration. Diabetologia 17: 291–295
30. Lauritzen T, Pramming S, Edwin AMG, Deckert D (1982) Absorption of isophane (NPH) insulin and its clinical implications. Brit Med J Vol 285: 159
31. Linde B (1986) Dissociation of insulin absorption and blood flow during massage of a subcutaneous injection site. Diabetes Care 9: 570–574
32. de Meijer PHEM, Luttermann JA, van't Laar A (1988) Insulin antibodies do not influence the absorption rate of sucutaneously injected insulin. Diabetic Med 5: 776–781
33. Olsson PO, Arnqvist H, von Schenck H (1987) Miscibility of human semi-synthetic regular and lente insulin and human biosynthetic regular and NPH insulin. Diabetes Care 10: 473
34. Owens DR, Jones IR, Birtwell AJ, Burge CTR, Luzio S, Davies CJ, Heyburn P, Heding LG (1984) Study of porcine and human isophane (NPH) insulins in normal subjects. Diabetologia 26: 261–265
35. Owens DR, Vora JP, Heding LG, Luzio S, Ryder REJ, Atiea J, Hayes TM (1986) Human, Porcine and Bovine Ultralente Insulin: Subcutaneous Administration in Normal Man. Diabetic Med 3: 326–329
36. Pickup J (1989) Human insulin. Br Med J 299: 991–993
37. Pramming S, Lauritzen T, Thorsteinsson B, Johansen K, Binder C (1984) Absorption of soluble and isophane semi-synthetic human and porcine insulin in insulin-dependent diabetic subjects. Acta Endocrinol 105: 215–220
38. Renner R, Vocke K, Hepp KD (1986) Wirkungsvergleich von protaminverzögertem NPH-Schweineinsulin und NPH-Humaninsulin bei Typ-I- und Typ-II-Diabetes. Dtsch Med Wochenschr 11: 1316–1320
39. Rizza RA, O'Brien PC, Service FJ (1986) Use of beef ultralente for basal insulin delivery: plasma insulin concentrations after chronic ultralente administrations in patients with IDDM. Diabetes Care 9: 120–123
40. Roland JM (1984) Need Stable Diabetics Mix their Insulins? Diab Med 1: 51–53
41. Spraul M, Chantelau E, Koumoulidou J, Berger M (1988) Subcutaneous or nonsubcutaneous injection of insulin. Diabetes Care 11: 733–736
42. Starke AAR, Heinemann L, Hohmann A, Berger M (1989) The action profiles of human NPH insulin preparations. Diabetic Med 6: 239–244
43. Thow JC, Johnson AB, Marsden S, Miller M, Home PD (1988) Delayed absorption of isophane insulin from palpably abnormal injection sites. Diabetic Med [Suppl 5] 2: 13
44. Turner RC, Philipps MA, Ward EA et al. (1983) Ultralente based insulin regimens – clinical applications, advantages and disadvantages. Acta Med Scand [Suppl 671] 213: 75–86
45. Volkholz HJ, Sailer D (1984) Therapie des insulin-abhängigen Diabetes. Münch Med Wochenschr 126: 969–972
46. Vora JP, Owens DR, Burch A, Dolben J, Atiea J, Dean J, Brange J (1987) Comparison of a monomeric insulin analogue and neutral soluble insulin in normal subjects. Diabetic Med 4: 558 A
47. Waldhäusl WK, Bratusch Marrain P, Kruse V et al. (1985) Effect of insulin antibodies on insulin pharmocokinetics and glucose utilization in insulin-dependent diabetic patients. Diabetes 34: 166
48. Wedemeyer HJ, v. Kriegstein E (1988) Ein Risiko des Humaninsulins. Dtsch Ärztebl 85: B 456–458
49. Young RJ, Hannan WJ, Frier BM, Steel JM, Duncan LJP (1984) Diabetic lipohypertrophy delays insulin absorption. Diabetes Care 7:479–482

50. Ziel FH, Davidson MB, Harris MD, Rosenberg S (1988) The Variability in the Action of Unmodified Insulin is More Dependent on Changes in Tissue Insulin Sensitivity than on Insulin Absorption. Diabetic Med 5: 662–666

Zusammenfassende Darstellungen

51. Berger M (1985) Insulin therapy conventional. In: Alberti KGMM, Krall LP (eds) The diabetes annual/1. Elsevier, Amsterdam, New York, Oxford, pp 111–128
52. Berger M (1986) Insulin therapy conventional. In: Alberti KGMM, Krall LP (eds) The Diabetes annual/2. Elsevier, Amsterdam, New York, Oxford, pp 69–80
53. Home PD (1987) Insulin injection therapy. In: Alberti KGMM, Krall LP (eds) The diabetes annual/3. Elsevier, Amsterdam, New York, Oxford pp 94–106
54. Home PD (1988) Insulin injection therapy, In: Alberti KGMM, Krall LP (eds) The diabetes annual/4. Elsevier, Amsterdam, New York, Oxford, pp 92–102
55. Brange J (1987) Galenics of insulin. Springer, Berlin, Heidelberg, New York
56. Moses AC, Jeffrey SF (1987) Unconventional routes of insulin administration. In: Alberti KGMM, Krall LP (eds) The diabetes annual/3. Elsevier, Amsterdam, New York, Oxford, pp 107–120
57. Williams G (1985) Subcutaneous insulin degradation. In: Pickup JC (ed) Brittle diabetes. Blackwell, Oxford, London, pp 154–166
58. Williams G (1985) Blood flow at insulin injections sites. In: Pickup JC (ed) Brittle diabetes. Blackwell, Oxford, London, pp 132–153

Proinsulin – oder Insulingabe?*

P. Bottermann

Summary

Through recombinant DNA technology sufficient quantities of biosynthetic human proinsulin have become available. Therefore it was obvious to look for therapeutic benefits of human proinsulin or the advantages of human proinsulin over human insulin. By in vitro studies it could be demonstrated that human proinsulin binds to the same receptor as insulin, but the binding of human proinsulin is one hundred times less than that of human insulin. After binding the postreceptor effects of human insulin and proinsulin are indistinguishable.

The pharmacokinetics of human proinsulin and human insulin are different. The dominant biologic half-life of human proinsulin amounted to 1.54 h, and the metabolic clearance rate to 120 ml/min. Corresponding to the longer half-life and lower clearance rate, the blood glucose-lowering effect of human proinsulin lasted longer than that of human insulin. In this sense, human proinsulin could be said to have an its own depot effect. After s.c. injection the duration of the blood glucose-lowering effect of human proinsulin is longer than that of regular human insulin, but shorter than that of a formulation of NPH-modified human insulin.

Some problems concern the dosage of human proinsulin, as human proinsulin is, like human insulin, standardized in the rabbit hypoglycemia test. However, in this test procedure the different pharmacokinetics of human insulin and proinsulin are not considered. Therefore, the potency of 4 IU per mg for human proinsulin – in comparison, human proinsulin has a potency of 28 IU per mg – seems to be a slight underestimate.

Whether human proinsulin inhibits hepatic glucose output more than human insulin or not is under discussion. Indeed, a pronounced inhibition of hepatic glucose output could be of interest in treatment of diabetics. The results of several groups working on this field and clinical studies with human proinsulin in comparison to human insulin are equivocal. In treatment with insulin delivery devices human proinsulin could have advantages over insulin if it is used for substitution

---

* Die Firma Lilly, die bisher Human-Proinsulin für klinische Studien zur Verfügung stellte, hat zwischenzeitlich weltweit alle klinischen Untersuchungen mit Proinsulin vorerst abgebrochen, da in einer von 5 Langzeitprüfungen in der mit Proinsulin behandelten Gruppe eine höhere Herzinfarktinzidenz als in der mit Insulin behandelten Vergleichsgruppe auftrat.

of the basal rate as, if the pump stops during the night, the longer half-life of human proinsulin will delay the glucose increase until the next morning.

(In the meantime, because of a suspected higher incidence of myocardial infarction in diabetics treated with human proinsulin, all clinical studies with human proinsulin have been interrupted).

Rezeptoraffinität und Wirkung

Die gentechnologisch gegebene Möglichkeit, Human-Proinsulin in ausreichender Menge herzustellen [8], legte nahe, Proinsulin hinsichtlich seiner Verwendbarkeit in der Diabetesbehandlung zu überprüfen und zu fragen, ob eine Proinsulinbehandlung evtl. Vorteile gegenüber einer Insulinbehandlung bieten könne. Bindungsstudien ergaben zunächst, daß Proinsulin hundertfach geringer an Monozyten bindet als Insulin [26]. In vitro-Untersuchungen an isolierten Adipozyten und Hepatozyten zeigten sodann, daß Proinsulin auf molarer Basis wesentlich schwächer wirksam ist als Insulin. An isolierten Fettzellen der Ratte wurde ebenfalls eine Rezeptorbindung von Proinsulin von nur 1% im Vergleich zu Insulin festgestellt. Entsprechend betrug der biologische Effekt, gemessen an der Lipogenese, ebenfalls nur 1% [24]. Andere Untersuchergruppen fanden dagegen bei ähnlichen Untersuchungen 3% [6] und 10 bzw. 11% Rezeptorbindung bzw. biologische Aktivität [25].

Proinsulin bindet langsamer als Insulin an den Rezeptor, dissoziiert aber genauso rasch wie Insulin. Ist der Rezeptor mit Insulin oder nach Zusatz der ca. hundertfachen Menge Proinsulin in gleichem Maße abgesättigt, besteht im Ausmaß der Rezeptor nachgeschalteten intrazellulären Wirkungen zwischen beiden Substanzen kein Unterschied. Ebenso klingt die bologische Wirkung mit gleicher Geschwindigkeit ab, wenn Insulin oder Proinsulin vom Rezeptor abgelöst werden.

Diese Gesetzmäßigkeiten gelten für den Adipozyten, der stellvertretend für das periphere Gewebe bzw. für die Glukoseaufnahme steht. Ähnlich sind die Verhältnisse am isoliertem Hepatozyten. Zur Stimulation der Glykolyse und zur Induktion der Schlüsselenzyme Glukokinase und Pyruvatkinase wurde ebenfalls die hundertfache Proinsulinmenge auf molarer Basis benötigt [27], ein Befund, der mit früheren Untersuchungsergebnissen über eine hundertfach geringere Bindung von Proinsulin im Vergleich zu Insulin an isolierten Leberzell-Plasmamembranen übereinstimmt [9, 10).

Weitere Untersuchungen zur Ketogenese, Glukoneogenese und Glykogensynthese durch Insulin und Proinsulin an kultivierten Leberzellen der Ratte zeigten, daß Proinsulin in 10–30facher Konzentration gleichermaßen wirksam ist wie Insulin [19]. Wieder andere Untersuchungen, die ebenfalls an isolierten Rattenhepatozyten mit Insulin und Proinsulin durchgeführt wurden, ergaben ein Verhältnis von 1:30 bis 1:50 für eine halbmaximale Hemmung der Glykogenolyse bzw. Abnahme der Glykogenphosphorylase [14]. Sie bestätigten vorhergehende, an der isolierten perfundierten Rattenleber und an der eviszerierten Ratte gewonnene Ergebnisse über eine bevorzugte Hemmung der Glukosefreisetzung aus der Leber durch Proinsulin nicht [19, 27].

Die an isolierten Zellen gewonnenen Untersuchungsergebnisse lassen sich daher dahingehend zusammenfassen, daß Insulin und Proinsulin den gleichen Rezeptor besetzen, die Rezeptorbindung von Proinsulin wesentlich schwächer als von Insulin ist, jedoch durch entsprechend höhere Proinsulinkonzentrationen kompensiert werden kann und daß die durch Insulin und Proinsulin ausgelösten Postrezeptoreffekte identisch sind.

Übereinstimmend mit den in vitro-Versuchen zeigten auch in vivo-Untersuchungen mittels Glukose-Clamp-Techniken sowohl im Tierversuch als auch an gesunden Probanden oder Diabetikern, daß ca. 15–50fach höhere Proinsulinspiegel auf molarer Basis im Vergleich zu Insulin benötigt werden, um einen bestimmten Blutzuckerspiegel zu erreichen bzw. im Clamp aufrecht zu erhalten. Dies entspricht einer Proinsulinwirkung von ca. 2–7% der Insulinwirkung [3, 12, 13, 22, 23, 29].

Auffällig, besonders interessant und mit den in vitro-Befunden nicht ohne weiteres in Einklang zu bringen sind in vivo gewonnene Untersuchungsergebnisse, die für eine überproportionale Suppression der hepatischen Glukoseproduktion durch Proinsulin sprechen [3, 12, 22, 29, 33]. Analysen von Dosis-Wirkungs-Kurven bei Clamp-Versuchen sprachen dafür, daß Proinsulin 8% der Insulinwirkung in bezug auf die Glukoseverwertung, aber 12% der Insulinwirkung in bezug auf die Glukosefreisetzung aus der Leber besitzt [12, 29]. Umgerechnet würde Proinsulin die Glukosefreisetzung aus der Leber also um 50% stärker hemmen als Insulin [12, 29], ein Effekt, der therapeutisch interessant wäre, wenn man bedenkt, daß z. B. beim Typ II-Diabetes die erhöhten Nüchternblutzuckerwerte durch eine vermehrte endogene Glukoseproduktion bedingt sind [4, 18, 28, 34]. Wie dieser relativ stärkere Effekt von Proinsulin auf die Glukosefreisetzung zustandekommt, ist letztlich nicht geklärt.

Bei den genannten Clamp-Versuchen wurden Insulin und Proinsulin meist über eine Versuchsdauer von 4–8 Stunden in der Regel in stufenweise steigender Dosis infundiert und die Euglykämie durch adjustierte Infusion 20%iger Glukoselösung aufrecht erhalten. Wurden dagegen bei Typ I-Diabetikern über mehr als 18 Std. adjustierte Infusionen von Proinsulin gegeben, um einen spontanen Blutzuckeranstieg zu verhindern, waren Glukoseverwertung und Glukosefreisetzung unter Insulin und Proinsulin nach 18 Std. nicht signifikant different. Glukagon führte bei diesen Versuchen sowohl unter Insulin- als auch Proinsulinsubstitution zu einer gleich starken Glukosefreisetzung [7].

In Abhängigkeit vom Aufbau der Versuchsanordnung scheinen sich also periphere Glukoseverwertung und hepatische Glukosefreisetzung unter Insulin und Proinsulin unterschiedlich zu verhalten. Ob hierfür bei non-steady-state Bedingungen der Versuchsanordnung die unterschiedlichen Halbwertzeiten und Clearance-Raten von Insulin und Proinsulin eine Rolle spielen, wie vermutet wurde [7], sei dahingestellt.

Bei bisher vorliegenden Untersuchungen mit Insulinpumpen wurde der basale Insulinbedarf durch Proinsulin ersetzt [2, 17, 20]. Auch bei s.c. Gabe von Proinsulin im Vergleich zu Normalinsulin und NPH-Insulin bei Typ II-Diabetikern wurde der Effekt in der postabsorptiven Phase, also unter Nüchternbedingungen untersucht [11].

Vorbehandlung mit Proinsulin

Weitere Untersuchungen zur Behandlung von Diabetikern mit Proinsulin befassen sich mehr mit der Frage eines synergistischen oder additiven Effektes von Proinsulin auf die Insulinwirkung bzw. den Effekt einer Vorbehandlung mit Proinsulin auf den Effekt einer nachfolgenden Insulingabe [2, 13, 16, 20, 29, 30]. Sie sprechen eher für einen additiven, denn für einen synergistischen Effekt von Insulin und Proinsulin.

Dosierung von Proinsulin

Der Einsatz von Proinsulin in der Diabetesbehandlung und die Frage nach der blutzuckersenkenden Potenz von Proinsulin wirft die Frage nach der Dosierung von Proinsulin auf.

Bei den genannten in vitro-Versuchen an isolierten Adipozyten und Hepatozyten wird die Rezeptorbindung und die biologische Effektivität von Insulin und Proinsulin auf molarer Basis verglichen. Bei der Insulinbehandlung des Diabeti-

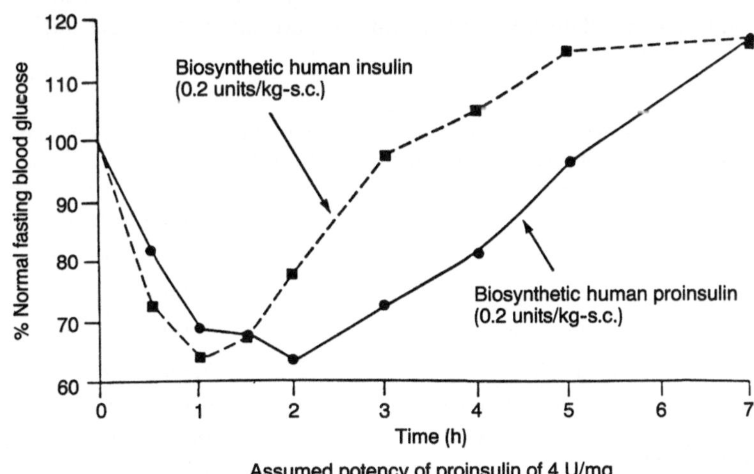

Abb. 1. Standardisierung des blutzuckersenkenden Effektes von Human-Insulin und Human-Proinsulin in biologischen Einheiten im Kaninchen-Hypoglykämietest (nach Angaben des Herstellers)

kers wird Insulin jedoch – historisch bedingt – in biologisch ermittelten Einheiten dosiert. In die Definition der Einheit geht aber lediglich der Nadir des Blutzuckerabfalles im Kaninchenhypoglykämietest ein (Abb. 1).

Andere Faktoren, so der Zeitpunkt, zu dem der Nadir erreicht wird, oder die Fläche unter der Kurve (in diesem Falle über der Kurve) des Blutzuckerabfalles bleiben unberücksichtigt. Auf dieser Basis ergibt sich eine biologische Potenz von 28 E/mg für Human-Insulin und 4 E/mg für Human-Proinsulin (Angabe der Herstellerfirma). Wird auf dieser Einheitenbasis Insulin mit Proinsulin verglichen, ist es nicht verwunderlich, daß z. B. bei der Behandlung mit Insulinpumpen Proinsulin als Basalinsulin stärker blutzuckersenkend wirkt als Insulin [17].

Der Versuch, Insulin und Proinsulin miteinander zu vergleichen, zeigt, wie mißlich im Grunde unsere biologische Standardisierung von Insulin ist, bei der ein Parameter eines biologischen Effektes von vielen biologischen Effekten herausgegriffen wird, um an einer Spezies (dem Kaninchen) Substanzen von anderen Spezies (nämlich Insulin vom Rind, vom Schwein oder vom Menschen) zu vergleichen und zu standardisieren und um dann die derart standardisierten Substanzen wiederum bei einer weiteren Spezies (bei Rinder- oder Schweineinsulin) oder bei der gleichen Spezies (bei Humaninsulin) anzuwenden. Würde man bei der Standardisierung von Proinsulin nicht den Nadir des Blutzuckerabfalles, sondern das Gesamtausmaß der Blutzuckersenkung als Maß der Effektivität zugrunde legen, käme man nicht auf einen Umrechnungsfaktor von 4 E/mg, sondern auf 5.7 E/mg [31] oder 5.84 E/mg [5].

Aber auch ein Parameter wie eine Fläche unter einer Kurve als Maß einer biologischen Aktivität würde nur ein numerisches Maß darstellen. Denn es berücksichtigt nicht den zeitlich-dynamischen Ablauf einer Wirkung. Klinisch relevante Vergleiche sind daher nur bei Betrachtung von Wirkprofilen möglich. Dies gilt nicht nur für den Vergleich von Insulin mit Proinsulin, sondern auch für den Vergleich von unmodifizierten Insulinen mit durch Depothilfsstoffe modifizierten Insulinen, bei denen Pharmakokinetik und davon abhängig auch Pharmakody-

Tabelle 1. Pharmakokinetische Daten von Human-Proinsulin nach intravenöser Applikation (N = 7) bei Annahme eines Dreikompartiment-Systems

α-Phase	0,053 ± 0,004 Std.
β-Phase	0,257 ± 0,087 Std.
γ-Phase	1,540 ± 0,100 Std.
totale Eliminationskonstante	2,270 ± 0,250 Std.$^{-1}$
zentrales Verteilungsvolumen	3,370 ± 0,340 l
Verteilungsvolumen im steady-state	9,250 ± 0,570 l
totale Clearance }	120,3 ± 6,760 ml/min. 1,700 ± 1,000 ml/kg/min.
Trapezoidfläche	4,780 ± 0,250
Integralfläche	5,660 ± 0,370

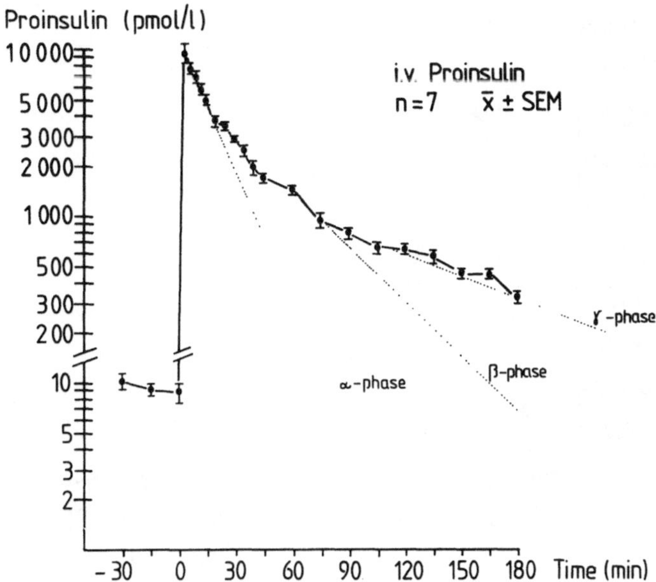

Abb. 2. Pharmakokinetik von Human-Proinsulin nach intravenöser Applikation bei Annahme eines Dreikompartiment-Systems

namik galenisch verändert worden sind. Proinsulin hat im Vergleich zu unmodifiziertem Insulin eine längere Halbwertzeit und eine geringere metabolische Clearance-Rate, wie von vielen Untersuchern, so auch von uns, gezeigt werden konnte [3, 12, 15, 21, 23, 29, 32, 35, 36] (Abb. 2, Tabelle 1).

Depot-Effekte

Vergleicht man das Verhalten der Serumspiegel von unmodifiziertem Human-Insulin, Human-Proinsulin und NPH-Human-Insulin nach s.c. Gabe und den blutzuckersenkenden Effekt dieser Substanzen, gemessen an der Dextroseinfusionsrate bei stoffwechselgesunden Probanden mittels einer speziellen Glukose-Clamp-Technik am BIOSTATOR, erkennt man, daß der Effekt von Proinsulin rasch einsetzt und länger anhält als der Effekt von unmodifiziertem Insulin. Proinsulin hat somit einen substanzeigenen Depot-Effekt. NPH-Insulin wirkt dagegen länger als Proinsulin [5] (Abb. 3).

Daß bei geeigneten Mischungen von unmodifiziertem Insulin und modifizierten Insulinen gleiche Wirkspiegelkurven erreicht werden könnten wie nach subkutaner Proinsulingabe, erscheint durchaus möglich. Der Vorteil einer Proinsulinbehandlung würde sich dann darauf reduzieren, daß ein bestimmter blutzuckersenkender Effekt ohne Depothilfsstoffe zu erreichen wäre.

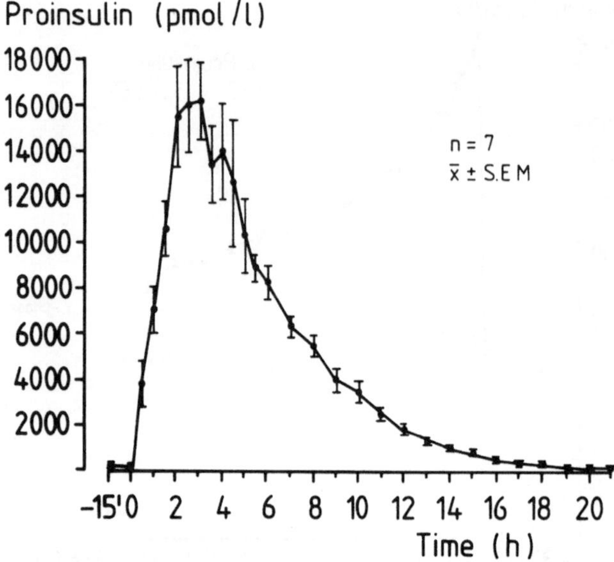

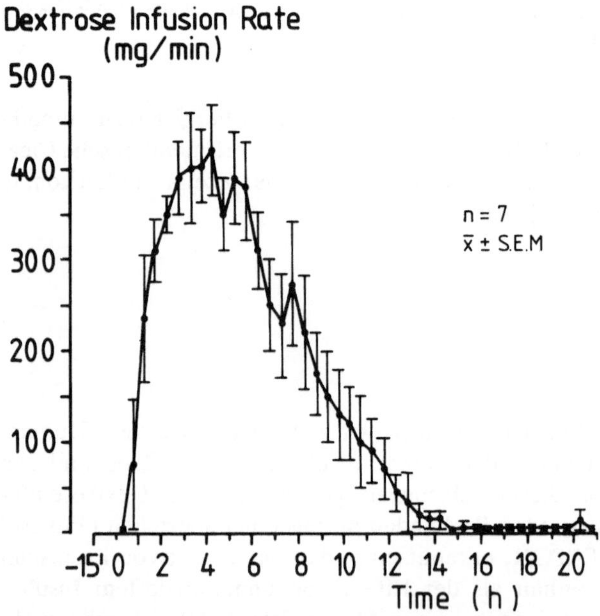

Abb. 3. Pharmakokinetik und Pharmakodynamik von Human-Proinsulin nach subkutaner Gabe im Clamp-Versuch am BIOSTATOR

Ob die beschriebene relativ stärkere Hemmung der Glukoseproduktion nach Proinsulingabe auf einem substanzeigenen Proinsulin-Effekt beruht oder unter non-steady-state Bedingungen nur durch die unterschiedliche Pharmakokinetik von Proinsulin und unmodifiziertem Insulin vorgetäuscht wird [7], müßte durch Untersuchungen von galenisch modifizierten Insulinen, die nach s.c. Gabe ähnliche pharmakokinetische Daten hinsichtlich Invasions- und Eliminationshalbwertzeit sowie mean transit time aufweisen wie Proinsulin, geklärt werden.

Schlußbemerkung

Faßt man zusammen, ergibt sich etwa folgendes Bild:

1. Proinsulin weist andere pharmakokinetische Daten auf als Insulin.
2. Proinsulin bindet an den gleichen Rezeptor wie Insulin. Die Rezeptoraffinität von Proinsulin ist geringer als von Insulin. Auf molarer Basis muß Proinsulin höher dosiert werden, um den gleichen biologischen Effekt zu erreichen. Die Dosierung von Proinsulin in Insulin-bezogenen Einheiten ist unbefriedigend. Sie suggeriert eine Äquivalenz von Proinsulin zu Insulin, die nicht gegeben ist.
3. Ob Proinsulin die hepatische Glukoseabgabe stärker hemmt als Insulin, wird widersprüchlich beurteilt.
4. Wieweit subkutane Proinsulingaben aufgrund des substanzeigenen Depoteffektes von Proinsulin gegenüber subkutaner Gabe galenisch modifizierter Insuline Vorteile bietet, ist nicht geklärt.
5. Bei der Pumpenbehandlung hat Proinsulin aufgrund seiner längeren Halbwertzeit Vorteile, wenn es zur Substitution des Basalbedarfes verwandt wird und die Pumpe zunächst unbemerkt, z.B. über Nacht ausfällt.

Fakten und Fragen stehen einander gegenüber!

Literatur

1. Agius L, Chowdhury MH, Davis SN, Alberti KGMM (1986) Regulation of Ketogenesis, Gluconeogenesis and Glycogen Synthesis by Insulin and Proinsulin in Rat Hepatocyte Monolayer Cultures. Diabetes 35: 1286–1293
2. Bellenberg S, Schröder KE, Schlüter KJ, Bottermann P, Zilker T, Grey P (1988) Clinical Investigation into the Modification of the Effects of Endogenous and Exogenous Insulin by Human Proinsulin in Type II and Type I Diabetics. Horm Metab Res Suppl Ser 18: 77–83
3. Bergenstal RM, Cohen RM, Lever E, Polonsky K, Jaspan J, Blix PM, Revers R, Olefsky JM, Kolterman O, Steiner K, Cherrington A, Frank B, Calloway J, Rubenstein AH (1984) The Metabolic Effects of Biosynthetic Human Proinsulin in Individuals with Type I Diabetes. J Clin Endocrinol Metab 58: 173–979
4. Bogardus C, Lillioja S, Howard BV, Reawen G, Mott D (1984) Relationships between insulin secretion, insulin action, and fasting plasma glucose concentration in nondiabetic and noninsulin-dependent diabetic subjects. J Clin Invest 47: 1238–1246

5. Bottermann P, Wahl K, Ermler R, Gray IP, Hales CN (1988) Action Profile of Biosynthetic Human Proinsulin. Trials with the BIOSTATOR in Metabolically Normal Subjects. Horm Metab Res Suppl Ser 18: 6–11

6. Ciaraldi TP, Bardy D, Olefsky JM (1986) Kinetics of Biosynthetic Human Proinsulin Action in Isolated Rat Adipocytes. Diabetes 35: 318–323

7. Cohen RM, Licinie J, Polonsky KS, Galloway JA, Frank BH, Cherrington AD, Rubenstein AH (1987) The Effect of Biosynthetic Human Proinsulin on the Hepatic Response to Glucagon in Insulin-Deficient Diabetes. J Clin Endocrinol Metab 64: 476–481

8. Frank BH, Pettee JM, Zimmerman RE, Burck PJ (1981) The Production of Human Proinsulin and its Transformation to Human Insulin and C-Peptide. In: Rich DH, Gross E (eds) Peptides: Synthesis-Structure-Function, Proceedings of the 7th American Peptide Symposium, Pierce-Rockford, Ill, pp 729–738

9. Freychet P (1974) The interactions of proinsulin with insulin receptors on the plasma membrane of the Liver. J Clin Invest 54: 1020–1031

10. Freychet P, Roth J, Neville DM (1971) Insulin receptors in the liver: specific binding of ^{125} J-insulin to the plasma membrane and its relation to insulin bioactivity. Proc Natl Acad Sci 68: 1833–1837

11. Glauber HS, Henry RR, Wallace P, Frank BH, Galloway JA, Cohen RM, Olefsky JM (1987) The Effects of Biosynthetic Human Proinsulin on Carbohydrate Metabolism in Non-Insulin-Dependent Diabetes Mellitus. N Engl J Med 316: 443–449

12. Glauber HS, Henry R, Schmeiser L, Wallace P, Koltermann OG, Cohen RM, Rubenstein AH, Galloway JA, Frank BH, Olefsky JM (1986) In Vivo Deactivation of Proinsulin Action on Glucose Disposal and Hepatic Glucose Production in Normal Man. Diabetes 35: 311–317

13. Glauber HS, Wallace P, Galloway J, Frank BH, Olefsky JM (1986) The Effects of Proinsulin Pretreatment on the Combined Actions of Insulin and Proinsulin in Normal Man. J Clin Endocrinol Metab 62: 785–788

14. Hartmann H, Probst I, Jungermann K, Creutzfeldt W (1987) Inhibition of Glycogenolysis and Glycogen Phosphorylase by Insulin and Proinsulin in Rat Hepatocyte Cultures. Diabetes 36: 551–555

15. Henriksen JH, Tronier B, Buelow JB (1987) Kinetics of circulating endogenous insulin, C-peptide, and proinsulin in fasting nondiabetic man. Metabolism 36: 463–468

16. Hübinger A, Randerath W, Toretti P, Schlüter KJ, Gries FA (1988) Effect of a Two Hour Proinsulin Infusion on the Glucose Lowering Potency of a Following Insulin Injection. Horm Metab Res Suppl Ser 18: 34–37

17. Kerner W, Wallmüller G, Beischer W, Pfeiffer EF (1988) Substitution of Basal Delivery of Insulin by Proinsulin in Type I Diabetic Patients under CSII. Horm Metab Res Suppl Ser 18: 74–77

18. Kolterman OG, Gray RS, Griffin J (1981) Receptor and postreceptor defects contribute to the insulin resistance in noninsulin-dependent diabetes mellitus. J Clin Invest 68: 957–969

19. Kramer U, Hartmann H, Creutzfeldt W (1988) Hypoglycemic Effect of Proinsulin and Insulin in Intact and Eviscerated Rats. Horm Metab Res Suppl Ser 18: 56–60

20. Landgraf-Leurs MMC, Hörmann R, Loy A, König A, Kammerer S, Landgraf R (1988) Human Proinsulin. Does it Improve the Treatment of Type I Diabetics? Horm Metab Res Suppl Ser 18: 83–89

21. Laube H, Pinter W, Federlin K (1988) Investigation of the Prolonged Hypoglycemic Effect of Human Proinsulin in Diabetes Mellitus. Horm Metab Res Suppl Ser 18: 12–15

22. Lavelle-Jones M, Scott MH, Kolterman O, Rubenstein AH, Olefsky JM, Moossa AR (1987) Selective suppression of hepatic glucose output by human proinsulin in the dog. Am J Physiol 252 (Endocrinol Metab 15): E 230–E 236

23. Nauck MA, Stöckmann F, Thiery J, Ebert R, Creutzfeld W (1988) Effects of Single and Combined Infusions of Human Biosynthetic Proinsulin and Insulin on Glucose Metabolism and on Plasma Hormone Concentrations in Euglycaemic Clamp Experiments. Horm Metab Res Suppl Ser 18: 60–67

24. Peavy DE, Abram JD, Frank BH, Duckworth WC (1984) In vitro activity of biosynthetic human proinsulin. Receptor Binding and Biologic Potency of Proinsulin and Insulin in Isolated Rat Adipocytes. Diabetes 33: 1062–1067

25. Podlecki DA, Frank BH, Olefsky JM (1984) In vitro characterization of biosynthetic human proinsulin. Diabetes 33: 111–118
26. Prager R, Schernthaner G (1982) Receptor binding properties of human insulin (recombinant DNA) and human proinsulin and their interaction at the receptor site. Diabetes Care [Suppl 2] 5: 104–106
27. Probst I, Hartmann H, Jungermann K, Creutzfeldt W (1985) Insulin - like Action of Proinsulin on Rat Liver Carbohydrate Metabolism in Vitro. Diabetes 34: 415–419
28. Revers RR, Fink R, Griffin J, Olefsky JM, Kolterman OG (1984) Influence of hyperglycemia on insulin's in vivo effects in Type II diabetes. J Clin Invest 73: 664–672
29. Revers RR, Henry L, Schmeiser L, Kolterman O, Cohen R, Bergenstal R, Polonsky K, Jaspan J, Rubenstein A, Frank B, Galloway J, Olefsky JM (1984) The Effects of Biosynthetic Human Proinsulin on Carbohydrate Metabolism. Diabetes 33: 762–770
30. Revers RR, Henry R, Schmeiser L, Kolterman O, Cohen R, Rubenstein A, Frank B, Galloway J, Olefsky JM (1984) Biosynthetic human insulin and proinsulin have additive but not synergistic effects on total body glucose disposal. J Clin Endocrinol Metab 58: 1094–1098
31. Rosak C, Boehm BO, Althoff PH, Schöffling K (1988) Biosynthetic Human Proinsulin, a new Therapeutic Compound for Diabetics? A Comparative Study of Biosynthetic Human Proinsulin with Biosynthetic Human Insulin. Horm Metab Res Suppl Ser 18: 16–21
32. Schatz H, Ammermann S (1988) Human Proinsulin: Bioactivity and Pharmacokinetics after Intravenous and Subcutaneous Administration. Horm Metab Res Suppl Ser 18: 1–5
33. Tompkins CV, Brandenburg D, Jones RH, Sonksen PH (1981) Mechanism of action of insulin and insulin analogues: a comparison of the hepatic and peripheral effects on glucose turnover of insulin, proinsulin, and three insulin analogoues modified at position A1 and B 29. Diabetologia 20: 94–101
34. Ward KW, Beard JC, Halter JB, Pfeifer MAM, Porte Dr (1984) Pathophysiology of insulin secretion in non-insulin-dependent diabetes mellitus. Diabetes Care 7: 491–502
35. Zilker Th, Gray IP, Hales CN, Wahl K, Ermler R, Lebender A, Heinzl G, Bottermann P (1988) Pharmacokinetics of Biosynthetic Human Proinsulin Following Intravenous and Subcutaneous Administration in Metabolically Healthy Volunteers. Horm Metab Res Suppl Ser 18: 37–43
36. Zilker Th, Rebel Ch, Kopp KF, Wahl K, Ermler R, Heinzl G, Hales CN, Bottermann P (1988) Kinetics of Biosynthetic Human Proinsulin in Patients with Terminal Renal Insufficiency. Horm Metab Res Suppl Ser 18: 43–48

Diskussion II (A)

Vorsitz: H. DITSCHUNEIT

G. Schernthaner:

Herr Bottermann, gibt es Erklärungsmöglichkeiten für die höhere Infarktrate unter der Proinsulingabe. Es gibt ja verschiedene Daten, die bisher erstellt wurden mit Bestimmung von Gerinnungsfaktoren, Plättchen, etc., die das eigentlich alles nicht sicher erklären. Gibt es direkte Effekte vielleicht von Proinsulin auf die Endothelzelle, die wir nicht kennen oder wieweit ist hier die Klärung?

P. Bottermann:

Ich kann nur dieses Rundschreiben, welches Sie alle bekommen haben, referieren. Mein Informationsstand geht trotz Nachfrage nicht darüber hinaus. Ich muß das ehrlich sagen, so ein bißchen erinnert mich dies an die Sulfonylharnstoff-Geschichte (UDPG-studies). Es sind wohl verschiedene Gruppen gewesen, und in einer Gruppe hat man eine etwas höhere Herzinfarktrate gesehen, also für mich ist noch keineswegs die Situation so klar. Nun, ein Gesichtspunkt, der immer wieder angesprochen wird, ist folgender: Wenn man sich das Proinsulinmolekül ansieht, und in der Strukturformel der Primärstruktur von IGF und EGF sind ja gewisse Ähnlichkeiten vorhanden, könnte man spekulieren, ob Proinsulin nicht auf diese Weise durch Fibroblastenstimulation stärker atherogen wirken würde als Insulin. Weiter könnte man sagen, wer einen gleichen biologischen Effekt bezüglich der Blutzuckersenkung mit Proinsulin erreichen möchte wie mit Insulin, muß ja wesentlich höher dosieren, vielleicht mag das eine Rolle spielen, aber ich glaube das sind alles Spekulationen.

S. Raptis:

Zum selben Punkt. Wir haben die Fotokopien der Krankengeschichten der Verstorbenen eingesehen. Viele Patienten wiesen ein Übergewicht und eine Hyperlipidämie auf und waren starke Raucher. Es kamen also mehrere Faktoren zusammen. Dies erinnert mich wieder einmal an die typisch amerikanische Hysterie, wie damals mit der UDPG Studie. Ich meine, diese Patienten wären auch ohne Proinsulin gestorben. Ein Patient hatte, glaube ich, Serumtriglyzeride in der Konzentration von 850 mg%.

E. F. Pfeiffer:

Ich finde sehr gut, was Herr Sauer angesprochen hat. Wir haben ja seinerzeit glaube ich zusammen mit der Kombinationsgeschichte angefangen mit dem NPH-Insulin und Zink-Protamin und ich muß sagen, es gibt ja kein wirkliches Basalinsulin und es ist eigentlich nicht richtig, daß die Industrie sich des Ausdrucks bedient hat, den wir mit den Insulininfusionssystemen ins Leben gerufen haben. Wir brauchen ein Basalinsulin, das tatsächlich so etwa eine halbe Einheit pro Stunde freisetzt, das wäre eine gute Basis der Diabetestherapie. Es würde viele Dinge, Infusionssysteme usw. ersetzen, wenn man dieses Insulin hätte. Es wird eine Sicherheit vorgegaukelt, die einfach nicht da ist.

H. Mehnert:

Am schlimmsten ist es natürlich, um diesen Punkt noch vollends auszuführen, mit den überlang wirkenden Insulinen wie mit dem Ultratard, wo angeblich über 24 Stunden eine Basalrate entsteht. Aber eine auch nur annähernd vergleichbare Wirkung wie mit Insulinpumpen können sie nicht bringen.

H. Sauer:

Ich kann nur nochmals bestätigen, was Herr Mehnert sagt. Vor allen Dingen beim Ultratard ist ja auch gegenüber dem Ultralente nachgewiesen, daß das sehr wohl ein Wirkungsmaximum hat, so daß von einer gleichbleibenden konstanten Wirkung über 24 Stunden nicht die Rede sein kann und wenn man Schwierigkeiten hat mit höherer Dosis, dies wird auch so empfohlen, ist man gezwungen, die Dosis aufzuteilen.

K. Federlin:

Ich wollte Herrn Bottermann noch etwas fragen, ich muß gestehen, ich weiß nicht, ob Sie es angeschnitten hatten. Hat man jemals daran gedacht, daß beim Proinsulin der Körper vielleicht ein Toleranzproblem bekäme im Hinblick auf die Immunologie. Der Organismus ist an sich sehr empfindlich, gegenüber bestimmten Stoffen reagiert er aber nicht, denken wir an das Thyreoglobulin. Wenn es ganz niedrig bleibt, gibt es keine Antikörper, steigt der Spiegel, dann ist die Toleranz durchbrochen und es gibt Antikörper und nun könnte bei solchen therapeutischen Versuchen auf die Dauer gesehen natürlich der Proinsulinspiegel Mengen erreichen, die ein ähnliches Phänomen dann zur Folge hätte. Weiß man hierüber etwas?

P. Bottermann:

Man hat darüber nachgedacht. Irgendwelche Daten hierzu habe ich in der Literatur aber nicht gefunden.

H. Ditschuneit:

Eine Frage an Herrn Schöffling, die häufige Verwendung von oralen Antidiabetika in der DDR betreffend. Ist das wirklich real? Wir wissen ja, daß auch unsere Patienten die Medikamente nicht einnehmen. Die holen die doch wahrscheinlich ab und nehmen sie gar nicht ein, ist das nicht so?

K. Schöffling:

Da wird sich also die staatliche Verteilungsstelle der DDR doch von unserer
Apotheke kaum unterscheiden. Umsatzzahlen zu oralen Antidiabetika muß man
ganz mühsam beschaffen. Die Tabelle von 1976 über den Umsatz von Therapeu-
tika auf dem Diabetessektor, das war die mühsamste Tabelle meines Lebens, bis
ich diese Zahlen zusammen hatte.

Use of Computer Systems in Treatment of Insulin-Dependent Diabetics

J. Beyer and J. Schrezenmeir

Zusammenfassung

Der Gebrauch von Computern hat neue Diagnose- und Therapiemöglichkeiten eröffnet. Computer ermöglichen sowohl eine ausführliche Datenerfassung und -registrierung, als auch eine umfangreiche Auswertung der gespeicherten Daten. Die unterschiedlichsten Darstellungsarten sind möglich. Zusätzlich ist es möglich, die Therapie mit Hilfe von selbsterstellten Programmen noch feiner zu regulieren und die Therapie noch effektiver zu handhaben als mit nicht-elektronischer Therapieanleitung. Dies ist deutlich bewiesen in Fällen von schlecht oder mittelmäßig eingestelltem Diabetes. Bei sehr gut und gut geschulten Diabetikern wird die Überlegenheit der Computertherapieführung ebenfalls ersichtlich. Hier kann sich dieses nicht in noch weiterer Verbesserung der Diabeteseinstellung ausdrücken ohne Risiken in Kauf zu nehmen. Hier zeigt die Reduktion der Frequenz von Hypoglykämien, daß die Stoffwechseleinstellung schon vorher gut eingestellter Diabetiker weiter verbessert werden kann durch eine Computeranwendung. Zusätzlich scheint der Computer weitere positive Auswirkungen auf das Lernverhalten der Diabetiker zu haben.

Introduction

Computer diagnosis now attains a precision of between 60%–80% for particular diseases, e.g., thyroid diseases. It is therefore to be expected that computer systems will also become established in various fields of highly specialized therapy. Their application will depend to varying extents on the particular problem under consideration and the nature of the disease. It is to be anticipated that diagnostic decisions may be made more simply and with lower risk with the assistance of computers and that they will be capable of making therapeutic decisions.

In general terms, diabetes therapy aims to enable individual patients to control their metabolic disorders by training and self-management. This presupposes that the diabetic is motivated to such an extent that he or she consistently carries out daily therapy without feeling that this is a punishment or a burden. Various media are available to convey these abilities. Depending on the nature of the knowledge or abilities to be conveyed, cognitive and emotional abilities or manual dexterity may be promoted in various ways. The greatest influence with regard to achieving the desired objective is exerted by the person acting as therapist, physician or diabetes advisor, or by group experience with fellow diabetics in the context of a self-help group. The "human" medium is able to address the emotional characteristics of the patients most intensively and can also impart cognitive abilities and manual skills. Instructional media such as films primarily address the emotional side. Cognitive knowledge is primarily imparted by means of computers, although their effects on emotional processes and on action are less.

The development of dry chemical methods for determination of blood sugar led to a more subtle therapy of diabetes. Diabetics were enabled permanently to control their own metabolic state at short intervals. The development of new strategies for therapeutic self-management (conventional insulin therapy, intensified insulin therapy, intensified meal-related insulin therapy, therapy with insulin pumps) which brought us nearer to the therapeutic objective of blood sugar compensation near to normal resulted as a consequence of this. These technical developments gave rise to the use of computers in therapy of diabetes. The prerequisites, possibilities, advantages, and possible risks of the latter development will be discussed in the present paper.

Use of Computer to Impart Knowledge About Diabetes

Computer systems have been used for years as training instruments for imparting specific information, as a rule in question and answer games. Their use is confined to imparting of additional knowledge to supplement a course of training.

Use of Computers as a Diary and as a Data Store

Keeping a diabetes diary is a precondition for meticulous diabetes therapy and guidance. By means of suitable minicalculators (pocket calculator, electronic logbook), it is becoming possible to collect, store, and process data which usually arise in great quantities and which become confusing when exclusively documented manually. The analysis and processing as well as documentation of this electronically gathered data is carried out by means of personal computers or similar systems with large storage capacities and possibilities of evaluation. In parallel with the amount of data obtained daily, the quality of the metabolic control by the diabetic patient is improved. Important items of information are the blood sugar level, the times it was measured, and its dependence on meals and injected insulin or other events of the day (sport, hypoglycemia, etc.). Also of importance is documentation of the amount and time of urinary sugar excretion, ketone bodies in the urine, amount and time of food intake, time and amount of insulin preparations administered, their activity profiles, time, extent and intensity of physical activity, the patient's weight, dietary errors, and a number of other factors. This means that a large amount of data must be noted and processed per day. Not all the factors listed have the same relevance for current therapy. It will thus be necessary to consider which of the recorded values (e.g., the level of blood sugar) is of current significance for therapy and which are more important for long-term decisions (body weight, etc.). When using such a documentation system, data which cannot readily be overviewed are produced on average every 4–12-weeks. It is understandable that such an amount of (in some cases mutually dependent) data cannot be assessed adequately during a medical ward round. Of necessity, a high proportion of the information must be neglected. This means that data processing must be by means of personal computers which collect and sort the profusion of data so that it can be rationally interpreted. This development is helped by the miniaturization of blood sugar measurement instruments and storage of data in units (Pepita, Glucofact^S, Camit in connection with Reflolux, Diva, etc.) which may be connected up to them. Depending on the configuration of the hardware and software, both individual values and data from a whole day can be selected on the monitor or printed out via printers. In this way, it is possible for the patient and doctor to leaf retrospectively through, as in a notebook, and to appraise values and correlations critically. Since larger-scale overviews cannot be represented and relationships cannot be analyzed with the mostly small monitors of these instruments, only connection to a personal computer can enables the desired analysis.

Systematic Evaluation

Electronic storage and data processing by mainframe and personal computers enable a systematic analysis and repeated access to the data as different questions are asked. Thus, representations of different use-adapted presentations can be selected. They enable the user to make a problem-oriented analysis, and results can be displayed on the monitor or printed out as a report or a graph.

The procedure introduced by Rodbard et al. 1984 has already led to programs for doctors' offices. A number of analysis programs are commercially available, corresponding to the Camit S from Boehringer Mannheim, Glucofacts from Bayer Diagnostics, and Homer from Diva.

If a randomly chosen follow-up period for a diabetic is considered with superimposed blood sugar levels from a long period arranged according to the time of day, the individual values at a particular time of day show the approximate range of variation. Trends are only indicated when the higher postprandial blood sugar values and lower preprandial blood sugar values are examined (Fig. 1).

Additional information can be provided by, for example, filtering out individual days. This allows more precise catogorization and corrections (Fig. 2), for instance

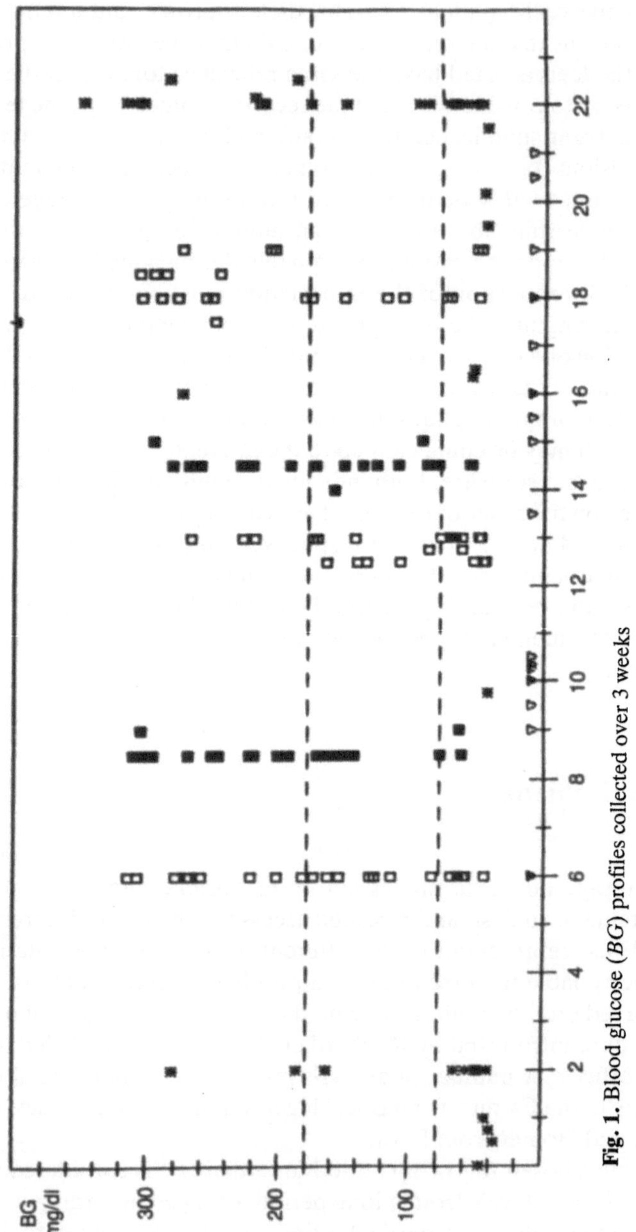

Fig. 1. Blood glucose (*BG*) profiles collected over 3 weeks

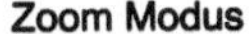

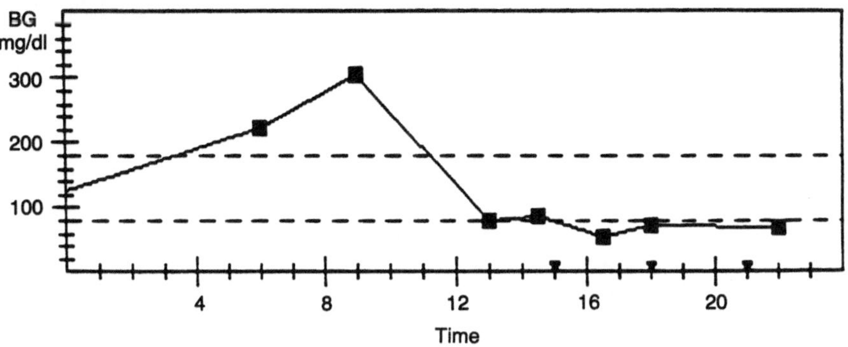

Mon 31.08.87

Time	Gluc	Ins	Event
6:00	222	12/5	12
9:00	306	0/0	20
13:00	80	4/5	12
14:30	87	0/0	20
15:00		0/0	1
16:30	54	0/0	91

Fig. 2. Blood glucose profile of a selected day

by selecting and graphically representing blood sugar curves of individual days and addition of such individual days to show systematic errors in the diurnal profile.

Weekly displays of mean values subdivided in to the individual days of the week are possible (Fig. 3). They allow analysis of problems at the weekends and during the week. Furthermore, it is possible to check therapy by displaying the mean blood sugar values, for example before and after breakfast, other before and after lunch, and after other meals. Exact knowledge, exact comparisons of the amounts of carbohydrates ingested are necessary for any further analysis (Fig. 4).

A system such as this consists of a peripheral storage unit and a central personal computer for the analysis. It provides information about the metabolic state in the past days and weeks and allows conclusions to be drawn from the results which can then be used prospectively for further therapy. This is a major advantage compared earlier to equipment, the disadvantage being that patients only alter their therapy via the roundabout route of notes their subsequent analysis.

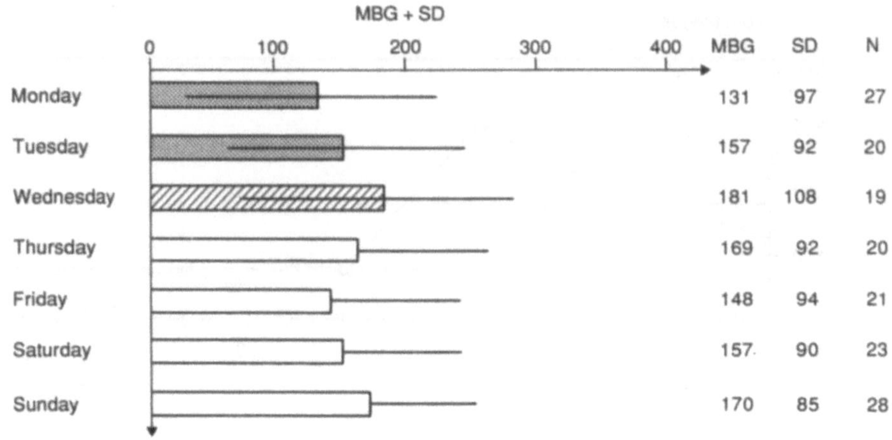

Fig. 3. Mean daily blood glucose values of one selected week

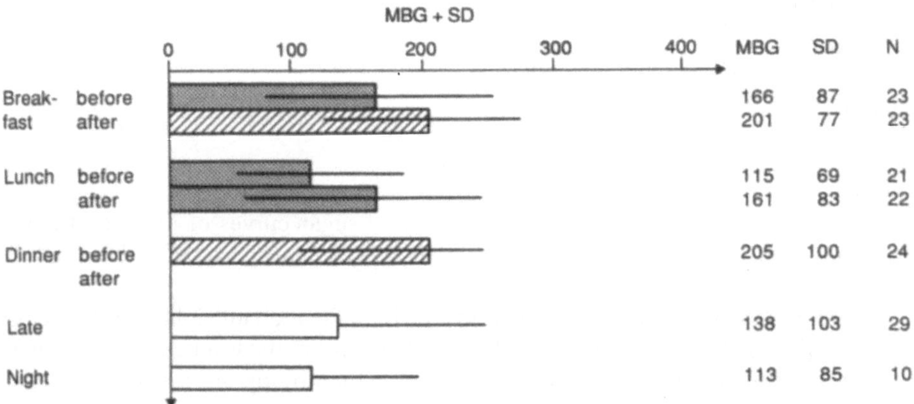

Fig. 4. Mean meal-dependent daily blood glucose determinations over a period of 29 days

Use of Portable Expert Systems

A futher major development in direct analysis of measurements and other data is expert systems in the form of pocket calculators which not only allow data analysis but also contains the algorithms to determine further therapy. The patient enters his or her blood sugar levels, food intake, planned sport activities, etc., into the pocket calculator containing the medical therapy algorithms. In addition, certain data relevant to therapy are initially entered by the doctor (body weight, daily insulin dose, distribution of the insulin doses over the day, maximum insulin doses, amount and distribution of carbohydrates, etc.). The calculator processes the entered information and supplies the patients with precise instructions on the dose of insulin and the amount of carbohydrate to be eaten, as well as warnings and other information.

In recent years, we as others have successfully developed and evaluated rules and algorithms for conventional insulin therapy (Beyer et al. 1981; Albisser et al. 1985; Schulz et al. 1985a; Strack et al. 1985a) meal-related intensified insulin therapy (Schrezenmeir et al. 1985a), and pump therapy (Schrezenmeir et al. 1985c; 1987; Selam et al. 1985; Strack et al. 1985a).

Diabetes Therapy Using a Portable Expert System. It has been shown by means of a simple control matrix that computer algorithms function in conventional insulin therapy with variable injection of rapidly and slowly acting insulin in the morning and evening with a fixed food intake (Albisser et al. 1985; Mihic et al. 1988; Schiffrin et al. 1985). Depending on the preprandial blood sugar level, supplementary doses of regular insulin and delayed-released insulin are recommended by the computer. Such a simple regulatory matrix has already led to prompt recompensation within a few days in inpatients (Fig. 5) (Schulz et al. 1984a, b+c; 1985a, b+c; Strack et al. 1985a)

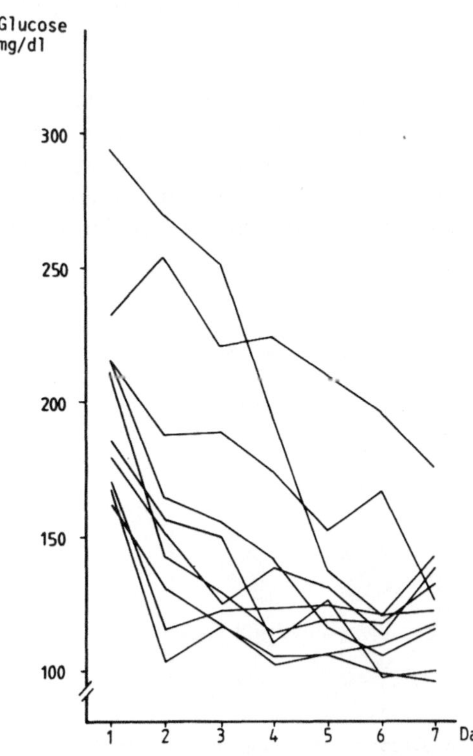

Fig. 5. Changes of blood glucose levels ($n = 10$) following computer assisted conventional insulin therapy (Schulz et al. 1985a)

Diabetes Therapy Using a Pocket Calculator Sized. The advantages of computer-guided therapy involve meal-related intensified insulin therapy. Conventional insulin therapy comprises a standardized diet plan with fixed amounts of carbohydrates allocated to the individual meals and only two or three injections of insulin per day. With meal-related intensified insulin therapy there is additional freedom in the daily intake of carbohydrates and in, for instance, sport activities the omission of a meal-related injection (three to four injections of insulin per day). With the development of further self-management algorithms using additional reference parameters, it became possible to arrive at more precise and individual diabetes compensation (Schrezenmeir et al. 1985a, b+c, 1987). The implementation of these more advanced algorithms in a pocket calculator also led to a significant improvement of the metabolic compensation in the patients concerned (Fig. 6). Even in patients who had already been familiar with intensified therapy over a long time, computer-guided therapy led to a further improvement of the metabolic state (Beyer et al. 1987). This was also shown by a decrease in the incidence of hypoglycemia (Fig. 7).

Learning Effect with Computer-Guided Therapy

Sustained good compensation of diabetes even without the computer suggested that learning effects also play a role. These learning effects were found with standardized questionnaires on knowledge about diabetes which were selected randomly from a large number of questions relating to diabetes. The number of questions answered correctly rose during the computer therapy and only leveled

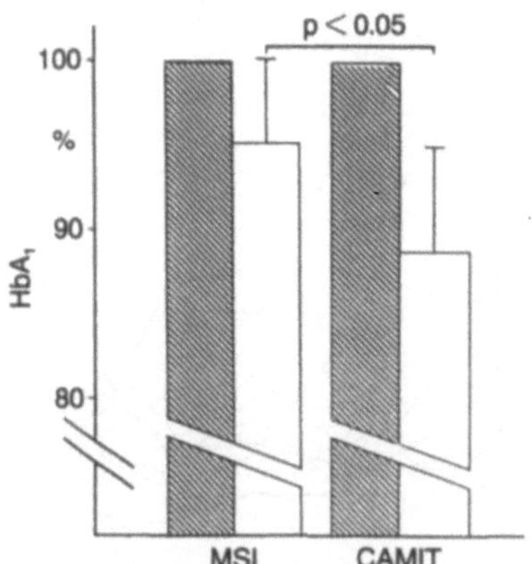

Fig. 6. Decrease of hemoglobin A₁ (*HbA₁*) after 3 months' treatment with multiple meal-dependent insulin injections (*MSI*) without and with computer assistance (*CAMIT*) ($n = 12$)
▨ before treatment, hatched bars = 100%
☐ after 3 months' treatment, open bars

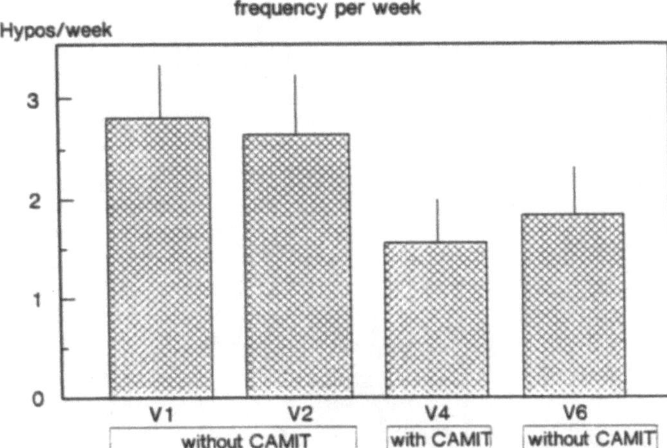

Fig. 7. Frequency of hypoglycaemias per week without and with computer-assisted meal-dependent insulin therapy (*CAMIT*)
V 1: Two weeks control phase with intensified (multiple) insulin injection therapy before additional teaching
V 2: Two weeks control phase with intensified (multiple) insulin injection therapy following an eight weeks intensive teaching in the therapy algosystems of the computers
V 4: Two weeks therapy phase at the end of the eight weeks phase of computers assisted insulin therapy
V 6: Two weeks control phase followed six weeks without computer assistance with the same therapeutic regime as before

off after the computer was taken away. It must thus be assumed that patients continue to deepen their knowledge of diabetes even when using the computer.

Role of the Computer in Treatment of Insulin-Dependent Diabetics

The computer can be used at two different levels in treatment of insulin-dependent diabetics.

The first level involves the patient having an expert system in pocket computer format linked to a glucose meter. Via a daily self-check of blood sugar and food intake, the patient interacts with his or her computer, in which the corresponding therapy algorithms are implemented. In this way, the patient obtains an immediate and direct reaction to alterations of his or her blood sugar and can directly enter the desired diet variations, which are in turn reflected in the answer about insulin dose. A feedback system thus results via the direct contact between the patient and the blood sugar measurement unit/pocket computer expert system which

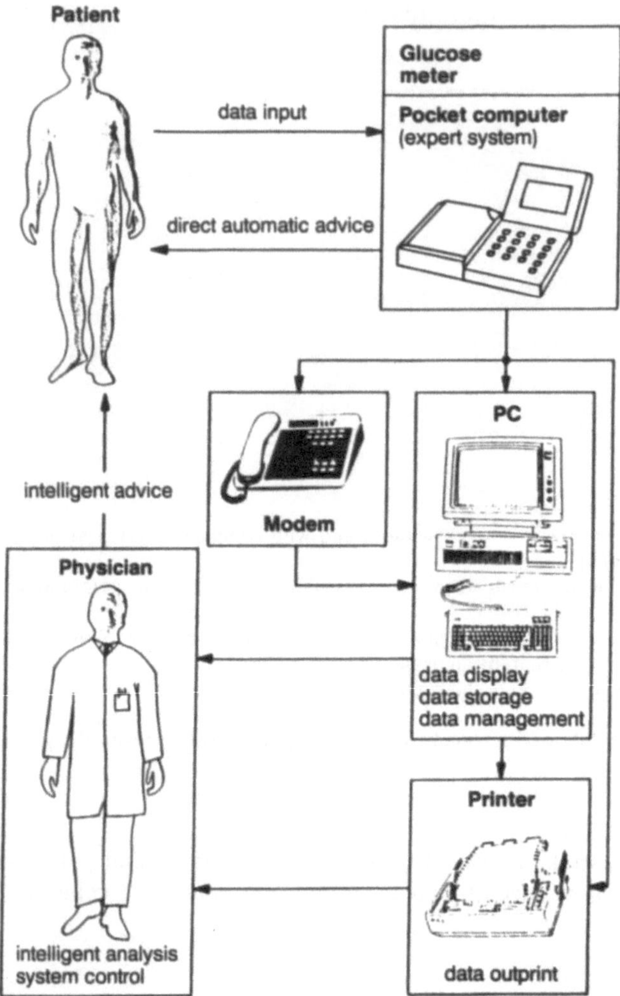

Fig. 8. Interactions between patient, glucosemeter and pocket size computer expert system, data management system (PC), physician and the patient

recommends the insulin dose required for a particular blood sugar level and food intake.

A storage unit in the expert system of the pocket calculator allows direct printout or transmission of all data to a central computer via the physician or a telephone modem system. This is the second level at which computers may be involved, and enalbes individual data collection and analysis and a selective display of certain critical times. This selective analysis by the doctor enables easier correction of insulin dosage by the patient because of the better overview and more rapid access to the multiplicity of data (Schrezenmeir, Beyer 1988). This in turn improves the quality of diabetes therapy (Fig. 8).

Advantages and Disadvantages of Computer Systems

The advantages and disadvantages of computer systems must be considered separately for the different types of system. The advantages of data storage devices (e.g. Diva, Homer, Glucocheck, etc.) are the simplicity of data recording and the systematic processing and interpretation of data with a personal computer. It is possible to discover and to correct systematic errors. In addition, there is a possible additional learning effect for the diabetic. Two major points must be mentioned as disadvantages. It is difficult for patients to retain an overview of their results over several days, and they lack direct instructions for immediate correction of the metabolic state.

Use of insulin dose computers provides patients with exact instructions about the correct therapeutic response to a particular blood sugar level and carbohydrate intake. This may motivate diabetics to measure blood sugar more frequently or regularly. As a consequence of the simplification, the situation may arise that a larger number of diabetics regularly carry out self-checks and determine themselves the insulin dose. By implementation of selfregulating algorithms, the instrument itself can adapt to the patient. Alarm algorithms recognize possibly wrong responses and can point these out. All the other possibilities for complete documentation, automatic evaluation, and data transmission that are found in the pure storage instruments are also available here.

References

Albisser AM, Mihic M, Leibel BS, Schulz M, Sperlich M (1985) Microprocessor aided self management of insulin dependent diabtes: a comparative computer study. In: Beyer J, Albisser M, Schrezenmeir J, Lehmann L (eds) Computer systems for insulin adjustment in diabetes mellitus. Panscienta, Hedingen, Switzerland, pp 23–28

Beyer J, Becker G, Schulz G, Gaberle E, Wolf E, Hassinger W, Cordes U (1981) Blutzucker-kontrollierte Insulin-Infusionssysteme zur Schnelleinstellung insulinpflichtiger Diabetiker. Dtsch Med Wochenschr 106: 1644–1649

Beyer J, Schulz G, Schrezenmeir J, Strack T, Achterberg H, Klausmann G, Hohleweg F (1987) Computer assisted insulin therapy. In: Brunetti P, Waldhäusl WK (eds) Advanced models for the therapy of insulin-dependent diabetes. Serono Symposia Publications, vol 37, Raven Press, pp 145–151

Mihic M, Pyper J, Albisser AM (1988) Conventional insulin therapy in private practice: a one year controlled prospective study. Diabetes Nutr Metab 1: 125–130

Rodbard D, Pernick N, Jaffe ML (1984) Diabetes data management program available for microcomputers. Diabetes Care 7: 401–402

Schiffrin A, Mihic M, Leibel BS, Albisser AM (1985) Computer-assisted insulin dosage adjustment. Diabetes Care 8: 545–52

Schrezenmeir J, Beyer J (1988) Computers in diabetes therapy. Int Diabetes Fed Bull 33: 94–99

Schrezenmeir J, Achterberg H, Bergeler J, Küstner E, Stürmer W, Hutten H, Beyer J (1985a) Computer-assisted meal-related insulin therapy (CAMIT). In: Beyer J, Albisser M, Schrezenmeir J, Lehmann L (eds) Computer systems for insulin adjustment in diabetes mellitus. Panscienta, Hedingen, Switzerland, pp 133–144

Schrezenmeir J, Achterberg H, Bergeler J, Küstner E, Stürmer W, Hutten H, Beyer J (1985b) Controlled study on the use of handheld insulin dosage computers enabling conversion to and optimizing of meal-related insulin therapy regimes. Life Support Systems, The journal of the European Society for Artificial Organs. Proceedings XII Annual meeting ESAO Athens, Greece, September 1985, vol 3, Suppl I, pp 561–567

Schrezenmeir J, Achterberg H, Bergeler J, Küstner E, Hutten H, Beyer J (1985c) Computer-assisted meal-related insulin therapy (CAMIT)-new approach to multiple subcutaneous injection (MSI) and continuous subcutaneous insulin infusion (CSII) regimes. Diabetes research and clinical practice. XII congress of the international diabetes federation, 1985a, Suppl I, Abstract 1310, p 503

Schrezenmeir J, Tato F, Tato S, Müller-Haberstock S, Achterberg H, Stürmer W, Hogan M, Beyer J (1987) Algorithms for CSII-quantified approach to basal rate and meal-induced requirements. In: Brunetti P, Waldhäusl WK (eds) Advanced models for the therapy of insulin-dependent diabetes. Serono Symposia Publications, vol 37 Raven Press, pp 191–197

Schulz G, Beyer J, Hohleweg E, Bergeler J, Hutten H (1984a) Optimierte Blutzuckereinstellung durch Anwendung eines Computerprogrammes zur Insulinadaptation bei subcutaner Insulintherapie. 18. Jahrestagung der Deutschen Gesellschaft für biomedizinische Technik Mainz, 13.–14. September 1984

Schulz G, Beyer J, Hohleweg E, Bergeler J, Küstner E, Hutten H (1984b) Die Entwicklung eines Computerprogrammes zur Blutzuckereinstellung auf der Basis der Blutzuckerselbstkontrolle. 19. Jahrestagung der Deutschen Diabetesgesellschaft, 30. 5.–2. 6. 1984 (abstract)

Schulz G, Beyer J, Hohleweg E, Bergeler J, Küstner E, Hutten H (1984c) Intensified subcutaneous insulin therapy using a computerized program for diabetes self adjustment. Third workshop on "Artificial Insulin Delivery Systems Pancreas and Islet Transplantation." February 5–7, 1984, Igls, Austria

Schulz G, Beyer J, Hohleweg E, Küstner E, Bergeler J, Hutten (1985a) Die Rechnergestützte Diabeteseinstellung. Klin Wochenschr 63: 1098–1101

Schulz G, Beyer J, Hohleweg E, Bergeler J, Hutten H (1985b) A computerized program for diabetes self-adjustment and its application in in- und outpatients. In: Beyer J, Albisser M, Schrezenmeir J, Lehmann L (eds) Computer systems for insulin adjustment in diabetes mellitus. Panscienta, Hedingen, Switzerland, pp 111–118

Schulz G, Beyer J, Hohleweg E, Bergeler J, Küstner E, Hutten H (1985c) Die Entwicklung eines Computerprogramms zur Diabeteseinstellung von Typ I-Diabetikern (abstract) 8. Internationales Donausymposium über Diabetes mellitus. 18.–21. 6. 1985, Bratislava

Selam JL, Coste F, Mirouze J, Hartmann K (1985) An individual pocket-, computer aid for pump-treated diabetic patients. In: Beyer J, Albisser M, Schrezenmeir J, Lehmann L (eds) Computer systems for insulin adjustment in diabetes mellitus. Panscienta, Hedingen, Switzerland, pp 145–151

Strack T, Bergeler J, Beyer J, Hutten H (1985a) computer assisted conventional insulin therapy. In: Computer systems for insulin. In: Beyer J, Albisser M, Schrezenmeir J, Lehmenn L (eds) Computer systems for insulin adjustment in diabetes mellitus. Panscienta, Hedingen, Switzerland, pp 119–127

Strack T, Bergeler J, Beyer J, Hutten H (1985b) A microcomputer based programme for CSII. In: Beyer J, Albisser M, Schrezenmeir J, Lehmann L (eds) Computer systems for insulin adjustment in diabetes mellitus, Panscienta, Hedingen, Switzerland, pp 153–159

Artifical β-Cell and Glucose Sensor

E. F. PFEIFFER

Dedication

It is a personal pleasure and privilege to congratulate my old associate and friend, Konrad Federlin, on his 60th birthday. For very many years we were marching in one line towards the final goal: to achieve academic independence for realizing what we had in mind to do in clinical research and, after having obtained that freedom, to fill the empty spaces which obviously lay ahead with fruitful ideas and productive work.

The common denominator which connected us scientifically, first when studying etiology and pathogenesis of kidney disorders, and then in experimental and clinical diabetology, had been the immunological background. Immune processes, which are behind so many human and animal diseases, have contributed more and more over the years to the understanding and to the treatment of a number of apparently far distant ailments. The same was true when jumping from glomerulonephritis to diabetes, first, as far as the antibodies to insulin were concerned, second when islet transplantation was attempted, and third when, surprisingly, the very beginning of special types of human diabetes appeared to be causatively related to antibodies. It was a special pleasure to observe how Konrad, after having obtained the chair in Giessen, and this very well-known and reputed department of medicine, continued the work we had started together, with a very fine group of devoted associates and collaborators.

Today we are honoring him and his beautiful and beloved wife, Geza, and his three now well grown-up children. However, most of all we are honoring friendship and joint dedication to the three big "Ds" of our profession and our lives:

1. Dedication to research,
2. Devotion to the medical profession, and
3. Deeds for the benefit of our trusting patients.

Continue the good work, for the many years we hope still lie ahead!

Zusammenfassung

Bei Säugern besteht ein positiver Rückkoppelungsmechanismus zwischen dem Anstieg der Glukosekonzentration im Blut und erhöhter Insulinfreisetzung, sowie dem Abfall des Blutzuckers und einer Hemmung der Insulinsekretion. Deshalb gewährleistet dieses Regelsystem ausreichende Mengen Insulin für die Nutzung der Kohlenhydrate aus der Nahrung, mit einer feinen Anpassung an die Bedürfnisse des Körpers. Bei allen Formen des Diabetes, dem Typ I und II-Diabetes, arbeitet dieses regulierende System nicht mehr. Konventionelle Insulinsubstitutionstherapie ersetzt nicht diese reziproke Feinabstimmung des Blutzuckers und der Insulinfreisetzung, und folglich ist auch die Nutzung und die Metabolisierung der aufgenommenen Nahrungsmittel nicht mehr optimal gewährleistet. Therapeutische Ausnahmen sind bis jetzt nur die erfolgreiche Transplantation von lebenden Langerhans'schen Inseln, segmentale oder Gesamtpankreasorgantransplantation einerseits, Anschluß des Patienten an ein artifizielles endokrines Pankreas oder die künstliche Betazelle andererseits. Letzteres System besteht immer aus einem Glukosesensor, einem Mikrocomputer und einer Insulininfusionspumpe, welche nach speziell entwickelten Algorithmen kontinuierlich Insulin und angepaßt an aktuelle Blutzuckerschwankungen insbesondere nach der Nahrungsaufnahme zur Verfügung stellt. Eine Kombination statischer und dynamischer Insulininfusionsabgaben ist notwendig, den bi-phasischen Typ der Insulinsekretion zu simulieren, – vorher anhand von Studien am isoliertperfundierten Rattenpankreas nachgewiesen – um den Rückkopplungsmechanismus zwischen Glukosekonzentration und Insulinsekretion wieder herzustellen, der eine Normoglykämie auch in den schwersten Fällen vom IDDM's garantiert.

Der Transfer von erfolgreichen Ergebnissen mit der großen künstlichen am Krankenbett stehenden Beta-zelle auf ein kleineres, tragbares vom Patienten selbst nutzbaren Gerät wurde bis vor kurzem erschwert durch das Fehlen eines implantierbaren Glukosesensors. Nach einigen Experimenten wurde eine amperometrisch-enzymatische Elektrode, die nach einem elektro-chemischen Prinzip arbeitet und eigentlich schon in der großen künstlichen Betazelle arbeitet, als die geeignetste Elektrode gefunden. Deshalb ist sie die am häufigsten verwendete Elektrode bei all den Gruppen, die mit diesen Systemen arbeiten.

Einige Probleme wurden in der Zwischenzeit gelöst. Die Glukosekonzentration im interstitiellen Gewebe, in das die Elektrode subkutan implantiert wird, wurde im Bereich der Plasmaglukosekonzentration gefunden. Man fand ferner heraus, daß das Enzym Glukose-Oxydase über Wochen und Monate hinweg aktiv bleibt. Ein leichter Anstieg und Abfall der Glukose, wie beobachtet nach Insulininjektion oder Glukagon oder Nahrungsaufnahme, wird sofort registriert, und auch die Algorithmen, die zur kontinuierlichen Glukosemessung im Blut und zur i.v. Insulintherapie entwickelt worden waren, sind weiterhin anwendbar, wenn die Glukosekonzentration im subkutanen Gewebe gemessen wird. Die erste klinische Anwendung offenbarte asymptomatische Hypoglykämien bei Typ I-Diabetikern unter intensivierter Insulintherapie. Ebenso traten bis dahin nicht beobachtete Hyperglykämien beeindruckenden Ausmaßes auf, trotz niedrige HbA1 Werte.

Eine verzögerte Normalisierung postprandialer Glukosewerte wurde schon bei nicht-diabetischen normalen und leicht übergewichtigen Probanden beobachtet, auch wenn nach der Nahrungsaufnahme leichte Bewegungsübungen erfolgten. Kontinuierliche Blut- und Gewebeglukosemessungen in einer dynamischen Art und Weise werden in der Zukunft nicht nur eine viel bessere Kontrolle jeglicher therapeutischer Maßnahmen sowohl bei Typ I und Typ II-Diabetes erlauben, sondern auch die Erfassung gestörter metabolischer Funktionen bei Personen, die bis jetzt als metabolisch absolut gesund galten.

Direkte Kombination des entweder subkutan oder intravenös implantierten Sensors mit einem Interface, einem Mikrocomputer, und einer der weiterentwikkelten modernen Insulininfusionspumpen, erlaubt eine Re-Normalisierung des Blutzuckers unter normalen Lebensbedingungen und ermöglicht dem Patienten, Insulin nach Belieben zum Zeitpunkt der Nahrungsaufnahme Bolus-ähnlich anzufordern, wogegen während der Mahlzeiten das System unter seiner eigenen Rückkopplungskontrolle arbeitet. In Intervallen von einigen Tagen werden Einweg-Glukosesensoren implantiert. Innerhalb dieser Zeit sollte die subkutan implantierte Nadel eine kontinuierliche Insulinversorgung und Normoglykämie gewährleisten, solange nicht eine permanente Implantation des gesamten Systems in einer Schrittmacher-ähnlichen Art und Weise zur Verfügung steht. Das wird erst in Zukunft möglich sein, wenn man besser die Abwehrreaktion des Organismus kontrollieren kann, die den Glukosesensor in einer Fremdkörperreaktion gegenwärtig noch neutralisiert.

Introduction

The motivation to develop an artificial β-cell and to assemble, about 15 years ago, the various parts constituting the artificial endocrine pancreas or artificial β-cell system was the realization that there appeared to be no other feasible way to renormalize blood glucose and, by doing so, to cure diabetes and prevent its complications.

In those days, we were deeply influenced by the experiences of continuous blood glucose monitoring or blood glucose sensing using the modified Technicon autoanalyzer and the continuous withdrawal of small amounts of heparinized blood by means of the Ferrari double-lumen catheter. The continuous recording of blood glucose concentrations, combined with frequent insulin determinations, more or less clearly revealed that there exists in the normal individual a complete parallelism between the two parameters (Fig. 1). Of course, in type I diabetes and, to a greater or lesser extent, also in type II diabetes, this parallelism is lost. This is a clear sign that the feedback mechanism works correctly only in nondiabetic subjects. No known strategy of conventional insulin substitution is capable of reestablishing, first, the stimulus effected by the increase of glucose on insulin secretion and, second, the negative feedback inhibiting mechanism which, following the fall in blood sugar stops, further insulin release. Also, intensified insulin

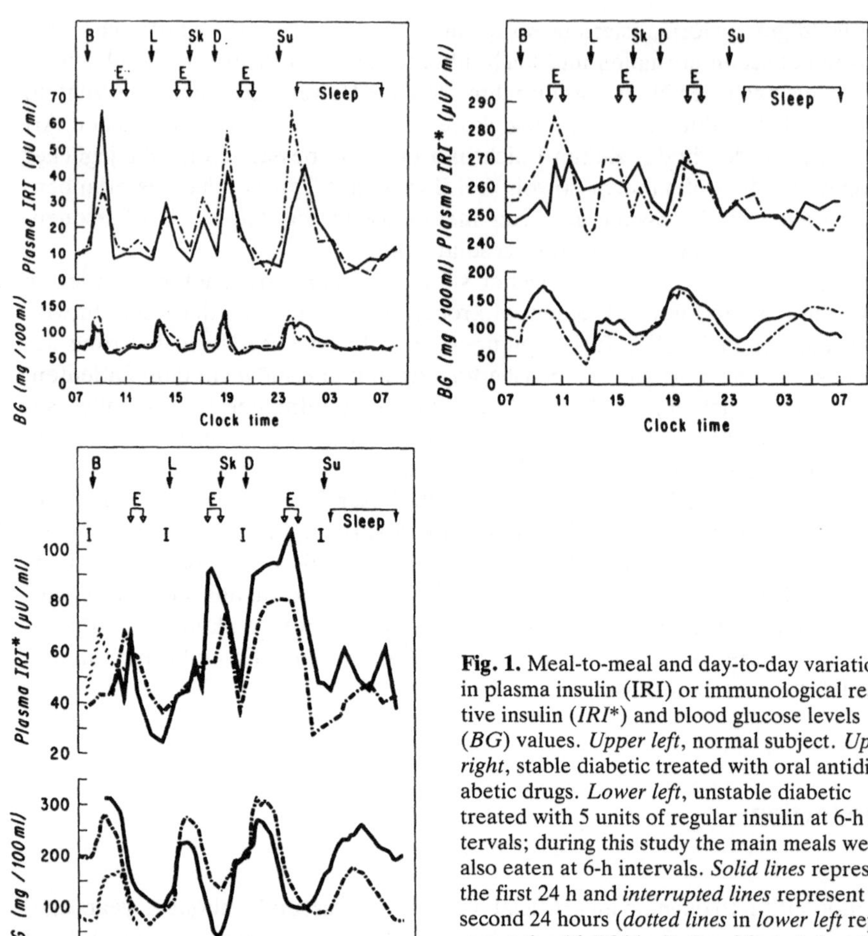

Fig. 1. Meal-to-meal and day-to-day variations in plasma insulin (IRI) or immunological reactive insulin (*IRI**) and blood glucose levels (*BG*) values. *Upper left*, normal subject. *Upper right*, stable diabetic treated with oral antidiabetic drugs. *Lower left*, unstable diabetic treated with 5 units of regular insulin at 6-h intervals; during this study the main meals were also eaten at 6-h intervals. *Solid lines* represent the first 24 h and *interrupted lines* represent the second 24 hours (*dotted lines* in *lower left* represent the third 24 h. *B*, Breakfast; *L*, lunch; *Sk*, snack; *D*, dinner, *Su*, supper; *E*, exercise. (From Molnar et al. 1972)

therapy where preprandial injections of shortacting insulin are given three times per day, does not prevent wide glucose fluctuations. Just at the right time, when the meaning of this hopeless situation became apparent, newly developed computers reached a size where they were of practical value for work in the laboratory. Within a short time, the University of Ulm in collaboration with A.H. Clemens (from Miles-Ames Co., Elkhart, Indiana) developed an artificial endocrine pancreas or artificial β-cell system consisting of a glucose Sensor and Monitor, a micro computer, and an insulin and glucose infusion pump (Fig. 2). This permitted withdrawal of blood for continuous blood glucose measurement and, by means of newly developed algorithms, the continuous infusion of metered amounts of insulin adapted to the changes in blood glucose levels, especially those occurring after food intake (Pfeiffer et al. 1974, a + b, 1977). Independently from 115 at

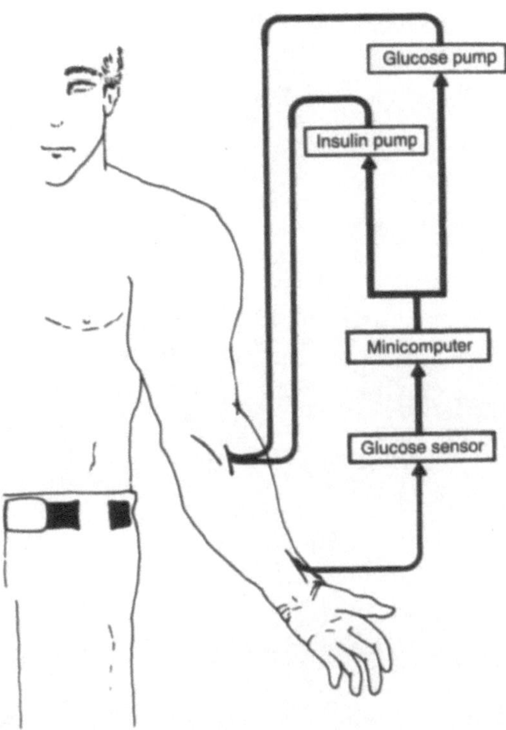

Fig. 2. The basic elements for feedback regulation of blood sugar. (From Pfeiffer 1987)

the same time, in Toronto B.S. Leibel and M. Albisser (Albisser et al. 1974) constructed an artificial endocrine pancreas on the same principles, although it was never given to the public. The three versions of this apparatus, the "Biostator" or glucose-controlled insulin infusion system, a blood glucose controller, and a blood glucose monitor, were built and did permit renormalization of blood glucose through reestablishing a regulatory feedback mechanism between blood sugar and insulin release (Fig. 3). The operational mode which did the trick was a combination of static and dynamic insulin infusion which took care of practically every excursion of blood sugar concentration. The clinical application ranged from diabetic ketoacidosis and coma down to organic hyperinsulinism, since glucose was also easily administered in cases of hypoglycemia (Table 1). Perhaps more important than the clinical applications was the use of the system for clinical research, as illustrated in Table 2. The variation insulin requirement due to circadian rhythms over the 24 h of the full day and night, the practical importance of the dawn phenomenon, the meaning of the self-inhibition of insulin effected by endogenous insulin, the prevention of blood sugar increases after meals by administering insulin at appropriate times before meals, and other problems were successfully attacked.

However, hidden behind all these efforts was the idea of transferring the results from the clinical research laboratory to individual diabetic patients under the conditions of normal life. This progress was not limited by the necessity to somehow miniaturize the artificial endocrine pancreas. The real problem was the

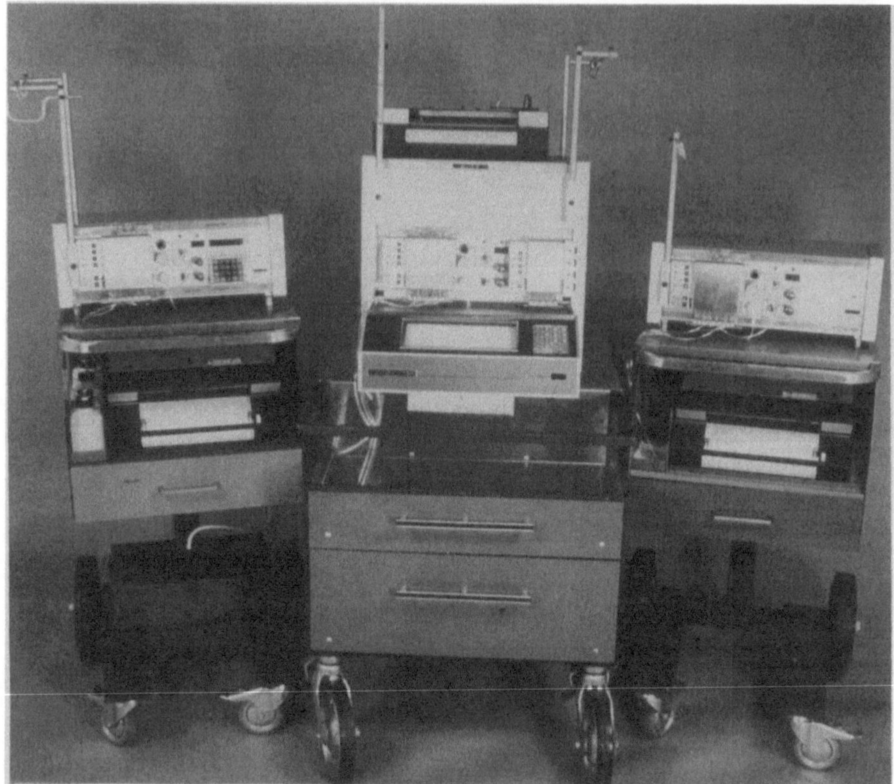

Fig. 3. Our artificial endocrine pancreas (Ulm-Elkhart version) and two simplified versions used as glucose controller and glucose monitor

Table 1. Applications of the artificial pancreas on clinical therapy. (From Pfeiffer 1987)

Diabetic coma
Surgery in diabetic patients
Total pancreatectomy
Delivery (diabetic mothers)
Organic hyperinsulinism
Hemodialysis in diabetic patients
Induction of the remission phase (honeymoon period)
Evaluation of insulin doses for subcutaneous therapy

irreplaceable part of the whole system, the glucose sensor, which in the bedside artificial pancreas existed in a flow-through glucometer, but now had to be transformed into an *implantable*, permanently working glucose sensor. The life-time of the Yellow Springs membrane working as a glucose sensor in the Biostator device was limited to 48–600 h despite continuous selective heparinization of the blood.

Table 2. Some applications of the artificial pancreas in clinical research. (From Pfeiffer 1987)

Blood glucose control applying different insulin infusion kinetics

Portal vs. peripheral insulin infusion

Glucose clamp studies
  Insulin feedback inhibition
  Insulin sensitivity
  Absorption kinetics of subcutaneously injected insulin

Diurnal rhythm of insulin requirement

Hormones, metabolites, lipids, and blood viscosity during short-term blood glucose
  normalization

Effect of drugs on insulin requirement
  Somatostatin and analogues of somatostatin
  Sulfonylureas
  Sugar substitutes
  Fiber diet
  Disaccharidase inhibitors

Table 3. Measures of blood glucose control in feedback-controlled insulin infusion and in pre-programmed insulin infusion. (From Pfeiffer and Kerner 1981)

Parameters of blood glucose control

	Feedback-controlled insulin infusion	Preprogrammed Insulin infusion	p[a]
MBG (mg/100 ml)	99.0 ± 37	113.3 ± 17.0	N. S.
MAGE (mg/100 ml)	47.6 ± 5.9	95.8 ± 10.3	0.001
M-Value	6.8 ± 0.9	30.3 ± 7.1	0.01

[a] Statistical significance calculated from Student's t test for paired data
MBG = mean blood glucose
MAGE = mean amplitude of glycemic excursions

As everybody knows, people did not wish to wait for this step to be taken, but were suggesting that in the meantime the insulin infusion part of the whole apparatus be employed as a "portable insulin infusion pump." Various types of these pumps were used. It was considered clinically of great importance that insulin be administered subcutaneously. However, as everybody also knows, the reestablishment of normoglycemia was just not perfect. Using the M value according to Schlichtkrull as a measure of comparison showed that results were extremely poor (Table 3). Perhaps because of the incomplete renormalization of blood sugar along with this type of intensified insulin therapy, the long-term results of continuous insulin infusion as regards secondary complications, e.g., retinopahy, were not satisfactory. This, however, was only one side of the coin. Hypoglycemic episodes were frequent, and even more frequent when continuous

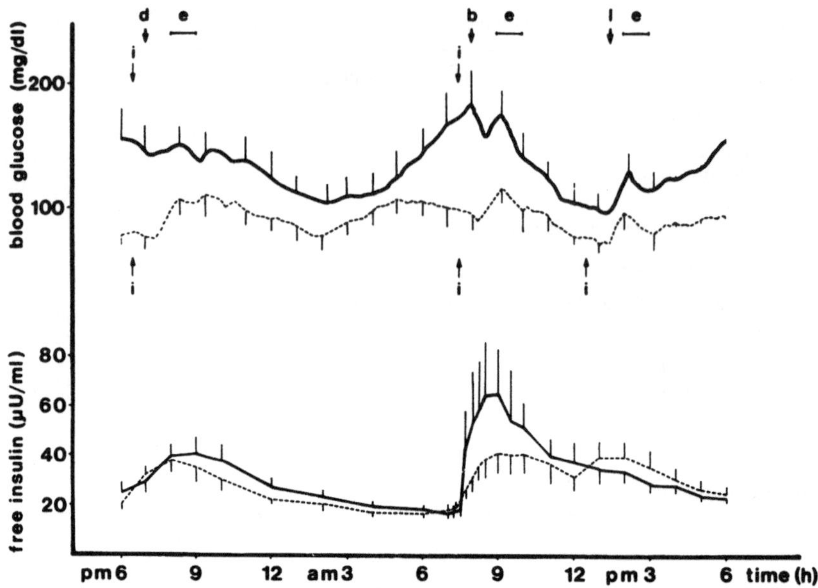

Fig. 4. Blood glucose levels and free insulin levels following continuous subcutaneous insulin infusion (*interrupted line*) and conventional intensified therapy (*continuous line*). (*b* = breakfast, *d* = dinner, *e* = exercise, *l* = lunch) (From Arias et al. 1985)

blood glucose monitoring was by some form of dynamic measurement. At least once per day in 9 out of 10 patients blood sugar levels below 40 mg% were measured (Fig. 4; Arias et al. 1985).

The combination of unsatisfactory results as far as inhibition, not to mention arrest, of progression of diabetic retinopathy was concerned, and the frequent hypoglycemic attacks induced our group to return to the problem of an implantable glucose sensor that could be used to enable glucose-regulated insulin infusions as part of intensified insulin therapy.

The Implantable Glucose Sensor, and The Portable Artificial Endocrine Pancreas

Ideally, a portable glucose sensor should be small, sensitive, implantable, work for an extended period of time, and allow patients to operate it themselves. This already practically excludes the intravenous blood glucose sensors used in the bedside artificial endrocrine pancreas or artificial β-cell which use diluted serum or plasma specimens. The sensor should be implanted in the interstitial tissue, either subcutaneously or intraperitoneally. This means we depend upon measuring the glucose content in the tissue fluid, i.e. the sensing must be done *in situ* not in aspirated fluid as is customary in clinical chemistry. This in turn means we must abandon most of the normal optical or enzymatic methods for blood, plasma, or serum glucose determinations and must rely upon modern bio- or electrochemical sensors using ion-selective electrodes and/or enzymes.

This field opened at the beginnung of this century when it was recognized that chemical reactions also generate an electrical potential. This can be measured by an ion-selective electrode always in comparison with an inert reference electrode that is also in contact with the sample. When an enzyme electrode is used, the enzyme provides the selectivity for the analyte and the chemical reaction. The enzyme, of course, must be continuously reusable. In any case, no blood has to be withdrawn. On the other hand, and this is true for all in vivo biosensors, various requirements must be met, such as stability in the position or biological fluid, reproducibility of the measurements, selectivity (i.e., specificity of the reactions), response of the reaction in the clinically relevant range (i.e., for glucose between 20 and 500 mg%), sufficiently fast response time (i.e., for glucose 1–2 min), relative independence from low oxygen levels (if oxygen levels are low in the tissue site selected for implantation), reasonable size to allow reimplantation, independence from stirring, for enzyme electrodes, reusability of enzymes, and, for long term implantation, good enough biocompatibility (i.e., producing no or little tissue reaction or irritation) to permit access of glucose and oxygen to the reaction site. The electrical energy generated by the chemical reactions with the particular anion can be measured either by potentiometry or by amperometry.

In general, in potentiometric sensors the ion-selective electrode responds to changes in ion activity; the sensing surface acts as a battery, generating a potential in proportion to the analyte concentration, and this is the so-called activity. Ion-selective electrodes are modified into enzyme electrodes by coating them with immobilized enzyme; the electrode then measures the product of the enzyme reaction. Happily, the selective enzymes can be immobilized into polymer such as PVC, so a complete dynamic package with an ion-selective electrode and the enzyme chanelling the chemical reaction can be given to the clinician. This explains the increased interest clinicians have recently taken in this field. The first enzyme electrodes did not appear before 1975. They were designed for urea measurements by Cammann in Ulm and were also used for measuring glucose in diluted blood. This electrode was incorporated into the Ulm version of the artificial endocrine pancreas (Clemens et al. 1977).

The amperometric sensors use an applied electrode potential to drive the reaction and then measure the resulting current. The best known is the Clark membrane electrode for measuring partial oxygen pressure in blood gas analyzers (polarographic sensors). This principle can also be used for determination of glucose. When a negative potential of 600–700 mV is applied to the platinum cathode, oxygen is reduced to peroxide and gluconic acid is produced. It is then possible to measure peroxide, oxygen consumption, or changes in the pH, and/or to use a number of other indicator techniques (Table 4).

In summary, the important parts of the amperometric sensors are the substrate, the immobilized enzyme which converts the substrate to products and reactants, and the detector. In the original work of Clark and Lyons (1962), and Updike and

Table 4. Methods used for continuous extracorporal blood glucose monitoring. (From Pfeiffer 1987)

I. Optical methods

1. Ferricyanide method
2. Enzymatic methods
a) Hexokinase
b) Glucose oxidase
c) Glucose-6-phosphate dehydrogenase

II. Electroenzymatic (electrochemical) methods

1. O_2 measurement
2. H_2O_2 measurement
3. Changes in pH
4. Exchange of electron acceptors (ferricyanide, benzochinon, ferrocene)
5. Enzyme competition (glucosedehydrogenase GDH and glucoseoxidase GOD) for glucose (NAD^+ variable)
6. Immunosensing, fluorine formation, biotin production, etc.

Hicks (1967), a traditional cation-selective glass electrode was coated with enzyme, polymerized acrylamide gel matrix being used for coverage. Now, PVC and polyurethane-based matrices do the job. Since commercial implantable sensors are not yet available, scientists still have to construct their own sensors.

When selecting a glucose sensor for implantation, either potentiometric or amperometric, the choice is similar to the one that had to be made between extracorporal electrochemical or enzymatic glucose electrodes, as happened in our case when we decided to switch from the large bedside artificial endocrine pancreas developed in the early 1970s in Ulm (Pfeiffer et al. 1974, Pfeiffer et al. 1977), to a portable automated artificial endocrine pancreas or a new "glucose-controlled insulin infusion system" (GCIIS). Early we were forced to abandon the Glucose-Oxidase (GOD), Peroxidase- and Hexokinase-based techniques for measuring glucose continuously in heparinized blood and to start with the glucose oxidase amperometric and enzymatic techniques since the time lag between blood aspiration, glucose measurement, and printing of the results amounted to 5–6 min. This was too long for glucose measurements used for algorithmic regulation of insulin administration. The electroenzymatic, electrochemical technique, the amperometric method described above, was doing well. The time lag amounted to not more than 1–1.5 minutes and so the sensor was built into the artificial endocrine pancreas proper. It was also subsequently used by Shichiri et al. (1988) in their attempts to determine glucose in subcutaneous tissue, and by all other people going into that field afterwards such as Abel and Fischer and their associates (Abel et al. 1988).

It can, therefore, easily be understood that after a period of experimentation with the various methods, we returned more or less ruefully to the technique we had already used before, aiming to develop an implantable glucose sensor based on the electroenzymatic, amperometric method. This method uses, as already mentioned, a glucose-sensitive membrane and a polarographic electrode. The sensor developed in our laboratory now consists of a central platinum wire (0.03 mm) surrounded by stainless steel tubing (1.0 mm outer diameter; 30–50 mm length). Using successive dip-coating procedures, layers of cellulose acetate, glucose oxidase (cross-linked with glutaraldehyde), and polyurethane are placed on its surface (Kerner et al. 1987 a, b, c, d; Kerner et al. 1988). The platinum wire is the anode, and is polarized to 700 mV against the steel. The potential of 700 mV between the platinum wire and the steel tubing drives the chemical reaction and peroxide, produced by the glucose oxidase reaction, is measured after oxidation. The measurement is therefore in nanoamperes. The 10–100 nA measured is proportional to the glucose content of the solution. The linear range extends up to 500 mg/dl glucose. Response time (T 90%) is < 100 s. The sensors do not depend on stirring, were insensitive to changes of pH, and also permit glucose measurement up to 42°C. The specificity for glucose (response set as 100% relative current) in comparison with other carbohydrates, i.e., mannose and glactose, is satisfactory. The only substances that interfere are uric acid and ascorbic acid, producing up to 158% and 106% relative current, respectively; impairment of glucose measurement in dissolved oxygen concentration is negligible at oxygen levels > 0.5 mg.

The enzyme is reusable, and even after more than 2 weeks of continuous measurement, rapid increases in the glucose concentration are recorded. Lifetimes of several months have been observed in the various sensors constructed.

After extensive in vitro experimentation, the sensors were placed subcutaneously in rats, sheep, and rabbits. The glucose content in the peripheral blood was continuously monitored with the miniaturized version of the Biostator, i.e., the monitor.

The most difficult problem which we were confronted with very soon was the delay in changes in the interstitial tissue glucose in comparison with blood glucose levels when glucose was injected intravenously. The delay observed in sheep and rats amounted to 10 and 15 min respectively and, to our minds, seriously interfered with the aim of the whole venture i.e., to use tissue glucose determination for automated feedback regulation of insulin supply (Pfeiffer 1987; Steinbach et al. 1987) (Fig. 5).

However, when the glucose levels in the circulation and subcutaneous tissue were increased slowly, e.g., by glucagon injection, the increases in the current indicating subcutaneous glucose content and the blood sugar rises were more or less parallel (Fig. 6) (Brückel et al. 1988). Identical results were obtained in rats when insulin was injected (Fig. 7) (Dolderer et al. 1987, Dolderer et al. 1987 a+b, 1988 a+b). This clearly indicated that slow increases and decreases of glucose, as occur normally after food intake or reactive insulin secretion from the endocrine pancreas, permit measurement of tissue glucose and evaluation of these data for the automated regulation of insulin delivery using the algorithms developed for the large artificial endocrine pancreas.

This conclusion was supported by measurement of the subcutaneous and interstitial cell glucose contents by conventional methods, i.e., using the "wick" or

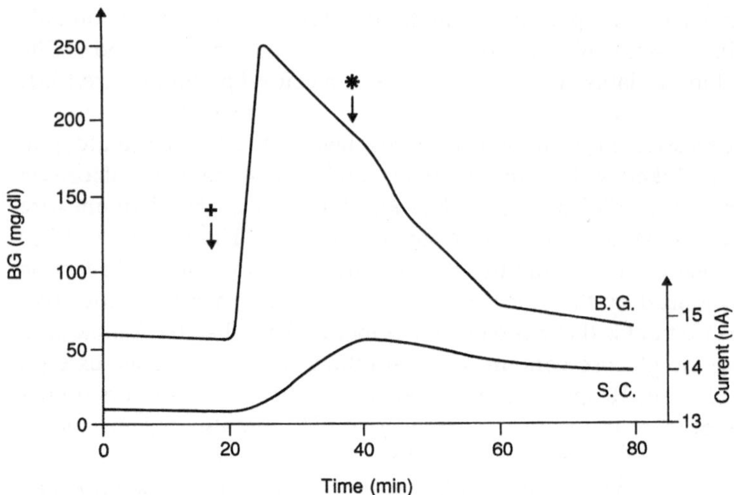

Fig. 5. Comparison of blood glucose (*B.G.*, *left ordinate*) and output from the glucose sensor implanted subcutaneously in 9 sheep (*S.C.*, *right ordinate*) following an intravenous glucose tolerance test (+, 1 g glucose/kg body weight; * 5 units insulin, intravenous). (From Pfeiffer 1987)

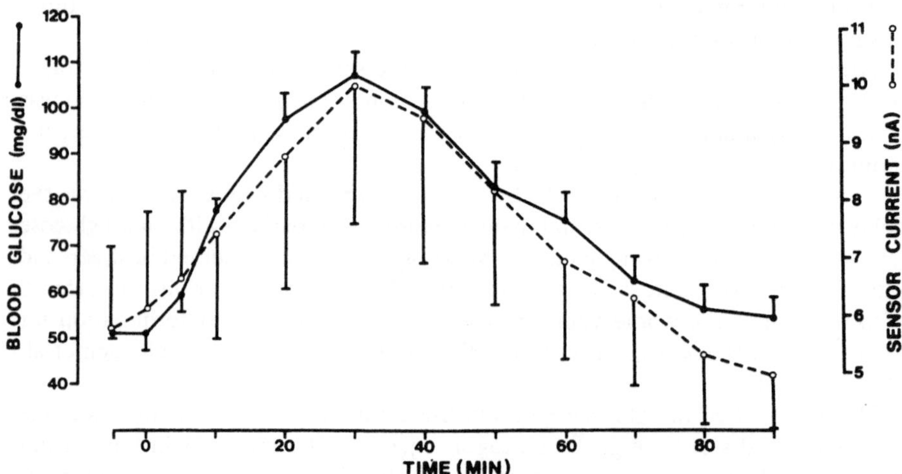

Fig. 6. Course of Blood glucose concentration (*continuous line*) and sensor signal (*interrupted line*) in a sheep following intravenous glucagon administration (1 mg). (From Kerner et al. 1988)

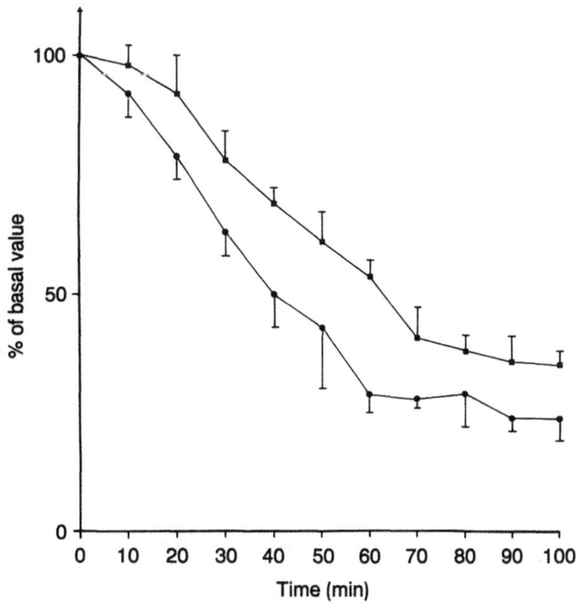

Fig. 7. Course of Sensor output (square) and blood glucose concentration (*circles*) in four diabetic rats following intravenous administration of insulin (8 U/kg). (From Dolderer et al. 1988c)

"thread" technique, which produced values within $\pm$ 10% of the blood glucose concentrations measured (Brückel et al. 1988) (Fig. 8).

In both rats and sheep, a steady decrease of the sensitivity of the electrode was seen over a period of 4 days, the capacity to measure glucose being lost after that time. Interestingly, the same needles which stopped working in situ in the tissue readily regained their activity after being removed in vitro experiments in the laboratory. This problem is obviously directly related to acute-type foreign body reactions which are seen in the first few days after implantation, independent of the material implanted. Exactly the same reactions were generally observed after subcutaneous and intramuscular injections. They were characterized by hyperemia, exudation, and neutrophil granulocyte accumulation. After implantation for several months, however, practically all material produced a more or less pronounced late-type reaction, i.e., accumulation of monocytes, macrophages, giant cells, fibroblasts, and collagen (Dolderer et al. 1987a, b; 1988c; Warhadpande et al. 1987a, b). Since clear differences existed between the various polymers as regards the strength of this foreign body reaction, further studies in this direction seem justified. This problem has not yet been overcome.

However, the needles used for the infusion of insulin from portable pumps must also be changed after 2–4 days of use, and so it should be possible to combine the glucose sensor with such insulin-infusion devices and exchange both devices together after several days. From the point of view of the patient, he or she still has the advantage of complete control of blood glucose, and the great benefit of piercing the skin, 5 or 6 times per month instead of 5 or 6 times per day.

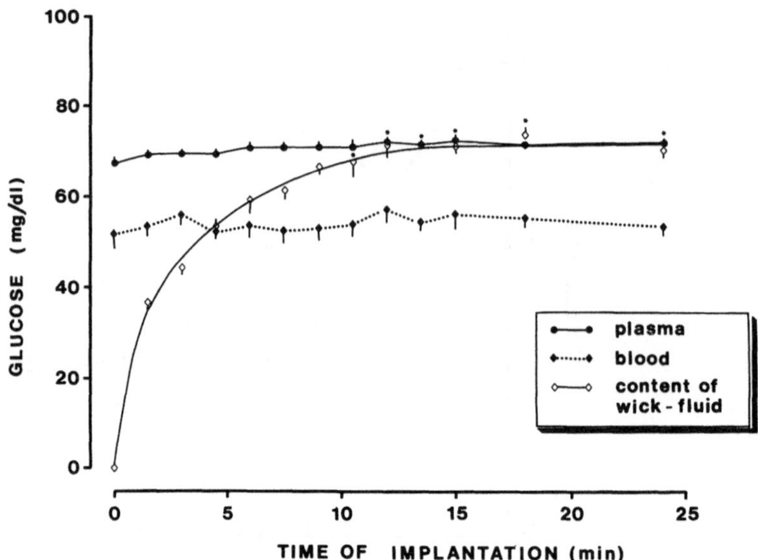

Fig. 8. Comparison of blood and plasma sugar concentrations with interstitial cell glucose concentrations measured using the wick technique. (From Brückel et al. 1988)

In rats, cannulas of refined steel, dip-coated with various polymers and used for amperometric glucose sensing in the tissues, were studied with regard to biocompatibility after up to 8 month of implantation (Dolderer et al. 1987a). In all species acute-type foreign body reactions characterized by hyperemia, exudation, and neutrophile granulocyte accumulation were seen in the first few days after implantation, independent of the material implanted. After implantation for some month, practically all materials produced a more or less pronounced reaction of the late type, i.e., accumulation of monocytes, macrophages, giant cells, fibroblasts, and collagen. Only one polyvinyl derivative produced a negligible foreign-body reaction after months. The same was true when using certain polyurethane models in rats (Dolderer et al. 1987a).

To our great regret, the same sensors that were used successfully in animals had a lifetime of no more than 12–24 h when implanted subcutaneously in human beings. Most probably, this is due to the special anatomy of human subcutaneous tissue, which is very similar to that of pigs in that it contains much more adipose tissue than the skin of sheep or rats. This results in more bleeding and so the lifetime of this type of sensor, already shortened because of the acute foreign body reactions, is further decreased.

Continuous Blood Glucose Monitoring with Portable Glucose Sensors: Implications for Automated Glucose Regulation

For the time being, continuous *blood* glucose determination by portable instruments has been done to (a) reveal the real pattern of blood sugar excursions in diabetic subjects under the conditions of normal life, over the 24 h of day and night; and (b) to observe whether, in conjunction with portable instruments, the algorithms developed for intravenous glucose determination and intravenous insulin infusions could also be employed for subcutaneous insulin infusions.

A miniaturized portable glucose sensor for *blood* glucose measurements was, therefore constructed, based on the same principles as the sensor designed for tissue glucose measurements. In contrast to the implantable glucose sensor, however, this sensor uses heparinized blood, about 12–25 ml per day. Details of this type of flow-through sensor and of the monitor used for continuous glucose determination in both the blood and the interstitial tissues have been given elsewhere (Kerner et al. 1988). The first apparatus was used in combination with the glucose sensor and monitor offered by Gambro, and with our own initial version of a mobile glucose monitor, which consisted of the modified glucose monitor of the artificial endocrine pancreas, the Biostator.

While the Gambro apparatus separates plasma and cells in heparinized blood and uses a Clark electrode for measurement of the oxygen (and weights 4.5 kg), the modified version of the Biostator was put on a mobile carriage and was moved by the patient outside the bed. Our own blood glucose sensor and monitor is a miniaturized (14×8×4 cm) portable analyzer which weighs 120 g, as described before (Kerner et al. 1988).

This analyzer is battery-operated and can store up to 7200 values of glucose levels. The evaluation done by a personal computer (Apple IIe) and blood is withdrawn with a portable roller pump developed by us by means of a double lumen catheter. The small accumulators used to supply power represent the largest part of this flow-through instrument. The apparatus permits continuous blood glucose monitoring in humans for up to 3 days (Zier et al. 1987a+b).

Our portable version was first used to check the results already obtained by the mobile version of the Biostator monitor as to the number of hypoglycemias appearing without clinical symptoms during 24 h under normal conditions in patients carrying the insulin infusion pumps. In the former study we took special note of levels below 40 mg%. In 9 out of 10 patients levels of below 40 mg% were observed during the 24 h; very clearly continuous insulin infusion produces much lower glucose values than intensified conventional insulin therapy, where combined short- and long-acting insulin is injected 2 or 3 times per day (Fig. 5) (Arias et al. 1985).

All the results obtained by means of the mobile Biostator modification were confirmed in full by the portable instrument. There is no doubt that conventional glucose measurement by repeated multiple determinations cannot establish the number and severity of hypoglycemic reactions caused by continuous insulin infusion using portable pumps. The real picture is only obtained by continuously measuring glucose using portable instruments in the venous blood or in the interstitial tissue fluid.

Furthermore, even in those patients who were perfectly controlled by continuous insulin infusions and who had hemoglobin A_1 levels of around 8.5% fluctuations and oscillations of blood glucose during the day and night amounting to up to 250 mg% were still seen. Obviously, these elevated levels were not reflected by the hemoglobin measurement, since the formation and/or reaction occurred to such an extent that over hours the decrease in blood sugar reversed the glycosylation of proteins caused by elevated levels. In other words, conventional blood glucose monitoring is capable neither of determining hypoglycemic periods over a 24-h-period nor of showing whether glycosylated hemoglobin levels are normal in a patient treated by intensive therapy (Pfeiffer 1987).

Only a small proportion of blood glucose levels measured over the 24 h were in accordance with the estimated glycosylated hemoglobin concentrations. On the other hand, on a number of occasions the normal blood glucose concentrations were in clear contrast to the elevated levels of hemoglobin A_1, found at around the same time.

The clinical value of this type of estimation of glucose metabolism was convincingly demonstrated in patients who were thought to be "borderline", or "latent" diabetics. These patients were always very impressed by following their own blood glucose concentrations over 24 h under various caloric intakes. It was easy to convince patients that it was only possible to avoid treatment with blood-sugar-lowering agents or even insulin by maintaining a low caloric intake.

It was also interesting to follow the real changes in glucose levels in nondiabetic "normal" and "ideal weight" patients and compare the changes in obese subjects with and without impaired carbohydrate tolerance. Even in "normal" weight nondiabetic subjects, when blood glucose was measured dynamically following food intake combined with exercise, an obvious delay in renormalization of postprandial blood glucose concentrations was found in comparison to ideal weight non-diabetic subjects (Fig. 9) (Dolderer et al. 1987a). In some of the really obese nondiabetic subjects hyperinsulinism caused postprandially elevated blood glucose concentrations to return to initial values but faster than in the normal weight subjects.

It was also possible to directly combine blood glucose monitoring with subcutaneous insulin infusion from portable pumps by using an interface and minicomputer and evaluating data using only slightly modified versions of the algorithms worked out for the large Biostator artificial endocrine pancreas. This, of course, means that by combination with various commercially available insulin infusion systems the apparatus can be used as a portable artificial endocrine pancreas.

In addition, when continuous blood glucose monitoring permanently indicated the actual glucose concentration to the patient, the diabetic subject himself was in a position to adjusting the insulin pulses necessary after meals in such a way that normoglycemia was achieved. This was only possible when insulin infusions were continuous between meals. Continuous blood or tissue glucose monitoring by the patient might therefore reestablish normoglycemia; this is in contrast to our earlier opinion, that insulin infusions have to be increased before the meals

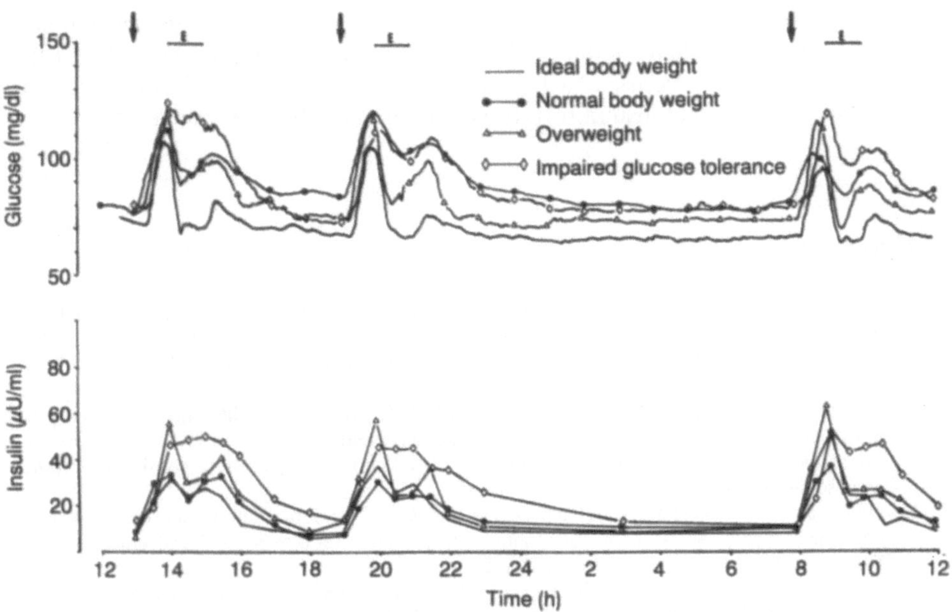

Fig. 9. Continuous blood glucose monitoring with the mobile version of the artificial endocrine pancreas in persons with ideal body weight (−), normal weight (● − ●), overweight (△ − △), and impaired glucose tolerance (◇–◇) (n = 8) (*arrows*, meals; *E*, exercise). (From Dolderer et al. 1987b)

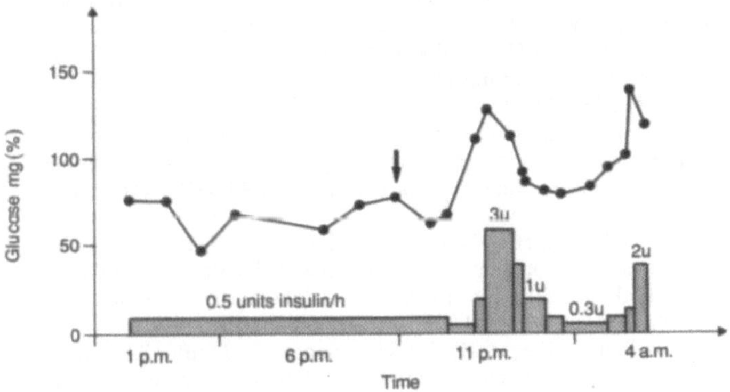

Fig. 10. Blood glucose monitored continuously during a combined kidney and pancreas transplantation (*arrow*, start of operation). Patient K. M., m, 51 yr.

to provide lower postprandial glycemic excursions (Kerner et al. 1982, 1984; Kraegen et al. 1981). Our former skepticism regarding tissue glucose monitoring in combination with subcutaneous insulin infusions is therefore not justified (Pfeiffer and Kerner 1985) when insulin pulses given in connection with the meals are regulated by the human brain and not by an automatic device, i.e., the computer. Interestingly enough, even the double operation of transplantation of the kidney and the whole pancreas, which lasts more than 8 h, was possible using only minimal amounts of insulin when continuous blood glucose monitoring was used (Fig. 10). The prerequisite for successful active and automatic regulation of insulin infusion with this system is that insulin be infused continuously between meals.

References

Abel P, Fischer U, Brunstein E, Ertle R (1988) The GOD-HO-electrode as an approach to implantable glucose sensors. Horm Metab Res [Suppl] 20: 26–29

Albisser AM, Leibel BS, Ewart TG, Davidovac Z, Botz CK, Zingg W (1974) An artificial endocrine pancreas. Diabetes 23: 389–396

Arias P, Kerner W, Zier H, Navascues I, Pfeiffer EF (1985) Incidence of hypoglycemic episodes in diabetic patients under continuous subcutaneous insulin infusion and intensified conventional insulin treatment: assessment by means of semiambulatory 24-hour continuous blood glucose monitoring. Diabetes Care 8: 134–140

Brückel J, Kerner W, Zier H, Steinbach G, Pfeiffer EF (1988) Subkutane Glukosekonzentrationen beim Schaf. Messungen mit einem enzymatischen Glukosesensor und einer Docht-Methode. Aktuel Endokrinol Stoffw 9: 115

Brückel J, Kerner W, Zier H, Steinbach G, Pfeiffer EF (1989) Subcutaneous glucose concentrations in sheep – measurement with an enzyme electrode and a wick-technique. Klin Wochenschr 67: 491–495

Clark LC, Lyons C (1962) Electrode systems for continuous monitoring in cardiovascular surgery. Ann NY Acad Sci 102: 29–45

Clemens AH, Chang PH, Myers RW (1977) The development of Biostator, a glucose controlled insulin infusion system (GCIIS) Horm Metab Res [Suppl] 8: 23–33

Dolderer M, Mohr W, Martin R, Zier H, Kerner W, Steinbach G, Pfeiffer EF (1987a) Biocompatibility of an implantable glucose sensor. Workshop at Schloss Reisensburg 1/87, abstract

Dolderer M, De la Fuente A, Kerner W, Zier H, Steinbach G, Pfeiffer EF (1987b) Mobile und transportable Blutglukosemonitoren: Bedeutung für Diagnose und Therapie des Diabetes mellitus. Verh Dtsch Ges Inn Med 93: 312–315

Dolderer M, Warhadpande RV, Zawadil C, Zier H, Kerner W, Steinbach G, Pfeiffer EF (1988a) Signal of a subcutaneously implanted glucose sensor and blood glucose following intravenous glucose load or insulin administration in normal and diabetic rats. 7th AIDSPIT Workshop, Igls 1988 (abstract)

Dolderer M, Warhadpande RV, Zawadil C, Zier H, Kerner W, Steinbach G, Pfeiffer EF (1988b) A subcutaneously implanted glucose sensor: sensor signal and blood glucose following intravenous glucose load or insulin administration in normal and diabetic rats. 32. Symposium der Deutschen Gesellschaft für Endokrinologie, Hamburg 1988 (abstract)

Dolderer M, Warhadpande RV, Zawadil C, Zier H, Kerner W, Steinbach G, Pfeiffer EF (1988c) Signal eines subkutan implantierten Glukosesensors und Blutzucker nach intravenöser Glukosebelastung und Insulingabe bei normalen und diabetischen Ratten. Aktuel Endokrinol Stoffw 9: 115

Kerner W, Schultz M, Schock D, Pfeiffer EF (1982) Variations of insulin requirements in insulin dependent diabetics for meals taken at different times of the day. Horm Metab Res [Suppl] 12: 228–230

Kerner W, Moll U, Navascues I, Pfeiffer EF (1984) Importance of early postprandial insulin delivery in insulin-dependent diabetics. Klin Wochenschr 62: 738–744

Kerner W, Zier H, Steinbach G, Haas J, Warhadpande RV, Brückel J, Pfeiffer EF (1987a) Measurement of subcutaneous glucose concentration in sheep with an amperometric enzyme electrode. Diabetologia 30: 539 A

Kerner W, Zier H, Steinbach G, Pfeiffer EF (1987b) Amperometric enzyme electrode for glucose measurement in biological fluids. 6th AIDSPIT Workshop, Igls, Austria, 1987 (abstract)

Kerner W, Zier H, Steinbach G, Pfeiffer EF (1987c) Amperometrische Enzymelektrode zur Glukosemessung in vivo. Aktuel Endokrinol Stoffw 8: 2 (abstract)

Kerner W, Zier H, Steinbach G, Brückel J, Warhadpande RV, Pfeiffer EF (1987d) Amperometrische Enzymelektrode zur Glukosemessung im subkutanen Gewebe. Aktuel Endokrinol Stoffw 8: 203

Kerner W, Zier H, Steinbach G, Brückel J, Pfeiffer EF, Weiß T, Cammann K, Planck H (1988) A potentially implantable enzyme electrode for amperometric measurement of glucose. Horm Metab Res [Suppl] 20: 8–13

Kraegen EW, Chisholz DY, McNamam ME (1981) Timing of insulin delivery with meals. Horm Metab Res 13: 365–367

Molnar GD, Taylor WF, Langworthy AL (1972) Plasma immunoreactive insulin pattern in insulin-treated diabetics: studies during continuous blood glucose monitoring Mayo Clin Proc 47: 709–713

Pfeiffer EF (1987) On the way to the automated (blood) glucose regulation in diabetes: the dark past, the grey present and the rosy future. Diabetologia 30: 51–65

Pfeiffer EF, Kerner W (1981) The impact of insulin infusion systems upon the theory and practice of diagnosis and treatment of diabetes mellitus. Diabetes Care 4 (1): 11–26

Pfeiffer EF, Kerner W (1985) Use of artificial pancreas and portable insulin infusion pumps in diabetes therapy: past, present und future. Artif Organs 9 (2): 129–137

Pfeiffer EF, Thum Ch (1974b): Die künstliche β-Zelle (The artificial β-cell). Naturwissenschaften 61: 455

Pfeiffer EF, Thum Ch, Clemens AH (1974a): The artificial beta-cell. A continuous control of blood sugar by external regulation of insulin infusion (glucose-controlled-insulin-infusion-system). Horm Metab Res 6: 339–342

Pfeiffer EF, Thum Ch, Beischer W, Clemens AH (1975) Die künstliche Beta-Zelle in Experiment und Klinik. Verh Dtsch Ges Inn Med 81: 602

Pfeiffer EF, Beischer W, Kerner W (1977) The artificial endocrine pancreas in clinical research. Horm Metab Res [Suppl] 7: 95–112

Schlichtkrull J, Munck O, Jersild M (1965) M-valve, an index of blood sugar control in diabetics. Acta Medica Scandinavica 177: 95–102

Shichiri M, Yamasaki Y, Nao K, Sekiya M, Ueda N (1988) In vivo characteristics of needle-type-glucose sensor-measurements of subcutaneous concentrations in human volunteers. Horm Metab Res [Suppl] 20: 17–20

Steinbach G, Kerner W, Zier H, Dolderer M, Pfeiffer EF (1987) In vivo experiments with a needle type glucose sensor. Workshop at Schloss Reisensburg 1/87 (abstract)

Updike SJ, Hicks G (1967) The enzyme electrode. Nature 214: 986

Warhadpande RV, Dolderer M, Zawadil C, Zier H, Kerner W, Steinbach G, Pfeiffer EF (1987a) Response of subcutaneously implanted glucose sensor to intravenous glucose load in normal and diabetic rats (abstract). Diabetologia 30: 595A

Warhadpande RV, Dolderer M, Zawadil C, Zier H, Kerner W, Bischof F, Steinbach G, Pfeiffer EF (1987b) Ein subkutan implantierter Glukosesensor bei normalen und diabetischen Ratten: Vergleich zwischen Sensorsignal und Blutzucker nach intravenöser Glukosebelastung (abstract). Aktuel Endokrinol Stoffw 8: 221

Zier H, Kerner W, Steinbach G, Pfeiffer EF (1987a) Ein miniaturisierter, tragbarer Glukosemonitor mit enzymatischem Glukosesensor (abstract). Aktuel Endokrinol Stoffw 8: 4

Zier H, Kerner W, Steinbach G, Pfeiffer EF (1987b) A miniaturized, portable analyzer for operation of glucose sensors. Biosensors, International workshop, 1987. Gesellschaft für Biotechnologische Forschung, Braunschweig

Diskussion II (B)

Vorsitz: W. TELLER

H. Ditschuneit:

Eine Frage zu Herrn Beyers Beitrag, aber auch den Vortrag zum künstlichen Pankreas betreffend.

Blutzucker und Insulin sind negativ korreliert miteinander. Aber das ist ja nicht eine einfache Gesetzmäßigkeit, sondern ein komplexes Geschehen, wie wir heute von vielen gehört haben und wir alle wissen. Wenn das so einfach wäre, dann könnte man das alles mit dem Computer machen. Ein Diabetologe, wenn er 20 Patienten behandelt, dann weiß er ungefähr, wieviel Insulin er heute zu geben hat, wieviel er morgen zu geben hat, wie dieser Patient reagiert und wie der andere reagiert. Und dieses hieße also für den Patienten, er müßte lange lernen an seinem Computer, um einigermaßen mit seinem Diabetes klarzukommen. Expertensysteme sind schön für Experten, aber nicht für Laien.

J. Beyer:

Wir dürfen Sie einmal zu einem Besuch einladen. Alles Schwierige löst sich irgendwann einmal genial einfach auf und ich glaube, daß es auch bei diesen Dingen so ist und wir haben zumindest zur Zeit die Möglichkeit, den Basalinsulinbedarf zu kalkulieren, den abhängigen Glukoseinsulinbedarf zu kalkulieren, den kohlenhydratabhängigen Insulinbedarf zu kalkulieren und das Gesamtsystem lernfähig zu machen, so daß der Computer lernt und darauf aufbauend weiter arbeitet. Das sind Gesetzmäßigkeiten, die 10 Jahre alt sind.

J. Dudeck:

Beim Einsatz von Computern hat man zunächst mal an die Diagnostik gedacht und es hat sich aber gezeigt, es gibt sehr hübsche Beispiele, diagnostizieren kann der Arzt relativ gut, das heißt in der Praxis haben diese wenig Anwendung gefunden. Dagegen haben solche Anwendungen, wie Sie sie gezeigt haben, im Sinne eines Monitorings, daß man also versucht interaktiv solche Prozesse zu beeinflussen, sich in vielen Bereichen bewährt und ich möchte im Gegensatz zu Herrn Ditschuneit sagen, ich glaube, daß dies der richtige Ansatz ist, solches Wissen in einer operationalisierten Form in einen Rechner zu bringen und das dem Patienten wirklich als Anleitung, als Hilfe zu geben. Es ist genau das gleiche, wie wenn man ihm ein Buch übergibt, nur in der operationalisierten Form kann das Wissen direkt angewendet werden, er muß es nicht erst nochmal intellektuell verarbeiten. Insofern meine ich, daß Sie auf dem richtigen zukunftsweisenden Wege sind und meine, daß man diese Arbeiten wirklich sehr intensivieren sollte.

W. Teller:

Schönen Dank für diesen Kommentar. Ich kann das in etwa bestätigen für juvenile Diabetiker, die natürlich intelligent sein müssen, Schüler, die sowieso mit Computern arbeiten, dann können sie diese Dinge etwas eher erfassen und besser verstehen und sich mehr engagieren hinsichtlich der Selbstkontrolle. Da ist etwas dran, dem stimme ich völlig zu.

E. F. Peiffer

Ich meine halt, der Unterschied ist doch minimal, ob ich nun dem Patienten eine Infusionsmaschine anhänge und er wählt sich nach den Mahlzeiten mit Drehungen seine 1, 2, 3 oder 4 E. Insulin. Das ist das Prinzip, welches die jetzigen Insulininfusionspumpen haben. Entscheidend ist, daß er zwischen den Mahlzeiten Insulin kontinierlich bekommt. Ob das nun pulsatil sein muß oder nicht, das kann dann vielleicht zu einer Reduktion der Insulindosis führen, das mag dahingestellt sein, aber im Grunde braucht er ununterbrochen eine gewisse Menge Insulin. Wenn die da ist und er nach den Mahlzeiten dann noch Insulin draufsetzt, hat man einen besseren Stoffwechsel als ohne das Verfahren. Das ist zweifelsfrei. Die Situation ist aber, daß wir hinter den Ereignissen herlaufen, wir können ihn praktisch nicht mehr einholen, weil er zu weit weg ist, bis er den Blutzucker selbst gemacht hat und dann nachspritzt, was er ja dann doch in der Regel nicht tut und nochmal sich mit der Nadel verletzen muß, das ist unser Problem. Wir sind einfach zu schlecht und zu insuffizient im Augenblick. Deswegen glaube ich, daß alles, was das versucht wegzuräumen, eine Besserung ist.

H. Ditschuneit:

Ich meine nur eines: Heute gelingt mit 6E. eine gute Stoffwechseleinstellung, der Blutzucker geht runter, morgen mit 4, übermorgen mit 10. Den Tag später folgt auf 4E. eine Hypoglykämie. Es ist täglich nicht dasselbe. Beim gleichen Blutzuckerausgangswert und das ist die Schwierigkeit.

W. Teller:

Nothing is perfect, es gibt überall Ausnahmen, das stimmt. Das ist das Problem. Natürlich.

H. Mehnert:

Ich wollte als Beispiel dafür, was gute Kooperation mit dem Patienten bei entsprechendem teaching und entsprechender Motivation vermag, die diabetischen Schwangeren anführen. Es wird immer wieder gesagt, daß diese Patientinnen Insulinpumpen brauchen. Ist überhaupt nicht nötig. Diese Patientinnen sind so kooperativ, sie lassen sich mit 4 – 5 Spritzen optimal mit HbA1-Werten von 6 % einstellen. Diese Patienten brauchen keinen Computer, das, was sie am ehesten haben könnten, das wäre die Sonde (Glukosesensor), um einfach die Kontrollen zu erleichtern. Aber, man soll wirklich die sonstigen apparativen Momente in der Diabetesführung nicht überschätzen, weil es das Problem meiner Ansicht nach in der Sicht verstellt, daß der Arzt sich um den Patienten zu kümmern hat und daß der Patient voll und möglichst ohne besondere apparative Hilfe aufgrund seines Wissens und seiner compliance mitarbeitet.

W. Teller
Danke Herr Mehnert, voll akzeptiert, ich glaube, dazu gibt es keinen Kommentar.

Die Bedeutung einer
dynamischen Insulinsubstitution
für Prophylaxe und Therapie
diabetischer Sekundärkomplikationen

Makroangiopathie beim Diabetes

E. Standl

Summary

Type II diabetics in particular suffer from macroangiopathy. However, type I diabetics may also have these complications, although microangiopathy is far more important in these cases. Only prophylaxis and follow-up can help avoid discovering consequences too late by learning form the late complications with which each diabetic has to reckon. In principle, therapy of macroangiopathic complications in diabetics does not differ from that in nondiabetics but the best therapy includes prophylaxis, early detection, and regular following. Physician working in private practice plays an important role in the long-term treatment of diabetics. Only prophylactic programs and regular follow-ups can help avoid the very late and untreatable complications which may affect every diabetic patient.

Einleitung

Nach wie vor erkranken die Diabetiker in ihrer großen Mehrzahl an charakteristischen Gefäßkomplikationen und sterben schließlich daran [2, 3, 4, 7, 8, 11, 12, 20, 23, 24, 28]. Grundsätzlich kann sich dieses zweite – vaskuläre – Gesicht der Stoffwechselkrankheit Diabetes bei allen Unterformen und -typen des chronischen Hyperglykämie-Syndroms einstellen, auch wenn die Ausprägung unterschiedlich akzentuiert ist. Dabei ist ganz vorwiegend der Typ II-Diabetes durch die Entwicklung von Makroangiopathien gekennzeichnet [20, 24, 28]. Es wäre aber ein Irrtum zu glauben, daß der Typ I-Diabetiker von der Makroangiopathie verschont bliebe. Allerdings steht beim Typ I-Diabetes die fast spezifische Mikroangiopathie weit im Vordergrund [4, 7, 8], wobei auch bei Typ II-Diabetikern durchaus diese mikrovaskulären Veränderungen an Auge und Niere sowie insbesondere an den Füßen und am Herz auftreten können [13, 14, 26, 38].

Epidemiologie

Drei von vier Diabetikern erliegen einem Gefäßleiden, jeder zweite stirbt an der koronaren Herzkrankheit [2, 11, 12, 20, 23, 24, 28]. Diese Mortalitätszahlen sind jeweils doppelt so hoch wie in der allgemeinen Bevölkerung. Die Morbidität der koronaren Herzkrankheit ist für diabetische Frauen auf das Fünf- bis Sechsfache, für diabetische Männer auf das Zwei- bis Dreifache erhöht [2, 11, 12, 20, 23, 24, 28].

Erkrankungen der hirnversorgenden Arterien sind zwei- bis dreimal, der extremitätenversorgenden Arterien fünfmal so häufig. Die Risikosteigerung für das Auftreten einer Fußgangrän beträgt mindestens das Zwanzigfache; jeder zehnte Diabetiker muß deshalb im Laufe seines Lebens amputiert werden.

Wie exzessiv die Häufung der Makroangiopathie bei Typ II-Diabetikern in der Bundesrepublik Deutschland ist, hat unsere Arbeitsgruppe kürzlich im Rahmen eines kooperativen Schulungsprojekts zwischen einem Diabeteszentrum und niedergelassenen Ärzten an rund 350 unselektierten Patienten unter 75 Jahren in Arztpraxen im Großraum München festgestellt [40, 43]. Jeder zweite Diabetiker wies koronartypische EKG-Veränderungen auf, 28% eine arterielle Verschlußkrankheit der Beine, 16% Veränderungen der hirnversorgenden Arterien.

Nach den Studien des Steno-Memorial-Hospitals in Kopenhagen beträgt die Makroangiopathiehäufigkeit für Typ I-Diabetiker nach 40jähriger Diabetesdauer 21% für den Myokardinfarkt, 10% für zerebrovaskuläre Komplikationen und 12% für schwerwiegende Komplikationen im Bereich der Extremitäten-versorgenden Arterien mit Auftreten einer Gangrän bzw. der Notwendigkeit einer Amputation [7, 8]. Selbst bei den Typ I-Diabetikern, die eine terminale Niereninsuffizienz infolge der Mikroangiopathie entwickeln, sterben ein Drittel an makrovaskulären Komplikationen [4].

Besondere Merkmale

Die Makroangiopathien bei Diabetes sind nicht als spezifische, wohl aber typische Komplikationen aufzufassen und dem Krankheitsbild der „normalen" Arteriosklerose zuzuordnen. Der Diabetiker ist davon nur besonders früh und ausgeprägt befallen. Es gibt jedoch, vor allem klinisch, einige Besonderheiten:

Diabetische Frauen sind – im Gegensatz zu Nichtdiabetikern – mindestens ebenso häufig betroffen wie diabetische Männer. Die Schwabinger Studie zur Makroangiopathie bei Diabetikern und die WHO-Studie über Gefäßkomplikationen bei Diabetikern belegen sogar, daß Frauen noch stärker als Männer gefährdet sind [2, 18, 21, 30].

Die Makroangiopathien bei Diabetes zeichnen sich anfänglich zumeist durch eine ausgesprochene Symptomarmut aus [16, 20, 24, 36, 37]. Selbst Ärzte bemerken u. U. nicht ihren Herzinfarkt oder ihre arterielle Verschlußkrankheit der

Beine. Dies mag zum Teil mit einer gleichzeitig bestehenden Neuropathie zu tun haben oder auch mit Abnormitäten bei der muskulären Laktatproduktion im Insulinmangel [35], zum Teil sicherlich auch mit der dritten Besonderheit, der besonders peripheren Lokalisation der Angiopathie.

Die Angiopathien bei Diabetes manifestieren sich bevorzugt an peripheren Gefäßabschnitten. Beispielsweise befällt die arterielle Verschlußkrankheit der Beine in zwei Dritteln das Unterschenkelsegment oder noch peripherer [1, 16, 36, 37] und eine Claudicatio projiziert sich deshalb nicht – wie sonst häufig – in die Wade, sondern in den Fuß und kann dann fehlgedeutet werden. Beim Nichtdiabetiker kommt Unterschenkelbefall nur in etwa 20 % einer arteriellen Verschlußkrankheit der Beine vor [1]. Ebenso sind bei der koronaren Herzkrankheit in 70 % auch intramurale Äste der Koronarien betroffen, wohingegen dies beim Nichtdiabetiker so gut wie nie der Fall ist.

Schließlich tritt beim Diabetiker in deutlicher Abhängigkeit von der Diabetesdauer eine Mediasklerose vom Mönckeberg-Typ auf [17, 20, 36, 37], d.h. eine röhrenförmige Verkalkung der Tunica media (Abb. 1). Eine obliterierende Angiopathie bzw. Intima-Veränderungen müssen dabei nicht vorliegen, sind aber nach Ergebnissen der Schwabinger Studie zur Makroangiopathie bei Diabetikern bei jedem zweiten Patienten vorhanden [16, 17, 20, 36]. Knapp 10 % aller unausgewählten Diabetiker leiden an einer Mediasklerose [17, 20, 36, 37].

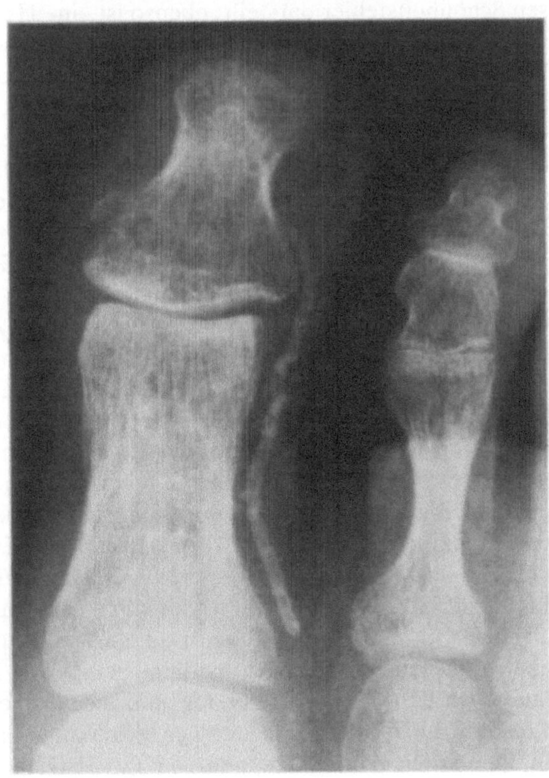

Abb. 1. Mediasklerose bei Langzeitdiabetes

Anzumerken ist, daß die diabetische Mikroangiopathie und Neuropathie die Symptomatologie und den klinischen Ablauf der Makroangiopathie bei Diabetes wesentlich mitprägen können. Infolge dieser Besonderheiten ist die Prognose makrovaskulärer Erkrankungen bei Diabetikern meist deutlich ungünstiger als bei Nichtdiabetikern.

Risikofaktoren und Risikoindikatoren

Hinsichtlich der für die horrende Massierung von Makroangiopathien bei Diabetikern verantwortlichen Risikofaktoren und -prädikatoren haben die verschiedenen epidemiologischen Untersuchungen, wie die Schwabinger Studie, die WHO-Studie und die Frankfurter PARD-Studie, kürzlich wesentliche neue Erkenntnisse gebracht [5, 18, 21, 30, 40]. Tabelle 1 bringt die Zusammenfassung von Multivarianzanalysen der Schwabinger- und der WHO-Daten. Es zeigt sich, daß (abgesehen vom Alter) Hypertonie, insbesondere die systolische Hypertonie, und Hypertriglyzeridämie die Risikoprädikatoren per excellence für den Diabetiker sind. Für die praktische Medizin erscheint besonders wichtig, daß eine ausschließlich systolische Hypertonie bei Diabetikern keineswegs einen harmlosen Schönheitsfehler darstellt, ebenso ist eine Hypertriglyzeridämie – im Gegensatz zu Nichtdiabetikern – vor allem bei diabetischen Frauen kein Kavaliersdelikt. Hohe Triglyzeride sind hier vermutlich als Indikator zu verstehen, daß der gesamte Lipidstoffwechsel, einschließlich LDL und HDL, in Richtung Atherogenese abläuft. Daneben scheint auch der Diabetes per se, d.h. die Diabetesdauer, eine nicht zu übersehende Rolle zu spielen (Tabelle 1).

Natürlich sind Rauchen, Adipositas oder Hypercholesterinämie auch für den Diabetiker ungünstig, stehen aber epidemiologisch gesehen nicht im Vordergrund. Wesentlich bedeutsamer jedoch sind in letzter Zeit weitere Prädikatoren und Risikomarker für die Makroangiopathien bei Typ II-Diabetikern in den Blickpunkt gerückt: Hyperinsulinämie, Thrombozytenaggregation, spezielle Gefäßwandfaktoren und Plasma-Viskosität sowie die sogenannte Mikroalbuminurie.

Erstaunlicherweise ist das Insulin selbst in jüngster Zeit in Verdacht geraten – sofern es in überhöhter Konzentration an der Gefäßwand wirksam wird – unabhängig von der Blutglukose kardiovaskulären Komplikationen Vorschub zu leisten [5, 45]. Man hat diese Beobachtung zunächst bei verschiedenen prospektiven epidemiologischen Untersuchungen an Nichtdiabetikern in Australien, Finnland und Frankreich gemacht [9, 31, 47]. Insulin hat Einfluß auf die Proliferation der Gefäßwand-Media, auch auf spezielle Gefäßwand-Wuchsfaktoren sowie auf den Lipidstoffwechsel der Gefäßwand, aber auch auf den Lipidstoffwechsel ganz allgemein [3, 29, 44, 45]. Hohe Insulinspiegel bei peripherer Insulinresistenz sind aber geradezu ein Charakteristikum bei Typ II-Diabetes. In der Schwabinger Studie wurden deshalb die endogenen Insulinspiegel, gemessen als C-Peptid, in Relation zum Vorhandensein einer Makroangiopathie analysiert [39, Tabelle 2]. In allen untersuchten Gruppen von Typ II-Diabetikern wie auch bei den nicht-

Tabelle 1. Prädiktoren und Risikomarker der Makroangiopathie bei Typ II-Diabetikern (Ergebnisse von Multivarianzanalysen: multiple logistische Regressionen)

| | Schwabinger Studie: 5-Jahres-Verlauf | | | | WHO-Studie | |
	Schwere Herz-Kreisl.-Kompl. Nur Tod (Typ I + II) Männer	Frauen	AVK		Männer	Frauen
Alter	××	××	××	××	×××	××
Syst. RR	××	×××	×××	×××	×××	×××
Triglyzeride	×		××	××	××[a]	××[a]
Diabetesdauer	×××		×		××	(××,
Rauchen				×		nur AVK)
BMI					××	××
Cholesterin					××	
Geschlecht						
Diast. RR						
Glukose						
Diabetestherapie						

[a] nur bei 1 Drittel gemessen

Tabelle 2. Nüchternkonzentration von C-Peptid (pmol/ml) bei Typ II-Diabetikern und Kontrollpersonen ($\bar{x} \pm$ SEM)

| | Makroangiopathie | | Signifikanz |
	ja	nein	p-Wert
Alle Typ II-Diabetiker (n = 323)	0,44 ± 0,02	0,36 ± 0,03	< 0,05
Typ II-Diabetiker ohne Insulinbehandlung (n = 154)	0,60 ± 0,04	0,45 ± 0,03	< 0,01
Typ II-Diabetiker mit Insulinbehandlung (n = 169)	0,31 ± 0,02	0,23 ± 0,03	< 0,05
Kontrollpersonen (n = 178)	0,43 ± 0,03	0,28 ± 0,03	< 0,01

diabetischen Kontrollen zeigten die Patienten mit Makroangiopathie signifikant höhere Nüchtern-Insulinspiegel. Die Gruppe der insulinbehandelten Typ II-Diabetiker spritzte überdies noch signifikant mehr exogenes Insulin [39]. Im prospektiven Ansatz bestimmten in der Multivarianzanalyse neben Alter und Triglyzeriden die Anzahl der Insulineinheiten das Auftreten bzw. die Verschlechterung einer arteriellen Verschlußkrankheit im Verlauf von fünf Jahren bei insulinbehandelten Diabetikern [21]. Ähnliche Beobachtungen über die Bedeutung der Hyperinsulinämie bei Typ II-Diabetikern liegen mittlerweile aus Oxford und Paris vor [10, 15].

Die Anzahl der täglichen Insulineinheiten – so die Schwabinger Daten [21, 39] – stand ihrerseits in signifikantem Zusammenhang mit der Höhe des systolischen

Blutdrucks, der Triglyzeride und der Blutglukose. Ferner war das endogene C-Peptid mit den triglyzeriden und – invers – mit dem HDL-Cholesterin korreliert. Das Syndrom von Hyperinsulinämie, Insulinresistenz, Hypertriglyzeridämie, HDL-Cholesterin-Erniedrigung, Hyperglykämie und Adipositas fördert demnach augenscheinlich das Auftreten der Makroangiopathien bei Typ II-Diabetikern und stellt womöglich den diabetestypischen Aspekt bei der Pathogenese dieser Angiopathien dar.

Hinsichtlich Thrombozyten- und Gerinnungsparametern hat die Schwabinger Studie ebenfalls signifikante Beziehungen zur Makroangiopathie aufgezeigt, insbesondere für das Faktor VIII-assoziierte Antigen, die Thrombozytenaggregation (PAT III) oder Fibrinogen im Blut aufwiesen [5]. Fibrinogen stellt die bestimmende Größe für die Blutplasmaviskosität dar. Analoge Befunde fanden sich für die diabetischen Frauen nicht. Hier traten die schweren kardiovaskulären Komplikationen hauptsächlich bei den insulinbehandelten Patientinnen auf [5].

Die Thematik der sogenannten Mikroalbuminurie ist vor allem von skandinavischen und englischen Arbeitsgruppen in den letzten Jahren bearbeitet worden [12, 26, 27, 46]. Bei einer Albuminausscheidung von wenigen Mikrogramm pro Milliliter spricht man von Mikroalbuminurie, die normalen Teststreifen-Methoden reagieren erst ab einer Eiweißausscheidung von 40 mg/dl. Je nach Diabetesdauer zeigen jeweils 10–20% der Typ II-Diabetiker eine Mikroalbuminurie. Mittlerweile ist klar, daß dieser Befund mit hoher prognostischer Aussagekraft Jahre vorher eine Makroalbuminurie und Niereninsuffizienz antizipieren läßt [26, 27, 46]. Das gänzlich Unerwartete aber war, daß bei Typ II-Diabetikern eine Mikroalbuminurie auch Herz-Kreislauf-Morbidität und -Mortalität prognostiziert [22, 26, 27]. Wie Tabelle 3 zeigt, lebten von Typ II-Diabetikern ohne Mikroalbuminurie 10 Jahre später noch 60 Prozent, mit Mikroalbuminurie aber nur noch 25 Prozent. Für diese Exzessmortalität war praktisch ausschließlich der Herz-Kreislauf-Tod [26, 27] verantwortlich.

Tabelle 4 mit Daten aus dem kooperativen Projekt Diabeteszentrum – niedergelassene Ärzte – demonstriert die Massierung von Risikofaktoren und -indikatoren bei unselektierten Typ II-Diabetikern in der Bundesrepublik Deutschland. Jeder zweite weist eine ungenügende Diabeteseinstellung auf mit HbA_{Ic}-Werten von 1.5 Prozentpunkten über dem Normbereich, zwei von drei Diabetikern haben jeweils eine Hypertonie bzw. Hypertriglyzeridämie. Überdies hat dieses Projekt einer Zusammenarbeit Klinik/Praxis bereits gezeigt, daß einfache, von einem Diabeteszentrum konzipierte Schulungsmaßnahmen, die in der Praxis vom Arzt und – eine Neuerung – von seinen Helferinnen durchgeführt werden, die Diabe-

Tabelle 3. 10-Jahres-Überlebensrate von Diabetikern mit und ohne Mikroalbuminurie. (Nach Mogensen, 1984)

Diabetestyp	Initiales Alter	Mikroalbuminurie	
		nein	ja
Typ I	ca. 25 J.	fast 100 %	ca. 80 %
Typ II	ca. 66 J.	ca. 60 %	ca. 25 %

Tabelle 4. BMFT-Projekt Zusammenarbeit Diabetes-Zentrum mit niedergelassenen Ärzten (Kardiovaskuläre Risikofaktoren bei 274 unausgewählten Typ II-Diabetikern unter 75 Jahren in der Praxis des niedergelassenen Arztes)

$HbA_{Ic} \geq 8\ \%$	49 %
Hypertonie (RR $\geq$ 160/95 mm Hg)	65 %
Hypertriglyzeridämie $\geq$ 200 mg/dl	64 %
Hypercholesterinämie $\geq$ 250 mg/dl	43 %
Übergewicht ($\geq$ Broca-Gewicht plus 10 %)	51 %
Raucher	16 %
Exraucher	9 %

und – eine Neuerung – von seinen Helferinnen durchgeführt werden, die Diabeteseinstellung, gemessen an den HbA_{Ic}-Werten, signifikant verbessern lassen [32].

Diagnostik

Sicherlich stehen die entsprechende Anamnese und der körperliche Untersuchungsbefund sowie EKG-Ableitungen nach wie vor an erster Stelle bei der Abklärung einer Makroangiopathie bei Diabetikern. Darüber hinaus haben die verschiedenen Ultraschall-Doppler-Verfahren der hirn- und extremitätenversorgenden Arterien die diagnostischen Möglichkeiten ganz wesentlich bereichert [16, 25]. Allerdings stellt die Ultraschall-Doppler-Untersuchung der hirnversorgenden Arterien besondere Anforderungen an die Erfahrungen des Untersuchers und sollte speziell angiologisch ausgebildeten Kollegen vorbehalten sein. Bei der Untersuchung der Beine wird der störende Einfluß einer u. U. vorhandenen Mediasklerose im allgemeinen überschätzt; sie ist ggf. durch einfache Zusatzuntersuchungen, z. B. akrale oszillographische Ableitungen, unschwer zu erkennen. Die Möglichkeiten der Echokardiographie, elektronische Oszillographie, Angiographie, einschließlich Koronar-, digitalen Subtraktions- und Vergrößerungsangiographie, sowie der Sonographie und Herzszintigraphie haben als weiterführende Untersuchungsmethoden auch bei den Angiopathien des Diabetikers ihren speziellen Stellenwert.

Therapie

Die Therapie der makroangiopathischen Komplikationen bei Diabetikern unterscheidet sich nicht prinzipiell von der bei Nichtdiabetikern. Ausgehend von der

Komplexität des Krankheitsgeschehens sind die Behandlungserfolge jedoch meist schlechter als bei Nichtdiabetikern. Gefäßchirurgische Maßnahmen, seien sie an den Koronarien, an den hirn- oder den extremitätenversorgenden Arterien, sind oft durch das Problem der diffusen und peripheren Lokalisation der Läsionen verkompliziert. Bei entsprechender Indikation kommen aber auch bei Diabetikern gefäßrekonstruktive Eingriffe und Bypass-Operationen aller Art in Frage, einschließlich der verschiedenen Verfahren einer perkutanen transluminalen Katheter-Angioplastie (PTA) und der lokalen Thrombolyse mit Strepto- bzw. Urokinase, Patienten mit Glaskörperblutungen sollten jedoch nicht lokal thrombolysiert werden. Nunmehr vorliegende Langzeitbeobachtungen nach Einsatz von PTA und lokaler Thrombolyse bei Diabetikern haben praktisch keine spezifischen Kontraindikationen erkennen lassen [42]. Immerhin ist auch bei jedem zweiten Diabetiker fünf Jahre nach dem Eingriff das rekanalisierte Gefäß noch durchgängig.

Bei den medikamentösen Maßnahmen sind die relativ geringen Glukosetoleranz-verschlechternden Effekte von nicht-selektiven Betablockern und Diuretika vom Thiazidtyp lange bekannt [20]. Sie spielen bei den heute verwendeten kleinen Dosen und Mehrfachtherapien im allgemeinen eine untergeordnete Rolle. Hinzuweisen ist, daß auch die kardioselektiven Betablocker gerade bei Diabetikern, vermutlich bei solchen mit latenter kardiale Neuropathie, beträchtliche Bradykardien auslösen und, speziell bei insulinspritzenden Patienten, die Hypoglykämie-Symptomatik maskieren können [20].

Angesichts der Ergebnisse der Frankfurter PARD-Studie verwundert es nicht, daß verschiedentlich bei diabetischen Männern über positive Erfahrungen mit Aggregationshemmern berichtet worden ist [6]. Diesbezüglich sind aber sicherlich weitere und bessere Studien erforderlich.

Zu den rheologischen Aspekten sei ausgeführt, daß Diabetiker recht häufig hohe Fibrinogenspiegel aufweisen, die im Bedarfsfall therapeutischen Maßnahmen zugänglich sind. Außerdem führt eine Hyperglykämie immer auch zu einer Hämokonzentration mit exponentieller Zunahme der Vollblutviskosität [41]. Allein schon aus diesem Grund können bei einer symptomatischen Makroangiopathie eine gute Hydrierung, eventuell unter Zuhilfenahme einer Insulintherapie, sowie eine isovolämische Hämodilution sinnvoll sein.

Vorsorgeprogramm

Wie immer liegt die beste Therapie im Vorbeugen und Früherkennen, gerade auch im Hinblick auf die häufig vorhandene Symptomarmut trotz oder bei bereits gravierenden angiopathischen Komplikationen. Für die Praxis würde es deshalb den größten Fortschritt bedeuten, wenn möglichst alle Diabetiker – zusätzlich zur Kontrolle der Glykämie – regelmäßig einfachen Laborkontrollen und klinischen Maßnahmen zur möglichst frühzeitigen Diagnose komplizierender Erkrankungen unterzogen würden. Eine solche Liste könnte umfassen.

1. Jährliche Kontrolle

a) Messung von Cholesterin und Triglyzeriden (evtl. von HDL-Cholesterin im Serum),

b) Augenärztliche Untersuchung – bei beginnender Retinopathie bzw. mehr als zehnjähriger Diabetesdauer in viertel- bis halbjährlichem Abstand,

c) Überprüfung des Harnstatus (einschließlich der Diagnose einer Mikroalbuminurie) und des Kreatinins im Serum.

2. Zweijährige Kontrolle

a) Gefäßstatus, einschließlich Blutdruckmessung, Auskultation des Herzens, EKG, Palpation und Auskultation der hirn- und extremitätenversorgenden Arterien (einschließlich von Ultraschall-Doppler-Untersuchungen),

b) Orientierende Untersuchung des peripheren Nervensystems.

Mit einem solchen „Vorsorgeprogramm" könnten rechtzeitig die Weichen gestellt werden, damit aus beginnenden Spätkomplikationen keine „Zu-spät-Komplikationen" werden. Dem niedergelassenen Arzt kommt hier eine zentrale Stellung bei der Langzeitbehandlung der Diabetiker zu.

Literatur

1. Alexander K (1970) Die diabetischen Angiopathien. Med Wochenschr 15: 690–696
2. Barret-Connor E, Wingard DL (1983) Sex differential in ischemic heart disease mortality in diabetics: a prospective population-based study. Amer J Epidem 118: 489–496
3. Biermann EL (1979) Atherosclerosis and lipoproteins in diabetes mellitus. Diabetes 28: 580–585
4. Borch-Johnson K, Andersen PK, Deckert T (1985) The effect of proteinuria on relative mortality in type I (insulin dependent) diabetes mellitus. Diabetologia 28: 590–596
5. Breddin HK, Krzywanek HJ, Althoff P, Schöffling K, Überla K (1985) PARD: Platelet aggregation as a risk factor in diabetics: results of a prospective study. Horm Metabol Res [Suppl] 15: 69–73
6. Colwell JA, Bingham SF, Abraira C, Anderson JW, Kwaan HC (1985) C. A. Cooperative Study on antiplatelet agents in diabetic patients after amputations from gangrene. Horm Metabol Res [Suppl] 15: 69–73
7. Deckert T, Poulsen JE, Larsen M (1978a) Prognosis of diabetics with diabetes onset before the age of thirtyone, I. Survival, causes of death, and complications. Diabetologia 14: 363–370
8. Deckert T, Poulsen JW, Larsen M (1978b) Prognosis of diabetics with diabetes onset before the age of thirtyone, II. Factors influencing the prognosis. Diabetologia 14: 371–377
9. Ducimetière P, Eschwege E, Papoz L, Richard JL, Claude JR, Rosselin GE (1980) Relationship of plasma insulin levels to the incidense of myocardial infarction and coronary heart disease mortality in a middle-aged population. Diabetologia 19: 205–210
10. Eschwege E, Richard JL, Thibult N, Ducimetière P, Warnet JM, Claude JR, Rosselin GE (1985) Coronary heart disease mortality in relation with diabetes, blood glucose and plasma insulin levels. The Paris Prospective Study – Ten Years later. Horm Metabol Res [Suppl] 15: 41–46
11. Fuller JH, Shipley MJ, Rose G, Jarrett RJ, Keen H (1983) Mortality from coronary heart disease and stroke in relation to degree of glycemia: the Withehall Study. Brit Med J 287: 867–870
12. Fuller JH (1985) Causes of Death in Diabetes Mellitus. Horm Metabol Res [Suppl] 15

13. Hasslacher Ch, Wolfrum M, Rall C, Stech G, Ritz E, Wahl P (1985) Nephropathie bei Typ II-Diabetikern. Akt Endokr Stoffw 6: 88

14. Hermann WH, Teutsch SM, Sepe SJ, Sinnock P, Klein R (1983) An approach to the prevention of blindness in diabetes. Diab Care 6: 608–613

15. Hillson RM, Hockaday TDR, Mann JI, Newton DJ (1984) Hyperinsulinaemia is associated with development of electrocardiographic abnormalities in diabetes. Diab Res 1: 143–149

16. Janka HU, Standl E, Mehnert H (1980) Peripheral vascular disease in diabetes mellitus and its relation to cardiovascular risk factors: Screening with the Doppler ultrasonic technique. Diab Care 3: 207–213

17. Janka HU, Standl E, Albert ED, Scholz S, Mehnert H (1980) Mediasklerose bei Diabetikern – eine Sonderform der Makroangiopathie. Vasa 9: 281–285

18. Janka HU, Grünwald P, Waldmann G, Standl E, Mehnert H (1982) Karotisstenosen, kardiovaskuläres Risikoprofil und assoziierte Makroangiopathie bei ambulanten Diabetikern: Die Schwabinger Studie zur Makroangiopathie bei Diabetikern. Vasa 11: 111–116

19. Janka HU, Standl E, Schramm W, Mehnert H (1983) Platelet enzyme activities in diabetes mellitus in relation to endothelial damage. Diabetes [Suppl 2] 32: 47–51

20. Janka HU, Haupt E, Standl E (1984) Gefäßkrankheiten bei Diabetes mellitus. In: Mehnert H, Schöffling K (Hrsg) Diabetologie in Klinik und Praxis, 2. Aufl. Thieme, Stuttgart, pp 505–429

21. Janka HU (1986) Herz-Kreislaufkrankheiten bei Diabetikern. Die Schwabinger Studie. Urban & Schwarzenberg, München

22. Jarret JR, Viberti GC, Argyropoulos A, Hill RD, Mahmud U, Murrells TJ (1984) Microalbuminuria predicts mortality in non-insulin-dependent diabetes. Diabetes Med 1: 17–19

23. Kannel EB, McGee DL (1979) Diabetes and cardiovascular risk factors: the Framingham Study. Circulation 59: 8–13

24. Krolewski AS, Warram JH, Christlieb AR (1985) Onset, course, complications and prognosis of diabetes mellitus. In: Marble A, Krall LP, Bradley RF, Christlieb AR, Soeldner JS (eds) Joslins's Diabetes mellitus, 12th edn. Lea & Febiger, Philadelphia, pp 251–277

25. Marshall M (1984) Praktische Dopplersonographie. Springer-Verlag, Berlin, Heidelberg, New York, Tokyo

26. Mogensen CE (1984) Diabetes and kidney function. A comparison between type I and type II diabetes. Medicographia 6: 28–32

27. Mogensen CE (1984) Microalbuminuria predicts clinical proteinuria and early mortality in maturity onset diabetes. N Engl J Med 310: 356–360

28. Panzram G, Zabel-Langhenning R (1984) Diabetes mellitus: Bedingte Gesundheit oder schicksalhafte Erkrankung? Med Klin 79: 282–289

29. Pfeifle B, Ditschuneit H (1986) Insulin reguliert die Synthese des insulinähnlichen Wachstumsfaktors I (IGF I) in glatten Muskelzellen der Rattenaorta. Akt End Stoffw 7: 87

30. Prevalence of small vessel and large vessel disease in diabetic patients from 14 centers. (1985) The World Health Organisation Multinational Study of Vascular Disease in Diabetics. Diabetologia 28 [Suppl]

31. Pyörälä K, Savulainen E, Kankola S, Haapakoski (1982) High plasma insulin as coronary heart disease risk factors. In: Eschwege E (ed) Advances in diabetes epidemiology, Inserm Symposium 22, Elsevier Biomedical, Amsterdam, pp 143–148

32. Rebell B, Helwig U, Past R, Standl R, Stiegler H, Ziegler AG, Schauer G, Standl E (1986) Metabolischer Verlauf bei Typ II-Diabetikern im Rahmen einer „Zentrums-unterstützten" Diabetikerschulung in der ambulanten Praxis. Akt End Stoffw 7: 99

33. Rett K, Wicklmayr M, Mickan C, Dietze G, Jauch KW, Hartl W, Günther B, Mehnert H (1986) ACE-Hemmung beim Typ II-Diabetes: Verbesserte periphere Insulinwirkung. Akt End Stoffw 7: 99

34. Silberbauer K, Schernthaner G, Sinzinger H, Pzia-Katzer H, Winter M (1979) Decreased vascular prostacyclin in juvenile onset diabetics. N Engl Med 300: 366–367

35. Standl E, Janka HU, Dexel T, Kolb HJ (1976) Muscle metabolism during rest and exercise: Influence on the oxygen transport system of blood in normal and diabetic subjects. Diabetes [Suppl 2] 25: 914–919

36. Standl E (1983) Der diabetische Fuß. Med Klin 78: 196–200

37. Standl E, Janka HU (1984) Der diabetische Fuß. In: Mehnert H, Schöffling K (Hrsg) Diabetologie in Klinik und Praxis, 2. Aufl, Thieme, Stuttgart, S 513–528
38. Standl E, Janka HU, Lander T, Stiegler H (1985) Diabetische Mikroangiopathie: Risikofaktoren und Möglichkeiten der Prävention durch gute Diabeteseinstellung. Akt End Stoffw 6: 121–128
39. Standl E, Janka HU (1985) High serum insulin concentrations in relation to other cardiovascular risk factors in macrovascular disease of type II diabetes. Horm Metabol Res [Suppl] 15: 46–51
40. Standl E, Stiegler H, Janka HU (1986) Diabetische Spätkomplikationen – neue Aspekte der Grundlagenforschung. Diagnostik und Therapie. In: X. Interdisziplinäres Forum der Bundesärztekammer, Fortschritt und Fortbildung in der Medizin, Dt Ärzte-Verlag, Köln, S 331–338
41. Standl E (1986) Kardiovaskuläre Komplikationen bei akuter Stoffwechselentgleisung des Diabetikers. In: Gleichmann U, Sauer H, Petzoldt R, Mannebach H (Hrsg) Herz und Diabetes – Diabetes und Herz, Steinkopff-Verlag, Darmstadt, S 61–71
42. Stiegler H, Standl E (1985) Nichtchirurgische Maßnahmen zur Wiederherstellung der Strombahn bei peripherer arterieller Verschlußkrankheit unter besonderer Berücksichtigung der lokalen Thrombolyse. Intern Welt 8: 135–144
43. Stiegler H, Rebell B, Ziegler AG, Standl R, Edelmann E, Janka HU, Lehmacher W, Roth R, Schulz K, Standl E (1986) Risikofaktoren und makrovaskuläre Komplikationen von unausgewählten Typ II-Diabetikern in der Praxis des niedergelassenen Arztes. Diabetes Kongreß Paderborn. Akt End Stoffw 7:106
44. Stout RW (1979) Diabetes and atherosclerosis – the role of insulin. Diabetologia 16: 141–150
45. Stout RW (1985) Hyperinsulinaemia – a possible risk factor for cardiovascular disease in diabetes mellitus. Horm Metabol Res [Suppl] 15: 37–41
46. Viberti GC, Hill RD, Jarett RJ (1982) Microalbuminuria as a predictor of clinical nephropathy in insulin-dependent diabetes mellitus. Lancet I: 1430–1431
47. Welborn T, Wearne K (1979) Coronary heart disease incidence and cardiovascular mortality in Busselton with reference to glucose and insulin concentrations. Diab Care 2: 154–160

Diabetische Neuropathie

F. A. Gries und D. Ziegler

Summary

In this survey we review the results of our recent studies on several aspects of diabetic neuropathy in type I diabetic patients, including the onset, the pattern of manifestations, the natural course, and the role of glycemic control. We provide evidence that a spectrum of subclinical peripheral and autonomic nerve function deficits may already be present at diagnosis of diabetes. The subsequent course of these dysfunctions is essentially determined by the degree of glycemic control: neural function is preserved by near normal glycemic control but further deteriorates under poor control. Such a progression of subclinical abnormalities seems to be of predictive value for subsequent clinically evident neuropathy. The latter may be favorably influenced by near-normoglycemia but improvement can obviously not be achieved in all cases and is mostly only partial.

Based on our current knowledge we suggest that a prevention of diabetic neuropathy over many years is possible by near normal glycemic control.

Einleitung

Neben der diabetischen Mikro- und Makroangiopathie gilt die diabetische Polyneuropathie als dritte wichtige chronische Komplikation des Diabetes. Der Begriff wird mit Selbstverständlichkeit gebraucht und den meisten, die ihn anwenden, scheint klar zu sein, was damit gemeint ist: Nervenschäden, die für den Diabetes typisch sind und mit zunehmender Diabetesdauer häufiger und stärker werden.

Das ist zwar nicht falsch, aber als Definition der diabetischen Polyneuropathie ungeeignet. Tatsächlich ist diese Komplikation nicht leicht zu definieren und diagnostisch abzugrenzen. Sie unterscheidet sich von anderen chronischen Komplikationen des Diabetes nicht nur durch das betroffene Organsystem.

Nosologische Probleme

Während die diabetische Nephropathie sich klinisch monoton präsentiert, in ihrem Verlauf regelhaft bestimmte Stadien durchmacht und morphologisch klar charakterisiert ist, erscheint die diabetische Polyneuropathie unter einer Fülle klinischer Bilder. Alle in der Literatur vorgeschlagenen Einteilungen und Klassifizierungen sind nicht ohne Willkür. Unser eigener Vorschlag bestätigt das [10] (Tabelle 1). Der Verlauf der Polyneuropathie erscheint eher launisch als regelhaft und wird in seiner Gesetzmäßigkeit erst klarer, wenn man die unterschiedlichen Manifestationsformen getrennt betrachtet. Die Morphologie der verschiedenen Stadien und Formen der diabetischen Polyneuropathie ist nicht eindeutig charakterisiert, und vielfältig bunt. Daraus ergeben sich weitere Probleme.

Definitorische und folglich diagnostische Schwierigkeiten resultieren aber auch aus der offenbar uneinheitlichen Pathogenese. Die Abhängigkeit von der Diabetesdauer legt einen Bezug zur diabetischen Stoffwechselstörung nahe [12]. Aber dieser ist offensichtlich komplex.

Folgt man den Modellvorstellungen von Greene, der die pathogenetischen Mechanismen zu einem logischen System fügen konnte [5, 6], so sollte die diabetische Polyneuropathie als eine Systemerkrankung verstanden werden können. Dieser Vorstellung entsprechen in der Klinik am ehesten die symmetrische distale Polyneuropathie und die autonome Neuropathie (Nr. 1 und 4 der Tabelle 1).

Demgegenüber sind Mononeuropathien, die unter dem Bild der asymmetrischen Oligoneuropathie auch mehrere Nerven betreffen können (Nr. 2 und 3 der Tabelle 1) nur schwer in die Vorstellung einer Systemerkrankung einzuordnen. Sie lassen eher an fokale [3], möglicherweise vasculäre Prozesse denken [2, 4]. Dazu paßt gut, daß sowohl das adhäsive als auch aggregatorische Potential der Thrombozyten bei Diabetikern mit Neuropathien erhöht ist [7, 9]. Diese Gruppe neuropathischer Phänomene, für die die Okulomotoriusparese ein typisches und häufig vorkommendes Beispiel ist, soll hier ausgespart werden und dafür im Folgenden näher auf den Teilaspekt der neuropathischen Störungen eingegangen werden, die sich in das Konzept einer Systemerkrankung einordnen lassen.

Um die distalen symmetrischen und die autonomen diabetischen Polyneuropathien zu diagnostizieren, sind wir auf Tests angewiesen, mit denen wir Funk-

---

Tabelle 1. Klassifikation der diabetrischen Polyneuropathie [nach 10]

1. Symmetrische diabetische Neuropathie
   - vorwiegend distale, sensible oder sensomotorische Reiz- und Ausfallerscheinungen

2. Mononeuropathie
   - einzelne oder wenige Nerven betreffende Ausfallerscheinungen

3. Asymmetrische diabetische Neuropathie
   - vorwiegend proximale motorische Ausfallerscheinungen
     Sonderform: diabetische Amyotrophie

4. Autonome diabetische Neuropathie

tionsdefizite nachweisen. Das Testarsenal für die Peripherie ist relativ überschaubar. Das Testarsenal für die autonome diabetische Neuropathie entzieht sich, auch wenn sich die Auswahl auf die gebräuchlichsten Verfahren beschränkt, einer rasch erfaßbaren Darstellung. In der Praxis gehen wir so vor, daß wir Normwerte bei Gesunden ermitteln, die in einigen Fällen, wie bei fast allen diesbezüglich untersuchten autonomen Funktionen, eine Altersabhängigkeit aufweisen. Werden beim Patienten die Normbereiche unter- bzw. überschritten, gilt eine Funktionsstörung als nachgewiesen. Der Nachweis einer solchen Funktionsstörung bei einem Diabetiker erlaubt allerdings nicht die Diagnose diabetische Neuropathie.

Die Funktionsstörungen als solche sind unspezifisch. Sie können viele Ursachen haben. Da wir in der Klinik bis auf die Histologie des Nervus suralis keine Möglichkeit einer Validierung durch externe Kriterien haben, kann die Diagnose nur per exclusionem gestellt werden, in dem zuvor die anderen möglichen Ursachen für eine solche Störung ausgeschlossen wurden. Hier offenbart sich ein Handikap der Neuropathiediagnostik, das angesichts der Anforderungen, die an die Validierung diagnostischer Tests zu stellen sind, schwer überwindbar ist.

Bei der weitverbreiteten Diagnostik der Neuropathie des Herzens hat Mayer versucht, diese Schwierigkeit durch Anwendung einer Batterie von Tests für überwiegend vagal gesteuerte Funktionen des Herzens zu überwinden, in dem er Konstellationen pathologischer Teste gesucht hat, die bei Gesunden fast nie, bei Diabetikern dagegen gehäuft vorkommen. Gemeinsam mit Cicmir hat er vorgeschlagen, 7 Tests einzusetzen und eine vagale Funktionsstörung dann als nachgewiesen anzunehmen, wenn 2 dieser Tests pathologisch ausfallen [8]. Dies erscheint z. Z. ein optimales definitorisches Arbeitskonzept für die vagale Neuropathie des Herzens.

Wir möchten die diagnostischen Probleme aber nicht vertiefen, sondern mit diesem Exkurs nur verdeutlichen, welche Probleme der Evaluation diagnostischer Verfahren speziell bei der autonomen diabetischen Neuropathie noch vor uns liegen.

Verläufe

Von größerem Interesse erscheint uns, daß sich bei den neurologischen Störungen, die wir als diabetesbedingte Systemerkrankungen auffassen, ein stadienhafter Ablauf abzuzeichnen beginnt, der auch Indikationen für therapeutische Interventionen nahelegt. Für den stadienhaften Verlauf möchten wir ein vorläufiges Schema vorschlagen, das in mancher Beziehung dem für die diabetische Nephropathie ähnelt (Abb. 1).

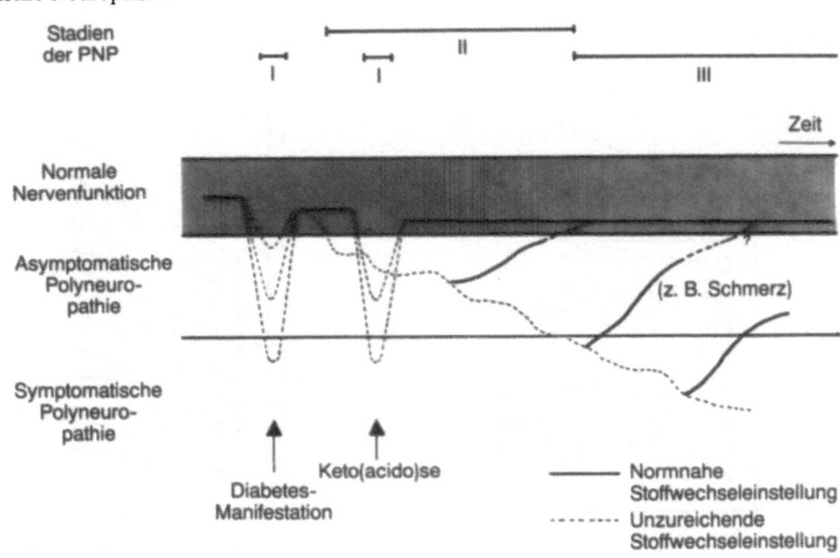

Abb. 1. Stadien der diabetischen Polyneuropathie

Stadium I

Die akute diabetische Stoffwechselstörung und hier offensichtlich nicht die Hyperglykämie, sondern die Ketose, möglicherweise auch die Azidose oder Elektrolytstörungen, führt u. a. zu schweren, jedoch in der Regel bei der Rekompensation des Stoffwechsels rasch reversiblen Funktionsausfällen, wie Petersohn u. Petersohn gezeigt haben [1] (Abb. 2). Dieses Stadium I, welches man auch als akute Neuropathie bezeichnen könnte, kann im Verlaufe des Diabetes wiederholt durchlaufen werden, es ist also nicht auf den Krankheitsbeginn beschränkt. Seine markanteste klinische Manifestation ist vielleicht die Atonie des Magendarmtraktes, die im Rahmen der schweren Ketoazidose regelmäßig beobachtet werden kann.

Stadium II

Möglicherweise als Residuen dieser akuten Stoffwechselstörungen sind bereits bei frisch manifesten Diabetikern – eingehend untersucht wurden bisher nur Typ I-Diabetiker mit klassischem Manifestationssyndrom – Funktionseinbußen nachweisbar, die im statistischen Mittel für fast alle peripheren und einige autonome Funktionen zu signifikanten Einbußen führen: Bis auf die Temperaturdiskrimination am Thenar und die Schmerzschwellen für Hitze und Kälte am Fuß sind alle Funktionen kleinkalibriger Fasern und bis auf das Vibrationsempfinden und die motorische Nervenleitgeschwindigkeit im Nervus medianus alle Funktionen der großkalibrigen Fasern im statistischen Mittel signifikant eingeschränkt [11,

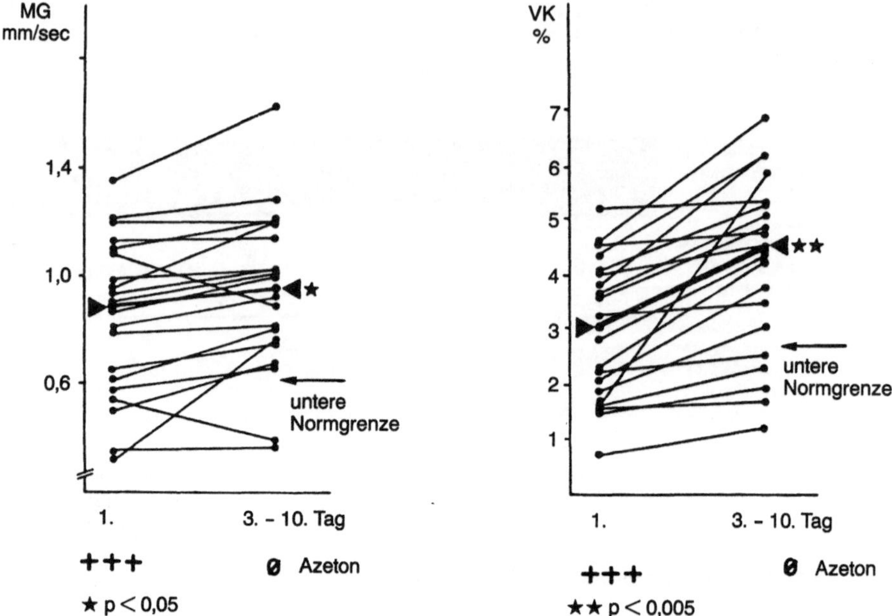

Abb. 2. Signifikante Besserung der Mydriasegeschwindigkeit (MG) und des Variationskoeffizienten (VK) der Ruheherzfrequenz nach Kompensation einer ketotischen Stoffwechselentgleisung [nach 1]

Tabelle 2. Funktion der klein- und großkalibrigen afferenten Nervenfasern bei frisch manifesten Typ I-Diabetikern (Dauer der Insulintherapie durchschnittlich 10,1 Tage) im Vergleich zu altersentsprechenden Kontrollpersonen. (Mittelwerte ± SEM) [nach 17]

		Diabetiker (n = 40)	Kontrollen (n = 48)	p
Temperaturdiskrimination (△ °C)				
	– Thenar	1.7 ± 0.5	1.9 ± 0.5	*NS*
	– Fuß	4.8 ± 2.5	3.7 ± 1.0	< 0.01
Temperaturschwelle (△ °C)				
Wärme	– Thenar	1.9 ± 0.9	1.3 ± 0.4	< 0.001
	– Fuß	4.7 ± 2.8	3.4 ± 1.7	< 0.05
Kälte	– Thenar	0.8 ± 0.2	0.6 ± 0.1	< 0.001
	– Fuß	2.3 ± 3.0	0.9 ± 0.4	< 0.01
Schmerzschwelle (°C)				
Hitze	– Thenar	45.8 ± 3.5	44.4 ± 3.2	< 0.05
	– Fuß	43.5 ± 2.3	44.1 ± 2.4	NS
Kälte	– Thenar	12.7 ± 8.4	15.2 ± 4.1	< 0.05
	– Fuß	14.1 ± 8.3	14.9 ± 5.0	NS
Vibrationsschwelle (μm)				
	– Metacarpal	0.26 ± 0.1	0.30 ± 0.1	NS
	– Malleolar	0.44 ± 0.2	0.39 ± 0.2	NS

NS = nicht signifikant

17] (Tabelle 2, Abb. 3). Bei den autonomen Funktionen findet man nur die Mydriasegeschwindigkeit (Sympathikus) und die Pupillenreflexlatenz (Vagus und Sympathikus), nicht jedoch die Herzfrequenzvariation (Vagus) statistisch signifikant verändert [11] (Abb. 4). Pathologische Funktionswerte der kleinkalibrigen Fasern kann man in Abhängigkeit vom durchgeführten Test in bis zu 27,5% der Fälle nachweisen [17] (Abb. 5), während die Nervenleitgeschwindigkeit als Parameter der großkalibrigen Fasern nur in 12% (motorisch) bzw. 14% (sensibel) pathologisch ausfällt [11]. Bei diesen Veränderungen handelt es sich bereits um chronische Störungen.

Der weitere Verlauf der neuralen Funktionen nach der Manifestation des Diabetes hängt entscheidend von der diabetischen Stoffwechsellage ab. Bei Patienten,

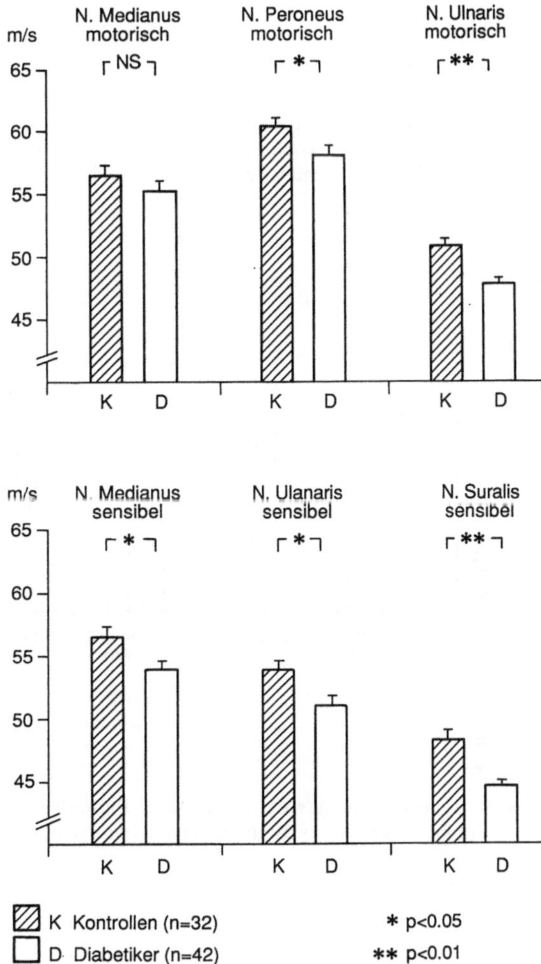

Abb. 3. Motorische und sensible Nervenleitgeschwindigkeit bei frisch manifesten Typ I-Diabetikern (Dauer der Insulintherapie durchschnittlich 18 Tage) im Vergleich zu altersentsprechenden Gesunden (Mittelwerte ± SEM) [nach 11]

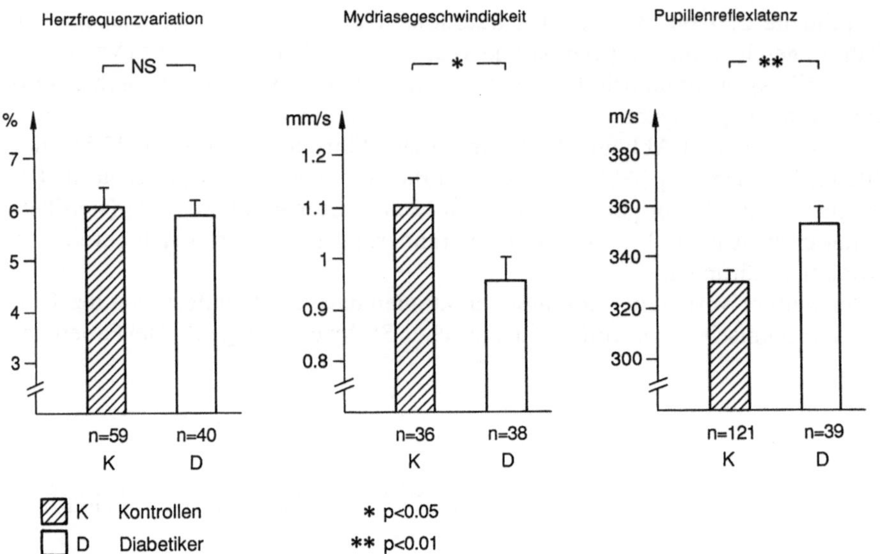

Abb. 4. Autonome Nervenfunktion an Herz (Herzfrequenzvariation in Ruhe) und Auge (Infrarotpupillometrie) bei frisch manifesten Typ I-Diabetikern (Dauer der Insulintherapie durchschnittlich 18 Tage) im Vergleich zu altersentsprechenden Kontrollpersonen (Mittelwerte ± SEM) [nach 11]

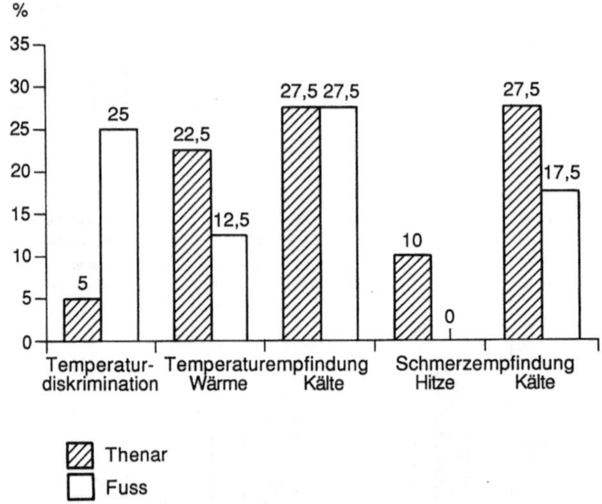

Abb. 5. Relative Häufigkeit pathologischer Befunde (>2 SD über der Normgrenze) verschiedener Funktionstests der Aδ- und C-Fasern bei frisch manifesten Typ I-Diabetikern [nach 17]

deren Stoffwechsel gut eingestellt ist – geprüft wurden bisher Verläufe über 2 Jahre – bleibt die Funktion erhalten. Bei schlechter Stoffwechseleinstellung kommt es dagegen zu einer weiteren Abnahme der peripheren und kardialen autonomen Nervenfunktion (Abb. 6), die teilweise progredient verläuft. Es entwickelt sich mit zunehmender Häufigkeit eine manifeste neuropathische Funktionsstörung, die klinisch zunächst asymptomatisch bleibt [13, 16].

Das Geschehen in dieser asymptomatischen Phase hängt wahrscheinlich von mehreren Faktoren ab, die noch unzureichend analysiert sind. Unter diesen scheint aber die Stoffwechseleinstellung von besonderer Bedeutung zu sein.

Untersucht man in dieser subklinischen Phase Langzeitdiabetiker, so findet man im statistischen Mittel hochsignifikante Einschränkungen aller Funktionen der kleinkalibrigen myelinhaltigen und myelinfreien Fasern mit Ausnahme der Kälteempfindung am Thenar sowie aller Funktionen der großkalibrigen Fasern [15] (Abb. 7, 8, 9 und 10). Auch der Vagus und der Sympathikus sind betroffen, allerdings deutlich seltener als die großkalibrigen motorischen und sensiblen Fasern [12].

Stadium III

Aus dem Stadium II kann sich allmählich eine symptomatische Polyneuropathie entwickeln, die wir als Stadium III bezeichnen. Neurophysiologisch ist dieses Stadium durch eine weitere Abnahme der Nervenfunktion charakterisiert. In unseren Studien bei Patienten mit schmerzhafter Neuropathie fielen besonders die weitere Einschränkung der Temperaturdiskrimination und der Vibrationsempfindung auf [15] (Abb. 7 und 10). Die Progredienz der autonomen Funktionsstörung ist derzeit noch nicht ausreichend analysiert. Ebenso nicht der zu vermutende Einfluß des Alters und peristatischer Faktoren.

Reversibilität

Von großem Interesse scheint uns der Nachweis, daß nicht nur in der Frühphase des Diabetes, sondern auch im späteren Verlauf in den Stadien II und III die Prognose der Polyneuropathie wesentlich von der Güte der Stoffwechseleinstellung abhängt. Wir haben in der Düsseldorfer prospektiven Studie Langzeitdiabetiker, die mindestens eine chronische Diabeteskomplikation am Augenhintergrund, den Nieren oder Nerven aufwiesen, prospektiv untersucht. Es zeigte sich, daß bei den Patienten, die auf Dauer normnahe eingestellt waren, die motorische und sensible Nervenleitgeschwindigkeit in 4 von 6 untersuchten peripheren Nerven nach einem Jahr signifikant besser war als bei den Patienten, die auf Dauer unzureichend eingestellt waren. Dieser Unterschied war ausschließlich auf die Patienten mit pathologischen Ausgangswerten zurückzuführen, bei denen sich die Nervenleitgeschwindigkeit gebessert, wenn auch nicht immer normalisiert hatte [14] (Abb. 11).

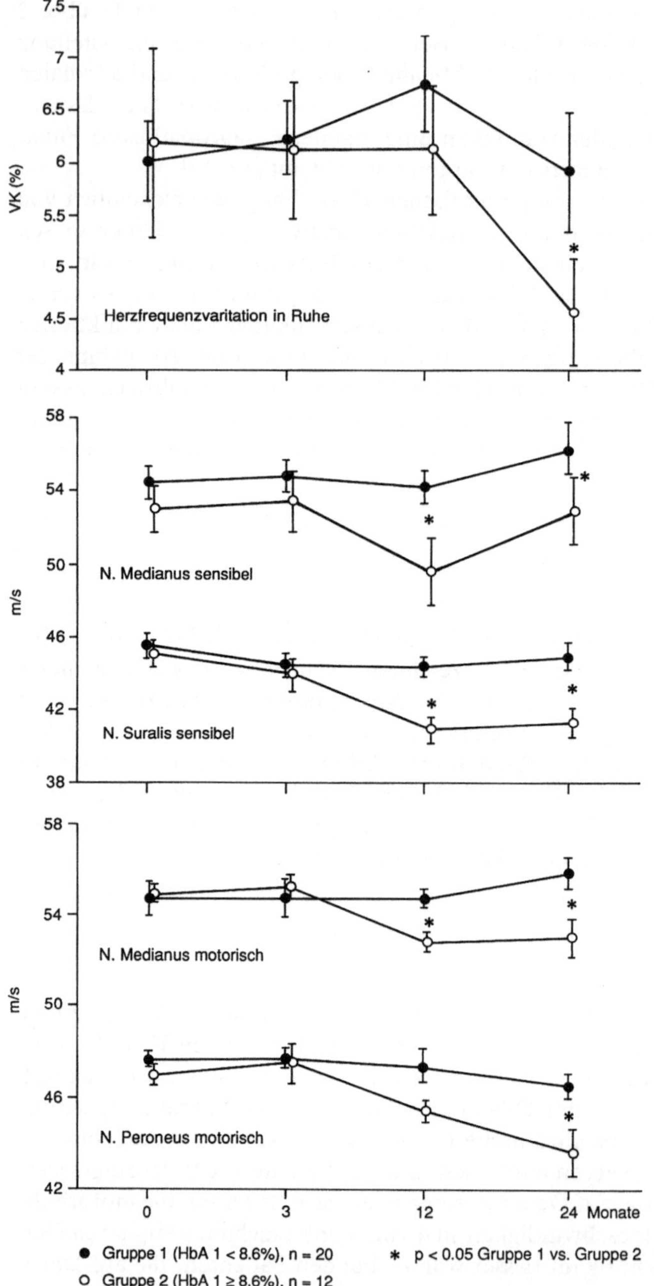

Abb. 6. Verlauf des Variationskoeffizienten (VK) der Ruheherzfrequenz und der sensiblen, sowie motorischen Nervenleitgeschwindigkeit während der ersten 2 Jahre nach Diagnose des Typ I-Diabetes bei Patienten mit normnaher Stoffwechseleinstellung (Gruppe 1; mittleres HbA$_1$ <8.6%; n=20) im Vergleich zu Patienten mit unzureichender Einstellung (Gruppe 2; mittleres HbA$_1$ ≥ 8.6%; n=12) (Mittelwerte ± SEM) [nach 16]

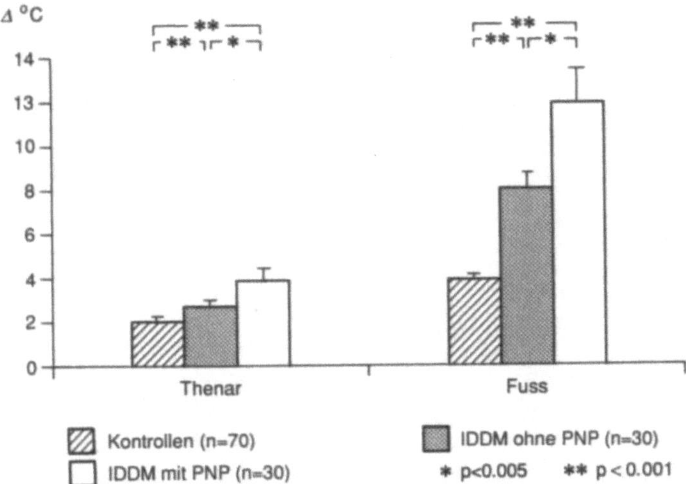

Abb. 7. Temperaturdiskrimination (Schwelle zwischen Warm- und Kaltempfindung) bei Langzeit-Typ I-Diabetikern mit (n = 30) und ohne schmerzhafte Neuropathie (n = 30) und altersentsprechenden Kontrollpersonen (n = 70) (Mittelwerte ± SEM)

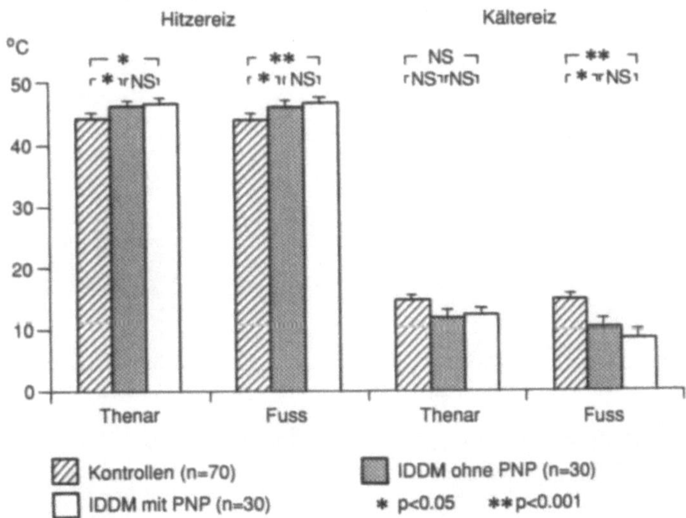

Abb. 8. Schmerzwellen nach Hitze- und Kältestimmulation bei Langzeit-Typ I-Diabetikern mit und ohne schmerzhafte Neuropathie und altersentsprechenden Kontrollpersonen (Mittelwerte ± SEM) NS = nicht signifikant [nach 15]

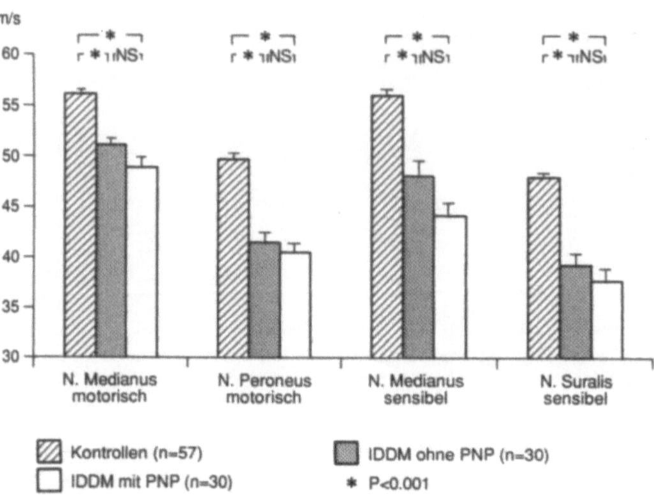

Abb. 9. Motorische und sensible Nervenleitgeschwindigkeit bei Patienten mit Langzeit-Typ I-Diabetes mit und ohne schmerzhafte Neuropathie im Vergleich zu altersentsprechenden Gesunden (Mittelwerte ± SEM) NS = nicht signifikant [nach 15]

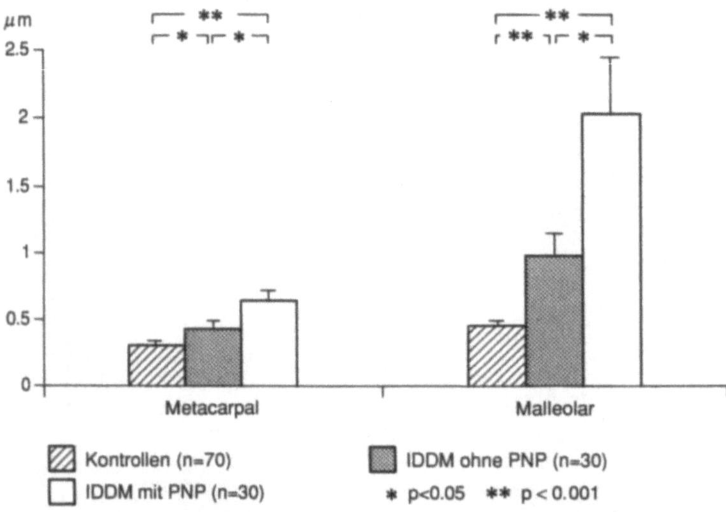

Abb. 10. Vibrationssensitivität bei Patienten mit Langzeit-Typ I-Diabetes mit und ohne schmerzhafte Neuropathie im Vergleich zu altersentsprechenden Gesunden (Mittelwerte ± SEM) [nach 15]

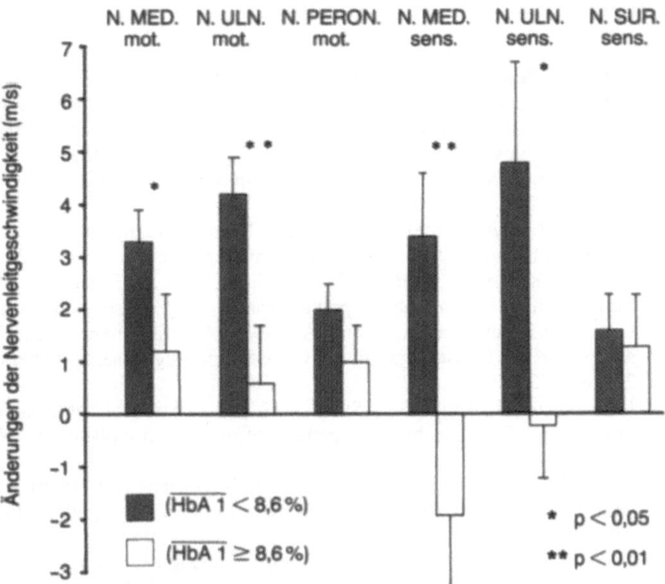

Abb. 11. Änderungen der motorischen und sensiblen Nervenleitgeschwindigkeit (NLG) nach einer einjährigen normnahen Stoffwechseleinstellung (mittleres HbA_1 <8.6%) im Vergleich zur unbefriedigenden Einstellung (mittleres HbA_1 ≥8.6%) unter intensivierter Insulintherapie. Dargestellt sind Patienten mit jeweils pathologischem Ausgangswert der NLG des betreffenden Nerven (Mittelwert ± SEM) [nach 14]

Wir möchten unsere bisherigen Studien so deuten, daß die chronische diabetische Neuropathie bereits mit der Manifestation des Typ 1 Diabetes beginnt. Sie ist zu diesem Zeitpunkt in aller Regel subklinisch, was nicht ausschließt, daß bei jeder ketotischen Stoffwechselentgleisung im Rahmen einer akuten Neuropathie (Stadium I) klinische Symptome auftreten können. Der Verlauf der zunächst subklinischen diabetischen Polyneuropathie (Stadium II) wird entscheidend durch die Stoffwechseleinstellung bestimmt: bei normnaher Einstellung bleibt die Funktion erhalten, bei unzureichender Einstellung kommt es zur Funktionsabnahme. Sie betrifft die großkalibrigen Fasern und vegetative Funktionen an Herz und Auge, wahrscheinlich auch die kleinkalibrigen Fasern. Aus diesem Stadium kann sich das Stadium III der diabetischen Polyneuropathie mit klinischer Symptomatik entwickeln. Sowohl im Stadium II als auch im Stadium III ist durch normnahe Stoffwechseleinstellung eine Besserung der Funktion zu erreichen. Sie gelingt jedoch nicht in allen Fällen und meist nur partiell. Eine Prädiktion über die Aussichten der Reversibilität ist derzeit nicht möglich. Dagegen scheint aufgrund von Verlaufsbeobachtungen eine Prophylaxe der diabetischen Neuropathie durch normnahe Einstellung über viele Jahre sicher möglich zu sein.

Literatur

1. Cicmir I, Petersohn A, Berger H, Petersohn HJ, Koschinsky T, Kashiwagi S, Gries FA (1984) Ursachen der rasch und langsam reversiblen Störungen der autonomen Nervenfunktion am Herzen bei Typ I-Diabetikern. Verh dtsch Ges Inn Med 90: 485–487

2. Dyck PJ, Hansen S, Karnes J, O'Brien P, Yasuda H, Windebank A, Zimmerman B (1985) Capillary number and percentage closed in human diabetic sural nerve. Proc Natl Acad Sci 82: 2513–2517

3. Dyck PJ, Lais A, Karnes JL, O'Brien P, Rizza R (1986) Fiber loss is primary and multifocal in sural nerves in diabetic polyneuropathy. Ann Neurol 19: 425–439

4. Dyck PJ, Karnes JL, O'Brien P, Okazaki H, Lais A, Engelstad J (1986) The spatial distribution of fiber loss in diabetic polyneurpathy suggests ischemia. Ann Neurol 19: 440–449

5. Greene DA, Lattimer SA, Sima AAF (1988) Are disturbances of sorbitol, phosphoinositide, and Na$^+$-K$^+$-AT Pase regulation involved in pathogenesis of diabetic neuropathy? Diabetes 37: 688–693

6. Greene DA, Lattimer SA, Sima AAf (1988) Sorbitol, phosphoinositides, and sodium-potassium-ATPase in the pathogenesis of diabetic complications. N Engl J Med 316: 599–606

7. Jennings PE, Dallinger KJC, Nightingale S, Barnett AH (1986) Abnormal platelet aggregation in chronic symptomatic diabetic peripheral neuropathy. Diabetic Medicine 3: 237–240

8. Mayer P, Cicmir J, Gries FA (1988) Optimierung der Computerdiagnostik der autonomen diabetischen Neuropathie (ADN) am Herzen mit Hilfe einer Testbatterie. Akt Endokrin Stoffw 9: 82

9. O'Malley BC, Timperley WR, Ward JD, Porter NR, Preston FE (1975) Platelet abnormalities in diabetic peripheral neuropathy. Lancet II: 1274–1276

10. Wiefels K, Gries FA (1988) Diagnostik der diabetischen Neuropathie. Dtsch med Wschr 113: 1067–1070

11. Ziegler D, Cicmir I, Mayer P, Wiefels K, Gries FA (1986) Peripheral and autonomic nerve dysfunction in newly diagnosed insulin-dependent diabetes. Transplant Proc 18: 1593–1594

12. Ziegler D, Cicmir I, Wiefels K, Berger H, Gries FA (1987) Peripheral and autonomic nerve function in long-term insulindependent diabetes. Diabetes Res 4: 9–14

13. Ziegler D, Cicmir I, Mayer P, Wiefels K, Gries FA (1988) Somatic and autonomic nerve function during the first year after diagnosis of type I (insulindependent) diabetes. Diabetes Res 7: 123–127

14. Ziegler D, Wiefels K, Dannehl K, Gries FA and the Düsseldorf Study Group (1988) Effects of one year of near-normoglycemia on peripheral nerve function in type I (insulin-dependent) diabetic patients. Klin Wochenschr 66: 388–396

15. Ziegler D, Mayer P, Wiefels K, Gries FA (1988) Assessment of small and large fiber function in longterm type I (insulindependent) diabetic patients with and without painful neuropathy. Pain 34: 1–10

16. Ziegler D, Cicmir I, Mayer P, Wiefels K, Gries FA (1988) The natural course of peripheral and autonomic neural function during the first two years after diagnosis of type I diabetes. Klin Wochenschr 66: 1085–1092

17. Ziegler D, Mayer P, Gries FA (1988) Evaluation of thermal, pain, and vibration sensation thresholds in newly diagnosed type I diabetic patients. J Neurol Neurosurg Psychiat 51: 1420–1424

Diskussion III

Vorsitz: R. ZIEGLER

H. Mehnert:
Vielleicht nur ein paar Anmerkungen, daß man die gleiche Sprache spricht. Ich
weiß nicht, ob man mit der frühesten Form der Neuropathie die Erbslöh und
Schrader als Neuropathie bei Diabetes mellitus bezeichnet hat, ob man das vergleichen kann mit der diabetischen Polyneuropathie. Das eine ist doch eine akute
Nervenstörung, die mit dem chronischen Krankheitsbild der diabetischen Polyneuropathie nichts zu tun hat und in gleicher Weise wie durch die Ketoazidose
die Stoffwechselentgleisung, die Exsikkose, die Elektrolytverschiebungen auch
durch Alkohol oder sonst was provoziert werden kann. Also ich glaube, das sollte
man nicht in die Polyneuropathie mit hineinnehmen und dann ist es natürlich
verlockend, was Herr Gries gesagt hat, bezüglich der Gefäßbeteiligung der Neuropathie in ihrer Ursache, Mikroangiopathie. Es gibt ja auch entsprechende Punk-
tionsbefunde von Fagerberg, wonach die kleinen Gefäße, die die Nerven ernäh-
ren, betroffen sind. Aber auch da muß ich sagen, sollte man doch bedenken, daß
die wirkliche chronische Polyneuropathie, also nicht die Neuropathie bei Diabetes, die ich in eine andere Ecke stellte, daß auch diese Neuropathie wesentlich
früher auftreten kann als die Mikroangiopathie, die Retinopathie in ihrer frühesten Form und die Nephropathie aufzutreten pflegt. Also ich glaube, es spricht
alles in allem doch mehr für die metabolische Theorie als die vaskuläre als Erklärung für die Pathogenese der diabetischen Polyneuropathie.

F. A. Gries:
Eine Reihe von Einwänden und Anregungen. Zunächst mal muß man sagen, bei
der Nephropathie hat man ja auch solche akuten Phasen, die auch relativ rasch
reversibel sind. Also die Steigerung des Glomerulumfiltrates ist eine Geschichte,
die kommt und wieder geht, auch bei dem Manifestationskoma hat man eine
Albuminurie und die verschwindet wieder und man spricht trotzdem von Früh-
stadien der Nephropathie oder zumindest wird dieses Konzept weniger von Kopenhagen, aber doch sehr deutlich von der Londoner Gruppe propagiert als ein
Frühstadium. Und die Frage ist natürlich sehr, ob das etwas miteinander zu tun
hat. Aber verblüffend ist natürlich auch, daß bereits bei der Manifestation Störungen nachweisbar sind und wie es dann so ist, wenn eine Arbeit draußen ist,
jetzt inzwischen sind unsere Daten ja schon bestätigt worden, tatsächlich, es gibt
also dieses sogenannte chronische Bild, das Herr Mehnert auch als chronisch
akzeptieren würde, bereits bei der Manifestation. Das zu dieser Sache. Zur zweiten Frage, der vaskulären Genese: Natürlich denke ich für die metabolische

Genese spricht alles bei diesen Systemerkrankungen, aber wie will man denn eine proximale asymmetrische, womöglich amyotrophische Störung, die jeder Neurologe beim Diabetiker als diabetische Schwerpunktneuropathie oder patchitype oder was auch immer da an Vokabeln fällt, diagnostiziert, wie möchte man die dann gerne in so eine Systemerkrankung einordnen. Ich denke, da kommt eben doch das Vaskuläre zum Tragen. Es spielt eine große Rolle unabhängig von Fagerberg und seinen Kapillarschäden, die er dann mit dem Stoffwechsel der Schwann'schen Zelle in Verbindung bringt. Das mag alles sein, aber ich denke, hier spielt auch noch etwas anderes eine Rolle, wahrscheinlich im Sinne einer Mikroangiopathie. Diese Neuropathien sind ja auch fast nicht reversibel, die sind extrem chronisch, im Gegensatz etwa zur Oculomotoriusparese. Dies ist also für mich ein sehr sehr buntes vielfältiges Feld, über das ich mit Absicht nicht sprechen wollte, weil ich denke, daß man es noch gar nicht in den Griff bekommt, sondern ich wollte jetzt von der autonomen und von der distalen symmetrischen Neuropathie sprechen, von der ich meine, daß dieser phasenhafte Verlauf regelmäßig nachweisbar ist.

H Mehnert:

Aber gerade die proximale, vorwiegend motorische Form, ist ja häufig reversibel. Aber das spräche doch sehr gegen die vaskuläre Komponente, die etwas Chronifiziertes, Dauerhaftes darstellt.

F. A. Gries:

Wir haben ja Revaskularisation, wir haben Umgehungskreisläufe. Warum sollten wir es nicht haben.

H. Mehnert:

Ob bei einem so ausgeprägten Krankheitsbild eine ganze Muskelgruppe befallen ist, das kann ich mir nicht vorstellen.

F. A. Gries:

Was schlagen Sie für eine Pathogenese vor?

H. Mehnert:

Die metabolische Pathogenese.

R. Ziegler:

Vielleicht können wir uns noch der einen oder anderen Frage widmen. Es tut mir leid, damit es nicht wirklich eine Überdiskussion einzelner Punkte wird.

F. Melani:

Wie kann man sich eine Mononeuropathie erklären. Durch vaskuläre oder metabolische Vorgänge?

F. A. Gries:

Vaskulär, z.B. durch Thromben, durch thrombozytäre Prozesse, die sich auch wieder auflösen können. Das ist ja schon seit mindestens 15 Jahren in der Literatur bekannt, daß man Thrombusaggregate findet und die können sich zweifellos wieder auflösen und dann kann eine vorübergehende Störung sich auch wieder regenerieren. Wenn man solche Biopsien im Tierexperiment ansieht, dann sieht man ja Remyelinisierungsprozesse, man sieht ein sprouting auch der Schwann'schen Zelle mit ihren Myelinscheiden und warum sollte so eine fokale Läsion nicht im Laufe von Wochen oder Monaten zurückgehen. Das ist etwas ganz anderes, als wenn ich einen ganzen Nerv zerstört habe oder eben der ganze Nerv metabolisch geschädigt ist und keine regenerative Kraft mehr hat. Also ähnlich wie bei der Neuropraxie, da kann ich ja auch Erholungsprozesse sehen.

R. Ziegler:
Meine Damen und Herren, zu meinem Bedauern möchte ich an diesem erfreulichen Punkte des Widerspruchs, der besonders der jüngeren Generation Ansätze für neue Forschungen bietet, unterbrechen, damit das Programm nicht ganz ins Schleudern kommt. Ich danke sehr den Rednern.

Pancreas and Islet Transplantation

Pancreatic Transplantation

C. F. BARKER, J. F. MARKMANN, D. C. DAFOE, L. J. PERLOFF, and A. NAJI

Zusammenfassung

Gegenwärtig werden ungefähr dreihundert Pankreastransplantationen pro Jahr durchgeführt, jeweils etwa die Hälfte hiervon in Europa und in Nordamerika. Die Ergebnisse haben sich innerhalb des letzten Jahrzehnts beachtlich verbessert und beginnen sich denen anderer Organtransplantationen zu nähern. Die Einjahresüberlebenschancen der zwischen 1986 und 1988 durchgeführten Fälle liegt bei 56 %, während sie für die Pankreastransplantationen zwischen 1978 und 1982 bei nur 20 % lag. Der letzte Bericht über die Fälle der Universität von Minnesota ist sehr ermutigend, wonach ein drei Jahre lang funktionierendes Pankreastransplantat ein Fortschreiten der diabetischen Retinopathie verhindert [32].

Introduction

It is a privilege and pleasure to be invited to contribute to this symposium and book honoring Dr. Konrad Federlin. Dr. Federlin is an outstanding investigator in the diabetes field and also a pioneer in islet transplantation who has been contributing to international symposia at least since 1974 when he presented his work at the first islet transplant symposium of the Transplantation Society [1]. A few years later during a visit to Philadelphia Konrad told me of his family connection with my city and he and our wives visited his uncles grave near Philadelphia. Since that time we have often exchanged ideas and advice on research projects and even have exchanged residents. Dr. Manfred Woehrle, who spoke earlier in this symposium, was sent by Dr. Federlin to work in our laboratories and in 1984–1985 was a very productive member of our group before returning to Giessen for further research training, and now clinical training, in Dr. Federlin's department.

Clinical Transplantation of the Pancreas

In discussing the current results in clinical pancreas transplantation, I will draw heavily on data on 1394 pancreas transplants which have been collected over a 22-year period from centers all over the world by Dr. David Sutherland of the University of Minnesota [33]. About half of these cases were from Europe and half from North America. Dr. Sutherland is the professional descendent in this field of Drs. William Kelly and Richard Lillehei, who in 1966 at Minnesota performed the first human pancreas transplant [15]. I will deal first with those technical aspects of the procedure which are thought to be influential in determining outcome:

(a) segmental vs. whole-pancreas transplants;
(b) inclusion of the spleen as a composite graft with the pancreas;
(c) various methods of handling the pancreatic duct and the exocrine secretions;
(d) methods and time of preservation.

Following this i will consider the biological factors, such as:

(a) tissue matching;
(b) immunosuppression;
(c) simultaneous pancreas and kidney transplants vs. sequential transplantation of the two organs vs. transplantation of the pancreas alone.

As we will see, the distinction of technical from biological factors is not simple since several of the technical factors appear to have a definite biological impact.

Technical Factors in Pancreas Transplantation

Technical factors were formerly considered the most important determinants of the outcome of the procedure.

Segmental vs. Whole Pancreas. The first consideration is whether to utilize only a portion of the pancreas or the entire pancreas (with or without an associated portion of duodenum). Factors which are possibly influential in the comparative results of segmental and whole pancreas transplants are:

(a) the amount of islet mass transplanted;
(b) the magnitude of blood flow to the transplant;
(c) donor availability

The difference in number of islets transplanted in a half as compared with a whole pancreas might seem unimportant since only 10% of normal islet mass should be sufficient to produce normoglycemia. However, since episodes of rejection may destroy some islets but eventually be reversed without loss of the entire graft there is a rationale for transplanting as many islets as possible.

It is evident that a whole-pancreas graft would have greater and thus more rapid blood flow than a smaller hemipancreas graft. This may be an important consideration since the pancreas is considered to have low and thus sluggish blood flow compared to other organs, such as the kidney [34]. This may be the underlying cause of the most frequent technical complication of pancreas transplantation, i.e., thrombosis of the graft's blood vessels in the early post-operative period which has been reported to occur in 12% of all cases. Thus, use of the whole pancreas might be advantageous in preventing thrombosis.

It has recently become evident that the most important aspect of the segmental vs. whole pancreas controversy is a practical rather than a the oretical one: donor availability. For the segmental or hemipancreas graft the splenic artery and vein are the donor vessels utilized. There is no competition for these vessels when the donor's other abdominal organs (i.e., the liver) are also to be transplanted. However, when a whole pancreas transplant is contemplated the portal vein, celiac axis (and superior mesenteric artery) and a Carrel patch of aorta are the donor vessels used for revascularization [34]. In this case, there is a major conflict with the liver transplant surgeon for the donor vessels, since these vessels are also used to revascularize the liver. Thus, it may be difficult or impossible to use both pancreas and liver from the same donor, at least without a reconstructive procedure on the pancreatic graft's vasculature. Although this is usually technically feasible, there is continued debate as to whether both liver and pancreas from the same donor should be used. The current outcome of this conflict is often the loss of a donor pancreas, which thus becomes an important consideration in selection of the segmental or whole-pancreas technique.

Surprisingly, despite these interesting theoretical and practical considerations, when one examines the results of the international experience as reported to Dr. Sutherland's registry, there appears to be no significant difference in the outcome of segmental and whole-pancreas grafts (46% vs. 47% 1-year graft survival) [33]. In recent years most United States centers have employed whole-pancreas grafts while in Europe the largest experience has been with segmental grafts. The present registry data indicate that with either technique there is about a 50% chance of pancreatic allograft function after 1 year.

Composite Pancreas-Spleen Transplants. Another interesting consideration is whether to transplant the donor spleen along with the pancreas. Such a composite graft would have an increased blood flow which might discourage thrombosis. The possibility that cellular elements of the splenic component might lead to a chimeric state and specific host unresponsiveness is an attractive theoretical possibility. However, splenic cells are highly immunogenic and, since they are also immunologically competent, could cause graft vs. host disease, a reported consequence of splenic transplantation. Dafoe et al. at the University of Michigan irradiated the donor spleen, finding that this prevented graft vs. host disease [7]. It is difficult to balance the positive and negative theoretical considerations of including the spleen with pancreas grafts. However, the international registry indicates quite clearly that the outcome was worse (by 20% at 1 year) when the spleen was included. Thus it presently seems unwise to do so.

Considerations Relating to Acinar Pancreas and Secretions. Factors relating to the pancreatic duct and pancreatic exocrine secretions have been considered to be the most important technical aspect of the operation and possibly the most important overall determinants of outcome. Ther are three general methods of handling the duct: drainage into the gastrointestinal tract; ductal obliteration; and drainage into the genitourinary system. Drainage into the gut has the important advantage that the alkaline pancreatic secretions are drained physiologically, allowing appropriate reabsorption of fluid and electrolytes. In the case of drainage into the urinary tract, acidosis requires administration of bicarbonate and is occasionally so sever that conversion to gut drainage is necessary. However, a major disadvantage of the gut drainage is opening the unsterile bowel in an immunosuppressed patient, which has been associated with an increased incidence of infection.

Ductal obliteration, a method commonly used in Europe, especially by the group at Lyons, is accomplished by inoculation of a polymer which, after filling the entire ductal system, hardens [10]. This appears to be the safest method since it results in fibrosis of exocrine tissue and is rarely if ever associated with fistula formation or electrolyte imbalance. Sterility is maintained since neither the donor nor the recipient gut is entered. It has the disadvantage that the fibrotic process induced for the purpose of destroying the exocrine pancreas may also damage islet tissue. It has been suggested that this is the cause of late graft failures which have been reported with this method. Dubernard and others, however, maintain that the incidence of either early or late failure from fibrosis of islets is rare [9].

The most popular technique presently, at least in the United States, is drainage of the pancreatic juice into the urinary tract. This strategy was advocated initially by Gleidman et al., who described a pancreatic duct to ureter anastomosis [12]. More recently it has been achieved with greater ease and success by drainage directly into urinary bladder. This can be accomplished by a pancreatic duct to bladder anastomosis, but usually utilizes a short segment of the duodenum transplanted along with the pancreas and anastomosed to the bladder [31]. Bladder drainage has the advantage of maintaining sterility and fistula formation is rare. The method has the disadvantage noted above of possible electrolyte imbalance.

Possibly the most important advantage of urinary drainage of pancreatic juice is that it allows serial monitoring of pancreatic enzymes which reflect the function of the exocrine pancreas (which usually parallels endocrine function). Detection of decreased pancreatic amylase as an early index of rejection can also be accomplished by draining the pancreatic duct of the transplant with a small catheter as advocated by Groth et al. in their pancreas to gastrointestinal tract anastomoses [13]. In either case, a major advantage is gained by monitoring changes in exocrine function, since hyperglycemia is not a sensitive index of rejection and may not occur until 90 % or more of islet tissue has been destroyed. In this advanced stage, rejection is often irreversible.

In spite of the fervor with which advocates of these various methods champion their causes, examination of the registry data surprisingly indicates no difference in outcome whether the ductal system is obliterated or whether either the gut or the bladder is used for drainage of exocrine secretions [33]. One-year graft survival of grafts done between 1982 and 1988 was 47% for ductal obliteration, 45% for intestinal drainage, and 51% for bladder drainage.

Preservation of the Pancreas. Another technical feature of importance is the *ex vivo* preservation time of the pancreas after removal from the donor and before revascularization. This has been a particularly difficult problem in pancreas transplantation as compared to those of kidney or even liver, presumably because the pancreas is highly vulnerable to ischemic damage. Fortunately, the latest registry analysis indicates that this has become a less severe problem, possibly because of the introduction of a new preservation solution from the University of Wisconsin [8]. Currently these seems to be little if any difference in outcome of pancreas transplants preserved less than 6 hours vs. those not vascularized for more than 12 h [33].

Biological Factors

Biological factors presently appear to be more important determinants of the outcome of pancreas transplants than technical ones. An important biological factor is histocompatibility matching, which according to Sutherland et al.'s most recent data has a significant influence on outcome [32]. A particularly favorable situation is a related donor pancreas transplant when the same donor has previously provided a kidney transplant. However, even with unrelated donors the outcome is significantly better (by about 10%) if four or more A, B, and DR antigens are matched than if not.

Immunosuppression also has a significant impact on the outcome of the pancreas transplants. Regimes which included both cyclosporin and azathioprene resulted in better outcome than those in which only one of these drugs was used [33]. However, it should be remembered that cyclosporin has been used only in the more recent transplants and since these may have had better results for reasons other than immunosuppresion, the true impact of the cyclosporin may be difficult to assess in the absence of randomized studies.

The biological factor which presently appears to be of greatest importance is whether or not a kidney is transplanted into the recipient simultaneously with the pancreas. The simultaneous kidney-pancreas transplant fares better (53% 1-year graft survival) than other groups including those patients who have previously received a successful kidney transplant (40%) [33]. The worst results by far are in those patients whose diabetes has not caused renal disease and who therefore received only a pancreas transplant (32% 1-year graft survival). There are several possible causes of this interesting finding. The first is that the immunosuppressive effects of uremia are not present in the latter group. Fortunately, this group also has the lowest mortality, making easier the justification of pancreatic transplantation in patients without severe vascular complications, such as nephropathy. Incidentally, although the graft survival is presently worst in this group, the rationale for transplantation prior to the onset of severe complications is attractive, since there is little evidence so far that vascular complications can be reversed by transplantation, once they are established.

An advantage of the simultaneous pancreas and kidney transplant wich may account for the best results being obtained in this group is the opportunity to monitor renal transplant function. Thus, early rejection of the pancreas may be diagnosed on the basis of increased creatinine or biopsy of the kidney graft, although rejection of kidney and pancreas are not always concurrent. Whatever the cause for the better results with simultaneous kidney and pancreas transplants, the superiority of the results in this group is perhaps the most consistent finding mentioned in this report.

Summary of Registry Results

Presently about 300 pancreas transplants per year are being performed, about half in Europe and half in North America. The results have improved considerably over the past decade and begin to approach those of other organs. One-year survival for transplants performed between 1986 and 1988 was 56%, while for 1978 to 1982 it was only 20%. Also very encouraging is the recent report from the University of Minnesota that a pancreas graft which functions for 3 years stabilizes diabetic retinopathy [32].

Experimental Islet Transplantation in Models of Insulin-Dependent Diabetes Mellitus

Although it is not surprising that the early development of pancreas transplantation has been concerned largely with overcoming technical problems, the most formidable obstacles to eventual clinical success of this or any other transplant are bound to be immunological. Therefore study of the immune response to the beta cell has been the major focus of our laboratory research for the last 16 years. Basic studies of this type have been facilitated by utilizing isolated islets or islet cells rather than whole pancreatic grafts in which technical complications and the biological response to the irrelevant acinar portion of the transplant are confounding features. The capability of manipulating of islets in vitro, in ways not feasible for the whole organ, has also allowed us to approach our ultimate goal: allograft survival without the use of chronic immunosuppression. The animal model used for most of the studies summarized in this report is the BB rat [25]. Use of these animals, which spontaneously develop a diabetes closely mimicking the human disease [18], has allowed us to study the immunological aspects not only of rejection but also of the autoimmune process which causes type I diabetes [3, 20].

Isolated pancreatic islet grafts share with most other tissues full susceptibility to rejection if transplanted across histocompatibility barriers [26]. In fact, early work from our laboratory established that isolated islets are even more sensitive to rejection than other endocrine tissues such as parathyroid, thyroid, or ovary [21]. A unique threat to transplanted islets- is- the immune response which has already eliminated the native pancreatic beta cells. The same concern in the case of kidney transplants was shown to have clinical relevance 30 years ago when Murray et al. noted that patients suffering from autoimmune glomerulonephritis were likely to exhibit autoimmune destruction of transplanted kidneys even when rejection was not a consideration, i.e., identical twin donor [19].

In 1979, we first examined whether autoimmunity alone would destroy transplanted islets [24]. Study of this question required an experimental model in which the autoimmune response to transplanted islets could be examined independently of allograft rejection. The system we devised was to render BB rats (known to be the future victims of autoimmune diabetes) immunologically unresponsive to the histocompatibility antigens of prospective islet donors by neonatal inoculation with donor strain bone marrow [23]. Since tolerance was confirmed by permanent acceptance of donor strain skin allografts, donor strain islets were also expected to be exempt from rejection. Thus, although islet transplantation temporarily reversed diabetes, the recurrence of hyperglycemia in these tolerant hosts could only represent autoimmune damage to islets. The results of experiments utilizing this approach in BB rats are shown in Table 1. In BB rats with autoimmune diabetes each of ten grafts was ultimately destroyed. This convinced us that transplanted islets are likely to be destroyed by autoimmunity in hosts whose original diabetes has an autoimmune pathogenesis. This finding has direct clinical importance and also provides a highly reproducible experimental model for examination of independent manipulation of either the donor tissue or the recipient and its autoimmune state.

We utilized this reproducible model for study of the immunopathogenic basis of diabetes itself. Specific questions we addressed were: (1) Do whole organ pancreatic grafts differ in their susceptibility to recurrent autoimmune damage from isolated islet grafts? (2) Is the autoimmune process confined to only transplanted islet cells which express the same MHC antigens as the BB rat recipients? (3) What subtypes of immune cell mediate beta cells damage? and (4) Does altering MHC antigen expression on transplanted beta cells affect their vulnerability to autoimmune attack?

Table 1. Survival of WF pancreatic or islet grafts in BB rats tolerant of WF

Type of allograft	Etiology of diabetes	Allograft survival (days)
Isolated islets	Spontaneous autoimmune	3, 6, 6, 9, 10, 10, 10, 11, 75, 85
Isolated islets	Induced by streptozotocin	$> 100 \times 4$
Whole pancreas	Spontaneous autoimmune	16, 27[a], 82, 100 $\times$ 4
Whole pancreas	Induced by streptozotocin	16[a], $> 100 \times 3$

[a] Died with a functioning graft

Vulnerability to Autoimmunity of Whole Organ vs. Isolated Islet Grafts

Several years after our demonstration that recurrent autoimmune diabetes destroyed islets transplanted to BB rats in only a few days, Sibley et al. reported that an analogous but more indolent process affected whole organ pancreatic grafts in human identical twins [29]. This suggested that a vascularized pancreas graft might differ in its immunologic vulnerabilitiy from that of a freely transplanted islet graft, a question we studied using a model of recurrent diabetes in immunologically tolerant rat recipients [27]. The results of these experiments are shown in Table 1. While each of ten isolated islet grafts was promptly destroyed by autoimmunity, only two of seven whole-organ recipients became diabetic within 100 days. Several explanations of this somewhat surprising observation are possible. First, the two types of allograft differ both in the quantity of islets transferred and in the amount and type of additional nonendocrine donor tissue transplanted. Secondly, the intact endothelium of the whole-organ graft may provide a physiologic barrier that prevents or retards infiltration by diabetogenic effectors. Finally, our previous work leads us to believe that islets have differing vulnerability to autoimmunity depending on their transplant site [2, 35, 28]. Isolated islets transplanted to certain sites such as the subcapsular space of the kidney or the testes may enjoy a degree of protection not afforded by other sites. Islets transplanted within a vascularized allograft may be similarly shielded. All of our experimental results indicate that the intraportal site may place transplanted islets in the most vulnerable location. Whether human islets are similarly influenced by the transplant site is not known but it is of considerable interest to us that virtually all human islet allografts have been placed in the "inhospitable" intraportal transplant site — and that they have all failed.

Is Recurrent Autoimmunity MHC Restricted?

The question of whether autoimmunity in BB rats is MHC restricted evolved from our studies of conventional islet allograft rejection. Because T-lymphocyte activation requires antigen to be associated with self-type MHC products, we had studied whether grafts either MHC compatible or incompatible with the recipient would be equally vulnerable to rejection following depletion of the allograft's native antigen presenting cells. We observed that with depletion of antigen presenting cells, MHC-*compatible* transplants of parathyroid, thyroid, and islets all paradoxically seemed to incite a more vigorous immune response than MHC-*incompatible* grafts [22, 4, 5]. This strongly implied that histocompatibility antigens of allografts were handled in an MHC-restricted manner [30], analogous to the viral antigens employed in the seminal restriction studies of Zinkerrnagle and Doherty in 1975 [37].

It therefore seemed logical to consider whether the yet undefined antigenic determinants on islets, which are the putative targets of autoimmune diabetes, were also dealt with by the hosts' immune system in an MHC-restricted fashion. Table 2 compares the survival of antigen presenting cell-free MHC-compatible

Table 2. Studies of MHC-restricted autoimmunity in spontaneously diabetic BB rats

Islet donor strain	Antigenic disparity	Islet graft survival (days)
WF	MHC-compatible	9, 12, 12, 14, 17
Lewis	MHC-incompatible	23, 39, > 100 × 4
BN	MHC-incompatible	49, 60, 81, > 100 × 2

and MHC-incompatible islet grafts in spontaneously diabetic BB recipients. The prolonged survival of the incompatible BN and Lewis grafts compared with MHC-compatible WF grafts is indicative of an MHC-restricted event [36]. Transposing these findings to clinical consideration suggests that if rejection can be prevented the use of an MHC-incompatible pancreas donor might avoid autoimmune recurrence.

What Immune Cell Type Mediates Recurrent Autoimmunity?

Definition of the immunological mediators of beta cell damage could lead to the development of specific strategies for avoiding autoimmune damage. Our model of autoimmune recurrence of diabetes after islet transplantation lends itself to study of this issue. We recently investigated the effect of a panel of specific immunosuppressive agents on recurrent autoimmunity in an attempt to define the specific cell types suspected of participation in this response [14, 16]. The monoclonal antibodies used were specific for: pan T cells (anti-CD5); class II restricted T helper cells (anti-CD4); class I restricted cytotoxic T cells, CTL (anti-CD8); and natural killer cells (also anti-CD8). In addition asialo GMI, a polyclonal antisera that binds both natural killer cells and CTL, was employed.

Diabetic BB rats which had been rendered tolerant to WF antigens were transplanted with WF islets and treated triweekly with injections of the various antibodies. Treatment with either anti-CD8 or anti-AGM1 (but not with anti-CD4 or anti-CD5) led to permanent survival of islet allografts (Table 3). Thus cells expressing these determinants (either CTL or natural killer cells or both) appear to be crucial to the process of recurrent diabetes. Immunosuppressive regimes directed at these effector mechanisms may prove useful in promoting clinical islet transplant survival.

Does Alteration in the MHC Antigen Expression of Beta Cells Affect Recurrent Autoimmunity?

Modulation of the level of MHC antigen expression is a phenomenon common to a variety of inflammatory states including graft rejection, graft vs. host disease, and certain autoimmune conditions. Bottazzo et al. recently make the intriguing

Table 3. Prevention of recurrent diabetes by immunosuppression

Islet donor	Islet recipient	Recipient treatment	Survival (days)
WF	BB tol. of WF	none	3, 6, 6, 9, 10, 10, 75, 85
WF	BB tol. of WF	anti-AGM1	28, > 100 × 4
WF	BB tol. of WF	anti-CD5	6, 8, 15, 17, 33[a]
WF	BB tol. of WF	anti-CD4	3, 21, 26, 26, 47
WF	BB tol. of WF	anti-CD8	> 100 × 5

[a] Died while normoglycemic

observation that during acute diabetes residual beta cells seen in the islets express elevated levels of class I MHC antigens and also express class II MHC antigens not normally found on the surface of beta cells [6, 11]. These observations prompted the hypothesis that abnormal expression of class II antigens by beta cells may permit them to function anomalously as antigen presenting cells since other cells which express class II antigens (macrophages, dendritic cells) have antigen presenting capability. Similarly, hyperexpression of class I antigens may render beta cells mor vulnerable by targeting them for attack by class I restricted T lymphocytes (CTL).

Pertinent to this question are recent experiments in our laboratory which utilized transgenic mouse islet donors in which beta cell class II expression is constitutive. We found with both in vitro assays and in vivo transplant experiments that the expression of class II antigens was not in itself sufficient to endow islet cells with antigen presenting capability [17]. We also examined the possibility that increased class I expression by islet cells might make them more efficient targets of recurrent autoimmunity. For these studies, we again exploited the model of recurrent disease in tolerant BB hosts (Table 4). Graft MHC antigen expression was increased prior to transplantation by culturing islets in the presence of the lymphokine interferon-γ. We had previously demonstrated that exposure of islet cells to interferon-γ for seven days increased class I expression approximately threefold. Whereas ten control grafts (cultured without interferon-γ) survived for a mean of 18.8 days in diabetic recipients, eight grafts exposed to interferon-γ prior to transplantation survived only 9.0 days ($p < .05$).

Table 4. Impact on recurrent autoimmunity of interferon treatment of transplanted islets

Donor strain	Islet treatment during in vitro culture	Recipient strain[a]	Islet transplant survival
WF	No interferon	BB tol. of WF	8, 9, 9, 13, 16, 20, 21, 25, 33, 34, (18.8[b])
WF	Interferon	BB tol. of WF	3, 7, 8, 8, 9, 9, 11, 15 (9.0[b])

[a] Recipients received 1 ml ALS on day of transplantation
[b] Mean

These findings substantiate in part the hypothesis of Bottazzo, verifying that hyperexpression of class I MHC antigens augments vulnerability to autoimmunity but arguing strongly that class II neoexpression is insufficient to endow cells with antigen presenting capability. Immunosuppression directed at reducing lymphokine-increased class I expression by islet grafts in tpye I diabetics may afford protection from damage by recurrent autoimmunity.

References

1. Barker CF (1975) Experimental clinical transplantation: Pancreas. Transplant Proc 7: 913–914
2. Barker CF, Billingham RE (1977) Immunologically privileged sites. In: Kunkel HG, Dixon FJ (eds) Advances in immunology. Academic, New York, pp 1–54
3. Barker CF, Naji A, Silvers W (1979) Immunological problems in islet transplantation. Diabetes 29: 86–92
4. Bartlett ST, Jennings AS, Yu C, Naji A, Barker CF, Silvers WK (1983) Influence of culturing on the survival of major histocompatibility complex compatible and incompatible thyroid grafts in rats. J Exp Med 157: 348–352
5. Bartlett ST, Naji A, Silvers WK, Barker CF (1983) Influence of culturing on the functioning of major histocompatibility complex compatible and incompatible islet grafts in diabetic mice. Transplantation 36: 687
6. Bottazzo GF, Dean BM, McNally JM, MacKay EH, Swift PGF, Gamble DR (1985) In situ characterization of autoimmune phenomena and expression of HLA molecules in the pancreas in diabetic insulitis. N Engl J Med 313: 353–360
7. Dafoe DC, Campbell DA, Marks WH et al. (1985) Karyotpic chimerism and rejection in a pancreaticoduodenal splenic transplant. Transplantation 40: 472–574
8. D'allesandro AM, Stratta RJ, Sollinger HW, Kalayoolum M, Pirsch JP, Belzer FO (1989) Use of UW solution in pancreas transplantation. Diabetes 38: 7–9
9. Dubernard JM, Monti LD, Faure JL et al. (1986) Report on 63 pancreas and kidney transplants in uremic diabetic patients. Transplant Proc 18: 1111–1113
10. Dubernard JM, Traeger J, Neyra P et al. (1978) A new method of preparation of segmental pancreatic grafts for transplantation: trials in dogs and in man. Surgery 84: 633
11. Foulis AK, Farquharson MA (1986) Aberrant expression of HLA-DR antigens by insulin containing B-cells in recent onset type I diabetes mellitus. Diabetes 35: 1215–1224
12. Gliedman ML, Gold M, Whittaker J et al. (1973) Clinical segmental pancreatic transplantation with ureter-pancreatic duct anastomosis for exocrine drainage. Surgery 74: 171–180
13. Groth CG, Tyden G, Ostman J (1989) Fifteen years experience with pancreas transplantation with pancreaticoenterostomy. Diabetes 38: 13–15
14. Jacobson JD, Markmann JF, Brayman KL, Barker CF, Naji A (1988) Prevention of recurrent autoimmune diabetes in BB rats by anti asialo GMI antibody. Diabetes 37: 838–841
15. Kelly WD, Lillehei RC, Merkel FC et al. (1967) Allotransplantation of the pancreas and duodenum along with the kidney in diabetic nephropathy. Surgery 61: 827
16. Markmann JF, Brayman KL, Kimura H, Barker CF, Naji A (1989) Prevention of recurrent autoimmune diabetes in BB rats by monoclonal antibody. Diabetes 38: 165–167
17. Markmann JF, Lo D, Naji A, Palmitter RD, Brinter RL, Hebrokaty E (1988) Antigen presenting function of class II MHC expressing pancreatic beta cells. Nature 336: 476–480
18. Marliss EB, Nakhooda AF, Poussier P, Sima AAF (1982) The diabetic syndrome of the BB Wistar rat: possible relevance to type I (insulin-dependent) diabetes in man. Diabetologia 22: 225–232
19. Murray JE (1982) Reminiscence on renal transplantation. In: Chatterjee SN (ed) Organ transplantation. John Wright, Littleton, pp 1–13
20. Naji A, Barker CF (1984) Animal models of human type I diabetes. In: Gupta S (ed) Immunology of clinical and experimental diabetes. Plenum, New York, pp 91–112

21. Naji A, Barker CF, Silvers WK (1979) Relative vulnerability of isolated pancreatic islets, parathyroid, and skin allografts to cellular and humoral immunity. Transplant Proc 560–562
22. Naji A, Silvers WK, Barker CF (1981) The influence of organ culture on the survival of MHC compatible and incompatible parathyroid allografts in rats. Transplantation 32: 296–298
23. Naji A, Silvers WK, Bellgrau D, Barker CF (1981) Spontaneous diabetes in rats: destruction of islets is prevented by immunological tolerance. Science 213: 1390–1392
24. Naji A, Silvers WK, Dafoe D, Barker CF (1979) Successful islet transplantation in spontaneous diabetes. Surgery 86: 218–226
25. Nakhooda AF, Like AA, Chappel CI, Murray FT, Marliss EB (1977) The spontaneously diabetic Wistar rat. Metabolic and morphologic studies. Diabetes 26: 100
26. Reckard CR, Barker CF (1973) Transplantation of isolated pancreatic islets across strong and weak histocompatibility barriers. Transplant Proc 5: 761–763
27. Roza A, Markmann J, Braymann K, Fox IJ, Naji A, Perloff LJ, Hickey WF, Barker CF (1987) Isolated islet cells are more vulnerable to recurrent diabetes than vascularized pancreas grafts. Surg Forum 38: 373–375
28. Selawry H, Fojaco R, Whittington K (1987) Extended survival of MHC compatible islet grafts from diabetes resistant donors in spontaneously diabetic BB/w rat. Diabetes 36: 1061–1067
29. Sibley RK, Sutherland DER, Goethe F, Michael AF (1985) Recurrent diabetes mellitus in the pancreas iso- and allograft. Lab Invest 53: 132
30. Silvers WK, Bartlett ST, Chen HD, Fleming HL, Naji A, Barker CF (1984) Major histocompatibility complex restrictions and transplantation immunity: a possible solution to the allograft problem. Transplantation 37: 28–32
31. Sollinger HW, Cook K, Kamps et al. (1984) Experimental experience with pancreaticocystostomy for exocrine pancreatic drainage in pancreas transplantation. Transplant Proc 16: 749
32. Sutherland DER, Goetz FC, Kennedy W, Ramsay R, Steffes MW, Mauer MS, Moudry-Munns KC, Dunn DL, Najarian JS (1989) A ten year experience with pancreas (PX) transplantation (TX) in more than 250 patients at a single institution. Ann Surg (in press)
33. Sutherland DER, Moudry KC, Fryd DS (1989) Results of Pancreas-Transplant Registry. Diabetes 38: 46–54
34. Sutherland DER, Moudry KC, Najarian JS (1987) Pancreas transplantation. In: Cerilli J (ed) Organ transplantation and replacement. Lippincott, Philadelphia, pp 535–574
35. Woehrle M, Markmann JF, Armstrong J, Silvers WK, Naji A (1987) Effect of transplant site on islet allograft survival in BB rats. Transplant Proc 19: 925–927
36. Woehrle M, Markmann JF, Silvers WK, Barker CF, Naji A (1986) Transplantation of cultured pancreatic islets in BB rats. Surgery 100: 334–340
37. Zinkernagel RM, Doherty PC (1975) H-2 compatibility requirement for T-cell mediated lysis of targets infected with lymphocytic choriomeninigitis virus. J Exp Med 141: 1427–1436

Metabolic Effects of Pancreas Transplantation in Humans

G. POZZA and A. SECCHI

Zusammenfassung

Eine Pankreas-Nierentransplantation kann als Therapie der Wahl bei urämischen Diabetikern angesehen werden. Wir berichten über die Stoffwechseleffekte einer Pankreas- und Nierentransplantation bei 23 urämischen Diabetikern. Das transplantierte Pankreas zeigt unmittelbar nach Re-Vaskularisation eine gute Funktion: das Serum-C-Peptid, vor dem Eingriff negativ, steigt an; ein klassischer Stimulus für die Insulinsekretion, Glukose, bewirkt eine dynamische Insulinfreisetzung bei intravenöser oder oraler Gabe der Glukose. Der Blutzuckerverlauf nach oraler Glukosebelastung zeigt aber eine verzögerte Rückkehr zur Normoglykämie. Das transplantierte Pankreas reagiert auch regelrecht auf andere Insulinstimulation, wie Aminosäuren. Die 24-Stunden-Profile für den Blutzucker und die freie Seruminsulinkonzentration und andere Faktoren beweisen, daß eine normale Blutzuckerhomöostase unter Alltagsbedingungen erreicht werden kann mit allerdings einer leichten Hyperglykämie in der postprandialen Phase und einer leichten Hyperinsulinämie während der Nacht. Die Gründe hierfür werden diskutiert. Die Langzeitauswirkungen der beobachteten dynamischen Insulinsubstitution auf die diabetischen Sekundärkomplikationen schließlich müssen noch untersucht werden.

Introduction

The goal in the treatment of insulin-dependent diabetes mellitus type I is the prevention of short- and long-term consequences of metabolic imbalance. This result cannot always be achieved since substitutive treatment with exogenous insulin cannot reproduce the physiologic variation of endogenous insulin release. Several methods have been proposed for achieving strict metabolic control such as multi-injection regimens, continuous subcutaneous insulin infusion, and intraperitoneal insulin infusion, but all these methods require the intervention of the operator: the loop remains open.

The aim of pancreatic transplantation is to provide a source of insulin autoregulated to blood glucose levels: from this point of view, it represents the ideal solution to the treatment of insulin-dependent diabetes. Nevertheless, several problems remain to be solved in pancreatic transplantation.

Historical Background

The first attempt to transplant pancreatic tissue was performed in 1894, several years before the discovery of insulin, by Williams [1], who implanted fragments of a sheep's pancreas subcutaneously in a young, ketosis-prone, diabetic patient. This first attempt was not successful.

The first attempt to transplant a vascularized pancreas was performed by Lillehei and his colleagues in 1967 [2]. They transplanted the pancreas and the duodenum in a diabetic patient, who also received a kidney graft. Only a few attempts to transplant a vascularized pancreas were performed in the following years. A new interest in this approach started at the end of the 1970s [3], when a new and safer surgical method, neoprene injection, and a new and powerful immunosuppressive agent, cyclosporin A, became available. As a consequence, pancreas transplantation became more widespread and an improvement in clinical results was observed.

Surgical Approach

Of the several surgical methods proposed, three of them are currently most widely used. These methods tackle the problem of handling or suppressing exocrine function using different approaches.

1. Injection of polymers. A segment of the pancreas (body and tail) is anastomosed to the iliac vessels. Exocrine function is suppressed by intracanalicular injection of polymers (usually neoprene or prolamine) [4]. This method, first described by Dubernard in 1978 [3], accounts for the increased use of pancreas transplantation in the late 1970s and a reduction of surgical sequelae. Among the disadvantages of this method is the fact that it provides patients with only a segment of the pancreas and that the sclerosis induced by neoprene on the exocrine part of the gland could also affect the endocrine part [5].

2. Enteric diversion. The transplanted pancreas is anastomosed in the normal way to the iliac vessels of the recipient. The exocrine secretion of the pancreas is not suppressed, but diverted into a jejunal Roux-en-Y loop of the recipient, through an anastomosis with a patch of the donor's duodenum (whole pancreas technique). Some groups, mainly the Stockholm group [6], apply this technique to segmental pancreas transplantation, by anastomosing the jejunal Roux-en-Y loop to the segmental pancreas. The latter approach simplifies vascular anastomosis. Among the disadvantages of this technique is the necessity for enteric anastomosis, which frequently leads to surgical complications.

3. Urinary diversion. The transplanted pancreas is anastomosed to the iliac vessels of the recipient in the normal way, while exocrine secretion is diverted into the bladder through an anastomosis of a patch of the duodenum with the recipient's bladder [7, 8]. The main advantage of this technique, which leads to exocrine secretion being passed into the recipient's bladder, is that it permits urine amylase concentration to be assayed, which can be useful in detecting pancreatic rejection [9].

Immunological Aspects

Pancreas transplantation is affected by the humoral and cellular immune response, as are all other organ transplantations [10]. As a consequence, a lower HLA mismatch is required to reduce the risk of rejection. The International Pancreas Transplantation Registry reports that 1-year graft survival rates were higher in patients sharing four to six HLA-A, -B, and -DR antigens with the donor (58%) than in patients sharing zero to three antigens (48%) [11]. These results were further improved when only the DR locus was considered (0 mismatch 71% versus 1–2 mismatch 45%), showing the importance of HLA-DR for pancreas transplantation. Nevertheless, some centers prefer to transplant only on the basis of patients' ABO blood group compatibility, since finding a high HLA match could mean a long period on a waiting list for the patients which would entail progressive deterioration of their clinical condition. As previously reported, the introduction of cyclosporin A led to an improvement in results of pancreas transplantation. The best results were achieved with combined administration of cyclosporin, azathioprine, and steroids (triple therapy). A further improvement was observed when antilymphocyte globulins or monoclonal antibodies (OKT3) were used for prophylactic immunosuppression [11].

Association with Kidney Transplantation

Survival rates are significantly higher if a pancreas and a kidney are transplanted simultaneously in uremic recipients than if pancreas transplantation is performed alone (1-year graft survival rate 58% vs 31%). The reasons for these results are probably related to several factors, mainly the possibility of treating pancreatic rejection at a preclinical stage while kidney rejection is being treated.

Metabolic Results

The transplanted pancreas functions well immediately after vascularization: serum C peptide, not detectable well before surgery, reaches 15 ng/ml 30 min after pancreas revascularization (Fig. 1) [12].

Complete insulin independence is achieved a few weeks after surgery. A classical insulinogenic stimulus such as glucose elicits prompt insulin release, with a peak at 3 min (43 ± 7 μU/ml) when glucose is administered i.v. and at 60 min (34 ± 7 μU/ml) when glucose is administered orally. The blood glucose response to oral glucose is a delay in the restoration of euglycemia (147 ± 17 mg/dl), reached at 180 min rather than at 120 min as in normal subjects (Figs. 2, 3) [13, 14].

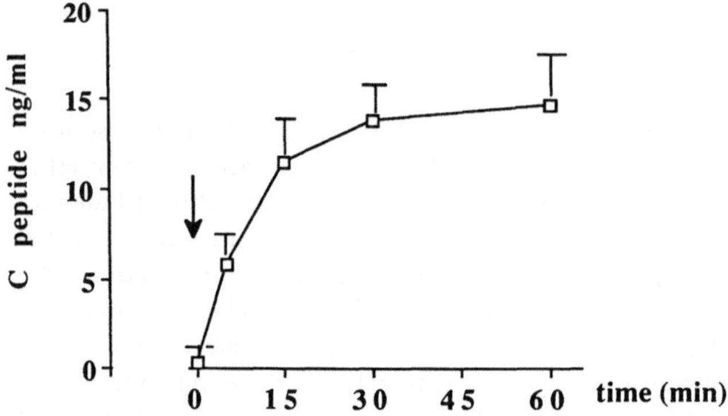

Fig. 1. Serum C peptide levels in 23 diabetic patients after revascularization of the transplanted pancreas

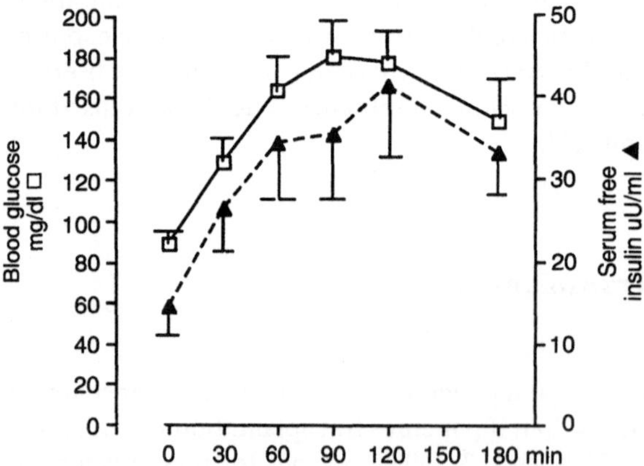

Fig. 2. Oral glucose tolerance test in 14 diabetic patients 3 months after a successful kidney and pancreas transplantation

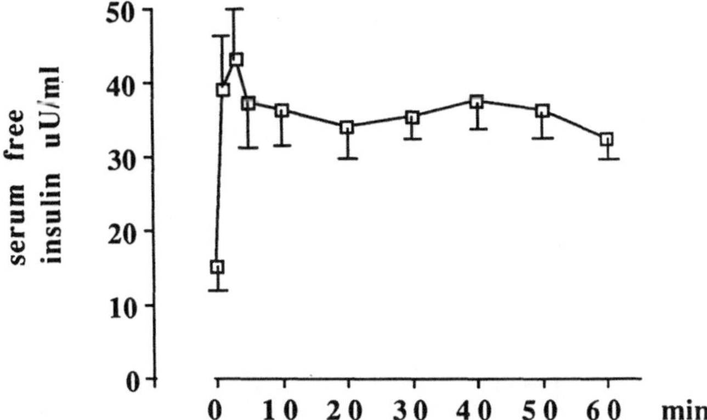

Fig. 3. Intravenous glucose tolerance test in 14 diabetic patients 3 months after a successful kidney and pancreas transplantation

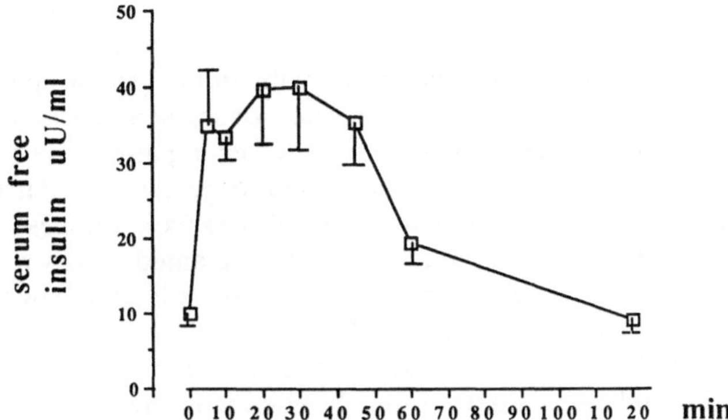

Fig. 4. Arginine infusion test in seven diabetic patients 3 months after successful kidney and pancreas transplantation

The transplanted pancreas also responds correctly to insulinogenic stimuli other than glucose, such as amino acids or oral hypoglycemic agents, as demonstrated by the arginine test (Fig. 4) which leads to biphasic insulin release, and by the tolbutamide test [13]. The 24-h metabolic profile for blood glucose, serum-free insulin, blood lactate, and β-OH-butyrate shows that normal glucose homeostasis is reached in everyday life, with mild hyperglycemia in the postprandial period (144 ± 11 mg/dl at 2 P M and 180 ± 17 mg/d lat 7 P M) and mild hyperinsulinemia: during the night (26 ± 5 μU/ml at 12 P M) (Fig. 5) [15].

The minor metabolic abnormalities observed, such as impaired glucose tolerance and mild hyperinsulinemia in the fasting state, can be explained by the fact

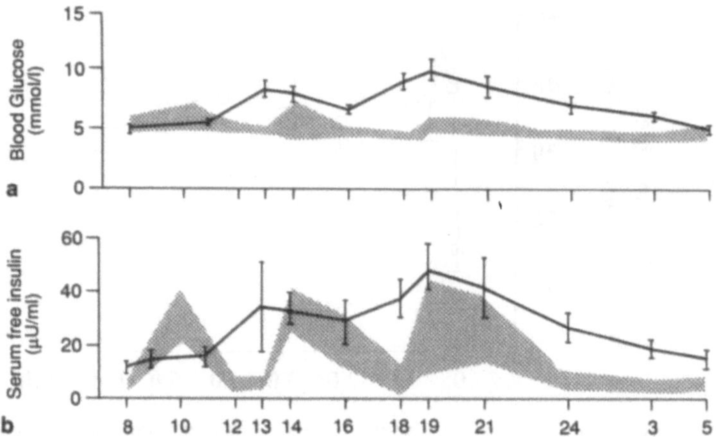

Fig. 5a, b. 24-h metabolic profile for **a** blood glucose and **b** serum-free insulin in 14 diabetic patients after a successful kidney and pancreas transplantation

that the majority of these investigations were performed in patients receiving a segmental pancreas. It was reported that the reduction of β-cell mass can lead to impaired glucose tolerance in animals. In fact, studies performed comparing the metabolic results achieved with whole or segmental pancreas showed that the rate of impaired glucose tolerance was lower in patients receiving a whole pancreas than in patients receiving a segmental pancreas [16]. Furthermore, the transplaneted pancreas is denervated and releases its hormones in the peripheral rather than in the portal circulation. The transplanted α-cells respond correctly to glucagonogenic stimuli: such as arginine and are inhibited by hypoglycemia as shown by the insulin-infusion test [17].

Peripheral insulin resistance, which occurs in uremic patients before transplantation and can be studied using the euglycemic hyperinsulinemic clamp, is reduced after pancreas transplantation to levels close to those found in normal subjects; in transplanted patients the mean value is 6.4 ± 0.5 mg/kg/min, in normal subjects 7.8 ± 0.2 mg/kg/min [18].

Hepatic glucose production and oxidation glucose disposal, which were studied using [^{3}H]glucose infusion and indirect calorimetry, were impaired before transplantation and returned to normal values 4 months after transplantation [18].

Effects of Pancreas Transplantation
on Degenerative Diabetic Complications

The treatment and the prevention of long-term degenerative complications of diabetes mellitus represents one of the aims of the therapy of this disease. Pancreatic transplantation, leading to near normalization of the metabolic milieu, could represent an ideal method for preventing degenerative complications. Several studies were performed on patients receiving a pancreas graft but no definitive conclusions were reached.

As regards diabetic retinopathy, no study has shown an improvement in the ocular lesions, while several studies have shown either progression or stabilization, mainly dependent on the degree of retinopathy at the moment of transplantation [19, 20].

Neurological complications, in the majority of cases peripheral neuropathy, show an improvement 2 years after pancreaticorenal transplantation. These results, however, seem to be the consequence of the treatment of uremia, rather than of the treatment of the metabolic imbalance caused by diabetes [21, 22].

An important result which demonstrates the strict relationship between metabolic control and degenerative complications and the efficacy of the transplanted pancreas in preventing the development of complications was achieved by studying diabetic nephropathy. In fact, renal biopsies of the transplanted kidney, performed in diabetic patients receiving a kidney transplant alone or a pancreaticorenal transplant, showed that 1 year after surgery early histological lesions caused by diabetic nephropathy were present in the former group, while they were absent in the latter group [23].

Conclusions

Pancreas transplantation accompanied by kidney transplantation can be considered the treatment of choice for uremic diabetic patients. Clinical results have improved in recent years. Metabolic investigations have shown that this surgical procedure can restore glucose metabolism to near normal, although some minor abnormalities are frequently observed. The effects of the transplanted pancreas on degenerative diabetic complications remain to be defined. The studies available gave different and contrasting results. These discrepancies appear to be mainly due to the lack of homogeneity of the patients studied and depend on the severity of the degenerative complications at the time of study.

References

1. Williams PW (1894) Notes on diabetes treated with extract and by grafts of sheep's pancreas. Br Med J II: 1303–1304
2. Kelly W, Lillehei RC, Merkel F, Idezaki Y, Goetz FC (1967) Allotransplantation of the pancreas and duodenum along with the kidney in diabetic nephropathy. Surgery 61: 827–837
3. Dubernard JM, Traeger J, Neyra P, Touraine JL, Tranchant D, Blanc Brunat N (1978) A new method of preparation of segmental pancreatic grafts for transplantation: trials in dogs and in man. Surgery 84: 633–639

4. Land W, Liebe W, Kuhlaman H, Eberhard E (1980) Simultaneous kidney and pancreas transplantation using prolamine for duct obstruction. Transplant Proc 12: 76–83

5. Di carlo V, Chiesa R, Pontiroli AE, Pozza G, Carlucci M, Staudacher C, Secchi A, Cristallo M (1984) Intraductal injection of neoprene to suppress native pancreatic exocrine secretion in humans: clinical and metabolic evaluation. Transplant Proc 16: 736–738

6. Groth CG, Collste H, Lundgren G, Wilczek H, Klintmaln G, Rindgen O, Gunnarson R, Ostman J (1982) Successful outcome of segmental human pancreatic transplantation with enteric exocrine diversion after modifications in technique. Lancet II: 552–524

7. Prieto M, Sutherland DER, Goetz FC, Najarian JS (1987) Pancreas transplantation results according to technique of duct management: bladder vs enteric drainage. Surgery 102: 680–691

8. Sollinger HW, Stratta RJ, Kalayoglu M, Pirsch JD, Beltzer FO (1987) Pancreas transplantation with pancreaticocistostomy and quadruple immunosuppression. Surgery 102: 672–676

9. Van Hoof JP, Leunissen KLM, Degenaar CP, Menhere CCPA, Beukers EKM, Koostra G (1987) Urine amylase and insulin reserve capacity are valuable tools for diagnosing pancreas allograft rejection. Third ESOT congress, Gothenburg 11–13 June 1987

10. Severyn W, Olson L, Miller J, Kyriakides G, Rabinovithh A, Flaa C, Mintz D (1982) Studies on the survival of simultaneous canine renal and segmental pancreatic allografts. Transplantation 33: 606–610

11. Sutherland DER (1987) Pancreas transplantation: an update. In: Alberti KGMM, Krall LP (eds) Diabetes Annual, vol 3. Elsevier, Amsterdam pp 159–188

12. Piatti PM, Traeger J, Dubernard JM, Bosi E, Finaz J, Mongin Long S, El Yafi S, Secchi A, Pozet N, Monti LD, Pozza G (1985) Hormonal evaluation of immediate pancreatic function in simultaneous kidney plus pancreas transplantation during artificial pancreas monitoring. Transplant Proc 17: 346–348

13. Pozza G, Traeger J, Dubernard JM, Secchi A, Pontiroli AE, Bosi E, Malik MC, Ruitton A, Blanc N (1983) Endocrine responses of type I diabetic patients following successful pancreas transplantation. Diabetologia 24: 244–248

14. Secchi A, Pontiroli AE, Bosi E, Piatti PM, Monti LD, Traeger J, Dubernard JM, Gelet A, Pozza G (1985) Effect of different immunosuppressive treatments on the endocrine function of segmental neoprene-injected pancreatic allografts. Transplant Proc 17: 136–140

15. Pozza G, Bosi E, Secchi A, Piatti PM, Touraine JL, Gelet A, Pontiroli AE, Dubernard JM, Traeger J (1985) Metabolic control of type I diabetes after pancreas transplantation. Br Med J 291: 510–513

16. Secchi A, Dubernard JM, La Rocca E, Melandri M, Monti L, Touraine JL, Faure JL, Lefrancois N, Pozza G (1988) Metabolic effects of total vs segmental pancreas allotransplantation. First international congress on pancreatic and islet transplantation, abstract 128, 27–29 March 1988, Stockholm

17. Bosi E, Piatti PM, Secchi A, Monti LD, Traeger J, Dubernard JM, Pozza G (1988) Response of glucagon and insulin secretion to insulin-induced hypoglycemia in type I diabetic patients after pancreatic transplantation. Diabetes Nutr Metab 1: 21–27

18. Luzi L, Secchi A, Facchini F, Spotti D, Staudacher C, Ferrari G, Martinenghi S, Di Carlo V, Pozza G (1988) Effect of combined kidney and pancreas transplantation on peripheral insulin sensitivity in type I insulin-dependent diabetic uremic subjects (abstract). 7th workshop of the AIDSPIT study group, 31. Jan–2. Feb 1988, Igls

19. Ramsay RC, Goetz FC, Sutherland DER, Mauer SM, Robison LL, Cantrill HL, Knobloch WH, Najarian JS (1988) Progression of diabetic retinopathy after pancreas transplantation for insulin-dependent diabetes mellitus. N Engl J Med 318: 208–214

20. Bandello F, Vigano C, Secchi A, La Rocca E, Spotti D, Caldara R, Staudacher C, Ferrari G, Carlucci M, Di Carlo V, Brancato R, Pozza G (1988) Diabetic retinopathy in patients submitted to successful kidney and pancreas allotransplantation. First international congress on pancreatic and islet transplantation, abstract 136, 27–29 March 1988, Stockholm

21. Solders G, Wilczek H, Gunnarsson R, Tyden G, Person A, Groth CG (1987) Effects of combined pancreatic and renal transplantation on diabetic neuropathy: a two-year follow-up study. Lancet II: 1232–1235

22. Di Carlo V, Secchi A, Staudacher C, Spotti D, Ferrari G, Bosi E, Carlucci M, Martinenghi S, Galardi G, La Rocca E, Torri G, Gallioli G, Valeri R, Perotti V, Pozza G (1988) Pancreas and kidney transplantation in diabetic patients: effects on metabolic control and degenerative complications. First international congress on pancreatic and islet transplantation, abstract 135, 27–29 March 1988, Stockholm
23. Bohman SO, Tyden G, Wiczek H, Lundgren G, Jaremko G, Gunnarsson R, Ostman J, Groth CG (1984) Prevention of kidney graft diabetic nephropathy by pancreas transplantation in man. Diabetes 34: 306–308

Islet Isolation and Cryopreservation in Rats and Dogs

R. V. Rajotte, M. G. Evans, G. L. Warnock, and N. M. Kneteman

Zusammenfassung

Wenn Methoden zur Isolation menschlicher Inseln immer mehr verbessert und klinische Versuche häufiger werden, wird irgendeine Art der Lagerung benötigt werden. Kryo-Konservierung würde viele Vorteile bieten: Lagerung in einer Gewebe-Bank, welche gewährleisten würde, daß genügend Inseln zur Transplantation für den einzelnen Empfänger zur Verfügung stehen, Immunmodulation des Gewebes, Anreicherung und Erleichterung des Versandes von Zentrum zu Zentrum. Seit 1976 hat man viele Erfahrungen auf dem Gebiet der Insel Kryo-Konservierung gemacht, mit Gefrierraten von 0.25°C/min bis 75°C/min, die jeweils als optimal beschrieben wurden. Wir stellten fest, daß bei Ratten langsames Einfrieren auf − 40°C und schnelles Auftauen von − 196°C die höchstmöglichen Überlebenschancen von Inseln gewährleistet, wie bei in-vivo und in-vitro Versuchen festzustellen war. Mit diesem Einfrier-Auftauprotokoll können ebenfalls lebensfähige pankreatische Mikrofragmente und reine Hundeinseln aufbewahrt werden. Mit beiden Präparationen kann nach Transplantation eine verlängerte Normoglykämie erreicht werden. Dieses Einfrierverfahren ergibt für Xeno-Transplantate verlängerte Überlebenschancen und reinigt die pankreatischen Mikrofragmente von ungewollten exokrinen Kontaminationen. Diese Erkenntnisse werden nun für menschliche Inseln genutzt. Niedrig-Temperatur-Lagerung von menschlichen Inseln wird in hohem Maß der klinischen Anwendung von Inseltransplantationen dienen.

Introduction

Methods for human islet isolation have improved to the extent that sufficient numbers of islets can now be collected to treat individual recipients (Scharp and Lacy 1985; Gray et al. 1984a; Rajotte et al. 1987; Warnock et al. 1987a; Alderson et al. 1987; Alejandro et al. 1987). To promote an effective islet transplant program, several forms of storage may be needed: cold storage of the pancreas during transport to a center for islet isolation; tissue culture to reduce immunogenicity; and cryopreservation for long-term storage. The ability to store islets in the frozen state would offer several advantages. A tissue bank containing islets with a wide variety of HLA types could be created, thus providing sufficient islets to treat individual recipients, while increasing the likelihood of matching donor and recipient for HLA (which would be desirable provided that the autoimmune response causing type I diabetes is not MHC restricted). Prolonged storage would allow induction of relative allograft unresponsiveness by renal transplantation, with transplantation of the stored islets from the same donor some time after acceptance of a renal graft (Gray et al. 1984b). Cryopreserved islets that are less immunogenic (Bretzel et al. 1986; Coulombe et al. 1987) and purified of the exocrine contaminants (Evans et al. 1987) could be transported between centers with ease (Rajotte et al. 1981a).

Since 1976 (Ferguson et al. 1976a, b; Rajotte et al. 1977), much work has been done on islet cell cryopreservation, when we showed that frozen-thawed transplanted islets were able to normalize the blood sugar in streptozotocin-diabetic rats. In experiments with adult rat islets, a number of different freezing protocols have been used with viability demonstrated both in vitro and in vivo (Federlin and Bretzel 1981; Bank 1983).

In vitro success with rodent islets has been with both slow and fast cooling rates (Rajotte et al. 1977, 1981a, b, 1983, 1984, 1989; Rajotte and DeGroot 1986; Ferguson et al. 1976a, b; Taylor et al. 1982, 1983; McKay and Karow 1983; Sandler et al. 1981, 1982, 1986; Weber et al. 1983; Bank et al. 1979; Bretzel et al. 1980, 1981; Andersson and Sandler 1983; Sandler and Andersson 1984; Wise et al. 1983, 1985). Postthaw culture was found to improve insulin release (Ferguson et al. 1976a, b; Rajotte et al. 1977; Federlin and Bretzel 1981), while Sandler and Andersson (1984, 1987) have shown similar results for prefreeze culture. Prefreeze culture, however, did not increase survival of the frozen-thawed islets in our transplantation experiments (Warnock and Rajotte 1987).

Cryopreserved islets can normalize the blood glucose after intraportal embolization into syngeneic diabetic rats. This was achieved by cooling the islets slowly to $-75\,^{\circ}$C with slow thawing from $-196\,^{\circ}$C (Rajotte et al. 1977, 1981a, b, 1983, 1984; Federlin and Bretzel 1981; Bank 1983; Taylor et al. 1983). Similar success has been reported when islets were cooled at $2\,^{\circ}$C/min to $-35\,^{\circ}$C, then at $7\,^{\circ}$C/min to $-100\,^{\circ}$C and abruptly to $-196\,^{\circ}$C (Bretzel et al. 1981). We have found that slow cooling to $-40\,^{\circ}$C with rapid thaw from $-196\,^{\circ}$C gave a high survival, with identical clinical response when 3000 frozen-thawed or fresh islets were implanted into the liver of diabetic recipients (Rajotte et al. 1984, 1986, 1989). The recipients of frozen-thawed tissue in these experiments had slightly abnormal, though nondiabetic, intravenous glucose tolerance tests (ivGTT) at 3 months posttransplant. In another study the clinical response and ivGTT was the same when the fresh or frozen-thawed islets were transplanted beneath the kidney capsule (Coulombe et al. 1988).

Cryopreserved pancreatic microfragments can normalize carbohydrate metabolism when autoimplanted into totally pancreatectomized dogs (Rajotte et al. 1983, 1984; Kneteman et al. 1986; Walsh et al. 1987) and partially pancreatectomized pigs (Wise et al. 1983, 1985). We found that 25 °C was important for equilibration of the 2 M dimethyl sulfoxide (DMSO) (Rajotte et al. 1983). Dogs autotransplanted with cryopreserved tissue have been rendered normoglycemic with non-diabetic glucose tolerance for up to 2.5 years posttransplant (Kneteman et al. 1986). Measuring the insulin and amylase content of the graft we found that cryopreservation purified the pancreatic microfragments by selectively destroying the unwanted exocrine tissue (Evans et al. 1987).

Recently, the methods used to isolate canine and human islets have improved to the point where it is now possible to obtain in excess of 110 000 islets from a single pancreas (Warnock and Rajotte 1988; Cattral et al. 1989; Scharp and Lacy 1985; Gray et al. 1984a; Alderson et al. 1987; Alejandro et al. 1987). When pure canine islets were frozen and then thawed they responded to glucose in vitro and were able to normalize the pancreatectomized recipient posttransplant (Evans et al. 1989). Frozen-thawed human islets also respond to glucose in vitro (Bretzel et al. 1981; Jutte et al. 1987; Kneteman and Rajotte 1986; Warnock et al. 1986, 1987b) and survived when transplanted beneath the kidney capsule of nude athymic rats (Warnock et al. 1986).

Methods

The methods used to isolate and cryopreserve canine and rat islets have been reported previously (Evans et al. 1989; Rajotte et al. 1977, 1981a, 1983; Rajotte and DeGroot 1986; Warnock and Rajotte 1988).

Isolation of Pure Islets

Dogs. Mongrel dogs weighing 18–25 kg were anesthetized with sodium pento-barbital 30 mg/kg body wt. The pancreas was mobilized with its major vascular connections preserved, and cannulas (PE90) were inserted into both main branches of the pancreatic duct and via a cut down into the left duct 5 cm from the distal end. The blood vessels were clamped, the gland was removed and weighed. Fifty milliliters of Hanks' solution (HBSS) containing collagenase (type XI, Sigma, St. Louis, MO; 1100 U/mL at 4°C) was injected slowly into each cannula. For digestion, each cannula was connected to a perfusion device and perfused with collagenase solution (6 mL/g of original pancreas weight, 1100 U/mL) at 4°C for 10 min. The perfusate was then warmed to 37°C and perfusion continued until the gland became mucoid (approximately 10–12 min). The digested tissue was cooled to 4°C by immersion in HBSS, then dissociated gently by teasing. The dissociated tissue was washed three times, then triturated through graded needles (14, 16, and 18 gauge). An aliquot of tissue was examined periodically by stereomicroscopy to judge the completeness of islet enucleation. Finally, the tissue was combined and resuspended in 120 mL medium 199 at 4°C. Aliquots of 4 mL were added to 50-mL conical tubes which contained 4.3 mL of Medium 199 (5 ×) and 16.7 mL Ficoll (Sigma, St. Louis, MO, density 1.125). Aliquots of

Ficoll (5 mL each, density 1.085, 1.075 and 1.045) were then layered successively over the tissue suspension and centrifuged at 550 g for 25 min at 22 °C (Alejandro et al. 1986). Purified islets were removed from the 1.045/1.075 and 1.075/1.085 interfaces, washed, combined, weighed, and then suspended in a final volume of 30 mL in medium 199 with 10% fetal calf serum, penicillin (100 U/mL) and streptomycin (100 μg/mL).

Rats. Islets were harvested from 2- to 3-months-old Wistar-Furth (WF) rats. Following collagenase digestion and Ficoll purification, islets were washed three times in medium 199 supplemented with 10% fetal calf serum (v/v), penicillin (100 U/mL), and streptomycin (100 μg/mL), and then transferred to a Petri dish. With the aid of a stereomicroscope, known numbers of islets (100–250 μm) were handpicked free of exocrine contamination.

Islet Cryopreservation

During freezing and thawing, three distinct steps were employed:

(1) a prefreezing phase during which the islets were incubated with the protective additive;
(2) freezing and thawing; and,
(3) return of the islets to a physiological medium.

Prefreezing phase. Following the isolation procedure, rat islets (1000–2000) were suspended in 0.2 mL fresh medium 199 with 25 mM HEPES (Gibco) supplemented with 10% fetal calf serum, penicillin (100 U/mL) and streptomycin (100 μg/mL), while dog islets (10,000–15,000) were suspended in 1 mL of the same medium.

To this suspension, DMSO was added stepwise at 25 °C to a final concentration of 1 M. This stepwise addition is used to minimize osmotic stress to the islets. Following the initial 30-min equilibration in 1 M DMSO, the concentration of the cryoprotectant was increased to 2 M and 15 min allowed for equilibration at 0 °C for rat islets and 25 °C for dog islets. The final 2 M volume was 0.8 and 4.0 mL for rat and dog islets respectively. Following this step the dog islets were placed in ice (4 °C) for 5 min.

Freezing and Thawing. Following the final 2 M DMSO equilibration period, the tubes were transferred to an ethanol seeding bath at -7.2 °C to supercool (5 min rodents, 10 min dogs), after which nucleation was induced. After release of the latent heat of fusion, the samples were transferred to an evacuated Dewar flask (Leibo and Mazur 1978) containing a calibrated volume of 95% ethanol (Rajotte et al. 1981a, 1983). Controlled cooling (0.25 °C/min) was used from -10 °C to -40 °C or -75 °C. The tubes were then transferred to liquid nitrogen for low-temperature storage. Following the desired storage period, the islets were thawed at 580 °C/min (rat) and 200 °C/min (dog) to 0 °C.

Removal of Protective Additive. The thawed tissue was placed in 0.75 *M* sucrose for 30 min at 0 °C (Rajotte et at. 1981a). The sucrose was then diluted by the stepwise addition of an isotonic medium for in vitro or in vivo testing (Rajotte et al. 1981a).

In Vitro and In Vivo Testing for Viability

We used two methods to assess viability after cryopreservation. The first was in vitro insulin release from islets perifused (Lacy et al. 1972) during three consecutive 60-min periods of low (50 mg/dL), high (500 mg/dL) and low (50 mg/dL) glucose. Islets in this group were cultured for 24 h postthaw. The second method was that of transplantation. WF rats were rendered diabetic with streptozotocin (65 mg/kg intravenously) and diabetes was monitored for 3 consecutive weeks. A known number of islets of constant size ($> 100 \mu$m) were implanted immediately postthaw into the liver via the portal vein (Rajotte et al. 1981a, 1983). The animals were examined daily and urine volume (UV), urine glucose (UG), plasma glucose (PG) and body weight were measured weekly.

Mongrel dogs were rendered diabetic by total pancreatectomy. Following islet isolation, defined numbers of fresh or cryopreserved islets were autografted by refluxing into splenic veins (Warnock et al. 1983). Function was assessed by measuring fasting PG using a Beckman glucose analyzer (Fullerton, CA) and compared with that of dogs receiving a similar number of freshly isolated islets.

Results

Perifusion

Figure 1 shows insulin secretion of frozen-thawed cultured rat islets during perifusion. For islets cooled at 2 °C/min to -35 °C and 7 °C/min to -75 °C, insulin secretion rose from a baseline of 0.13 μU/islet $\cdot$ min to 0.2 μU/islet $\cdot$ min after glucose challenge. The first phase insulin secretion was lost and the second phase was smaller than the other four groups. When the islets were returned to low glucose, they continued to secrete insulin at around 0.3 μU/islet $\cdot$ min. When 75 °C/ min was used to -75 °C, the insulin secretion during high glucose rose from a baseline of 0.14 to 0.39 μU/islet $\cdot$ min but the first phase release was lost. During the second low glucose period, these islets also continued to secrete insulin at a rate that reached 0.61 μU/islet $\cdot$ min by the end of 180 min. When 25 °C/min was used to -75 °C, the insulin secretion during baseline was higher at 0.20 μU/ islet $\cdot$ min and again the first phase was lost, but the second phase reached a maximum of 0.50 μU/islet $\cdot$ min during high glucose. During the final period of low glucose, these islets continued to secrete insulin at a rate that reached 0.61 μU/islet $\cdot$ min. When slow cooling of 0.25 °C/min was used to -40 °C or -75 °C

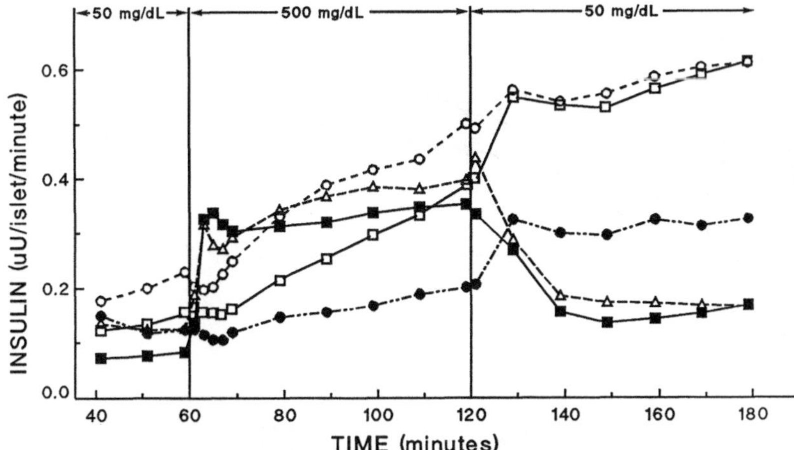

Fig. 1. Insulin secretion during three 60-min periods of low (50 mg/dL), high (500 mg/dL) and low (50 mg/dL) glucose. The groups tested are: two-step cooling of 2 °C/min to -35 °C and 7 °C/min to -75 °C ($n = 12$) (●—···—●); fast cooling of 75 °C/min to -75 °C ($n = 16$) (□—□); 25 °C/min to -75 °C ($n = 16$) (○- - -○); and slow cooling of 0.25 °C/min to -40 °C ($n = 16$) (△- - -△) or -75 °C ($n = 12$) (■—■). All groups were cultured for 24 h postthaw before perifusion

with rapid thawing from -196 °C, a biphasic secretion of insulin occurred. When slow cooling was used to -40 °C basal secretion was 0.13 μU/islet·min, which rose to a first phase of 0.32 and a sustained second phase of 0.38 μU/islet·min during the high glucose. During the final period of low glucose, insulin secretion returned to baseline by 20 min. When this cooling rate was to -75 °C, basal secretion was 0.08 μU/islet·min, which rose to a first phase of 0.38 and a second phase of 0.32 μU/islet·min. During the final period, insulin secretion returned to baseline.

Transplantation

Rats. Figure 2 shows the clinical reponse of rats transplanted immediately post-dilution with 3000 frozen-thawed islets into the liver. When slow-cooling was used to -75 °C with rapid-thawing the diabetic animals ($n = 6$) became partially normalized. PG posttransplant fell from 580 to 500 mg/dL and stabilized around this level throughout the 12-week follow-up period. This slight improvement was also seen in the other clinical parameters, UV and UG. The UV fell from 110 mL/day pretransplant to 70 mL/day posttransplant, but at 5 weeks posttransplant, these animals became more diabetic and returned to their pretransplant level. These animals, however, immediately gained weight posttransplant and levelled off at 280 g.

When slow cooling was used to -40 °C with rapid thawing the 3000 frozen-thawed islets normalized the animals ($n = 9$). By 2 weeks posttransplant the

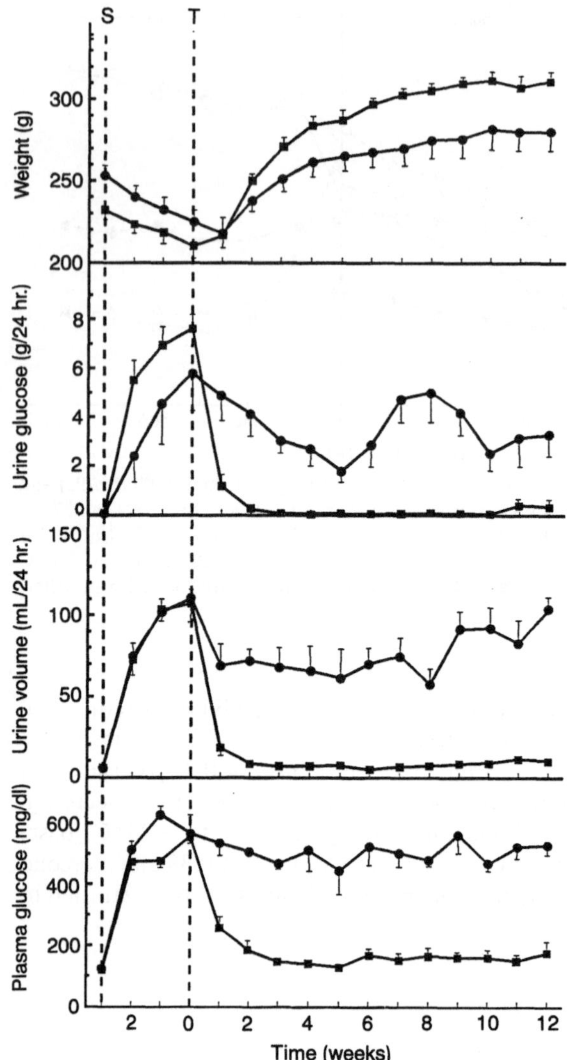

Fig. 2. The mean ± SEM clinical response of diabetic rats transplanted with 3000 frozen-thawed islets, >100 μm diameter, into the portal vein. The groups are: slow cooling to −75 °C ($n = 6$) (●——●) or −40 °C ($n = 9$) (■——■). Both groups were thawed at 580 °C/min. *S*, Induction of diabetes with streptozotocin; *T*, transplantation

animals' PG returned to baseline and remained normal throughout the 12 weeks. The UV and UG also returned to baseline levels. The weight gain in these animals was larger and continued to increase throughout the 12 week follow-up period.

Dogs. Seven dogs received 171 000 ± 10 000 cryopreserved islets (7868 ± 665/kg) while an equal number of dogs were engrafted with 143 000 ± 15 000 freshly isolated islets (6811 ± 653/kg). The mean diameter of islets in both groups was 95

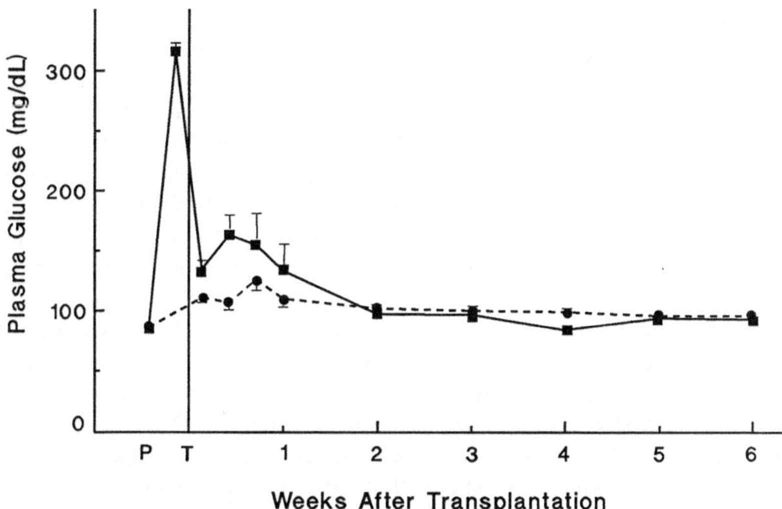

Fig. 3. Fasting plasma glucose of dogs engrafted with cryopreserved islets (■——■) was compared to that of control dogs receiving freshly isolated islets (●– – –●). Dogs receiving cryopreserved islets had higher plasma glucose than control dogs 1 and 3 days following implantation ($p < 0.05$). The frozen-thawed islets were immediately autografted postdilution. P, Pancreatectomy; T, transplantation

μm in a graft weighing 0.4 ± 0.1 g. Cryopreserved islets reversed hyperglycemia promptly with fasting PG of 133 ± 23 mg/dL 1 week postimplantation in six dogs (Figure 3). One recipient of cryopreserved tissue remained hyperglycemic despite receiving 8756 islets/kg and another normoglycemic dog died 3 weeks postimplantation due to complications arising from a small bowel volvulus (PG = 84 mg/dL). All seven recipients of freshly isolated islets were normoglycemic 24 h posttransplantation, with PG of 111 ± 4 mg/dL. One dog became hyperglycemic 14 days postimplantation, while another normoglycemic dog in this group died 4 weeks after engraftment, also due to a volvulus (PG = 103 mg/dL). PG of dogs receiving cryopreserved islets was significantly higher than that of control dogs receiving fresh islets 1 and 3 days postimplantation ($p < 0.05$). Subsequently, however, the PG of dogs receiving cryopreserved islets remained equal to that of control dogs for up to 6 weeks postimplantation.

Discussion

In the last decade considerable work has been done on islet cryopreservation. Valid comparison of previous studies has been difficult because of the large variation in the protocols and lack of detail given. Assessment of islet viability with in-vitro techniques should be interpreted cautiously since islet function in vitro has not always agreed with in vivo function (Taylor et al. 1983; Sandler et al. 1986). We have found that islets cooled slowly to $-40\,°C$ or $-75\,°C$ responded similarly in vitro, but failed to reverse indices of diabetes after implantation (Rajotte et al. 1989). For these reasons we have used transplantation as our main index of viability. With these limitations in mind, insulin secretion by perifusion gives valuable insight into islet viability during the stimulatory and nonstimulatory periods. In this study, islets cooled faster than $0.25\,°C/min$ were incapable of biphasic insulin release and regulation of secretion to basal during the return to low glucose. This indicates some damage, but this may be reversible with a longer postthaw culture period or following transplantation. Slow cooling to $-40\,°C$ in combination with rapid thawing from $-196\,°C$ gave the best response. This freezing procedure has also worked for pure dog islets. The viability of the cryopreserved canine islets was confirmed by the prompt reversal of hyperglycemia in six of seven pancreatectomized dogs receiving autografts. These dogs have remained normoglycemic for up to 6 weeks with function equal to that of dogs receiving freshly isolated tissue. This shows that rat and dog islets subjected to cryopreservation are viable and are able to promptly reverse hyperglycemia after transplantation. Cryopreservation is a realistic method for tissue banking of purified islets of Langerhans.

Acknowledgements. This work has been supported by the Edmonton Civic Employees' Charitable Assistance Fund, the Alberta Heritage Foundation for Medical Research, the Medical Research Council of Canada and the Muttart Diabetes Research and Training Centre. The authors are grateful to Organon Canada Ltd. for their donation of Cotazyme, to T. DeGroot and D. Ellis for their technical assistance and to C. Gardner for typing this manuscript.

References

Alderson D, Scharp DW, Kneteman NM (1987) The isolation of purified human islets of Langerhans. Transplant Proc 19: 916–917

Alejandro R, Cutfield RG, Shienvold RL, Polonsky KS, Noel J, Olson L, Dillberger J, Miller J, Mintz DH (1986) Natural history of intrahepatic canine islet cell autografts. J Clin Invest 78: 1339–1348

Alejandro R, Mintz DH, Noel J, Latif W, Koh N, Russell E, Miller J (1987) Islet cell transplantation in type I diabetes mellitus. Transplant Proc 19: 2359–2361

Andersson A, Sandler S (1983) Viability tests of cryopreserved endocrine pancreatic cells. Cryobiology 20: 161–168

Bank HL (1983) Symposium on cryobiology of isolated islets of Langerhans. Cryobiology 20: 119–245

Bank HL, Davis RF, Emerson D (1979) Cryogenic preservation of isolated rat islets of Langerhans: effect of cooling and warming rates. Diabetologia 16: 195–199

Bretzel RG, Schneider J, Dobroschke J, Schwemmle K, Pfeiffer EF, Federlin K (1980) Islet transplantation in experimental diabetes of the rat. Cryopreservation of rat and human islets. Preliminary results. Horm Metab Res 12: 274–275

Bretzel RG, Schneider J, Zekorn T, Federlin K (1981) Cryopreservation of rat, porcine and human pancreatic islets for transplantation. In: Federlin K et al. (eds) Islet isolation, culture and cryopreservation. Thieme, Stuttgart, pp 152–160

Bretzel RG, Blum BE, Hoel E, Hering BJ, Federlin K (1986) Rat islet allograft survival following different immunomodulative and immunosuppressive treatment. In: Jaworski MA et al. (eds) The immunology of diabetes mellitus. Elsevier, Amsterdam, pp 181–186

Cattral MS, Warnock GL, Kneteman NM, Rajotte RV (1989) Transplantation of single-donor purified canine islets to the spleen or renal subcapsular space with cyclosporine immunosuppression. Transplant Proc 21 (1): 2695–2696

Coulombe MG, Warnock GL, Rajotte RV (1987) Prolongation of islet xenograft survival by cryopreservation. Diabetes 36: 1086–1088

Coulombe MG, Warnock GL, Rajotte RV (1988) Reversal of diabetes by transplantation of cryopreserved rat islets of Langerhans to the renal subcapsular space. Diabetes Res 8: 9–15

Evans MG, Rajotte RV, Warnock GL, Procyshyn AW (1987) Cryopreservation purifies canine pancreatic microfragments. Transplant Proc 19: 3471–3477

Evans MG, Rajotte RV, Warnock GL, Kneteman NM (1989) Viability studies on cryopreserved isolated canine islets of Langerhans. Transplant Proc 21(2): 3368–3370

Federlin K, Bretzel RG (eds) (1981) Islet Isolation Culture and Cryopreservation. Thieme, Stuttgart pp 124–164

Ferguson J, Allsopp RH, Taylor RMR, Johnston IDA (1976a) Isolation and long-term preservation of pancreatic islets from mouse, rat and guinea-pig and human pancreas. Br J Surg 63: 767–773

Ferguson J, Allsopp RH, Taylor RMR, Johnston IDA (1976b) Isolation and long-term preservation of pancreatic islets from mouse, rat and guinea-pig. Diabetologia 12: 115–121

Gray DW, McShane P, Grant A, Morris PJ (1984a) A method for isolation of islets of Langerhans from the human pancreas. Diabetes 33: 1055–1061

Gray DW, Reece-Smith H, Fairbrother B, McShane P, Morris PJ (1984b) Isolated pancreatic islet allografts in rats rendered immunologically unresponsive to renal allografts: the effect of the site of transplantation. Transplantation 37: 434–437

Jutte NHPM, Heyse P, Jansen HG, Bruining GJ, Zeilmaker GH (1987) Vitrification of human islets of Langerhans. Cryobiology 24: 403–411

Kneteman NM, Rajotte RV (1986) Isolation and cryopreservation of human pancreatic islets. Transplant Proc 18: 182–185

Kneteman NM, Rajotte RV, Warnock GL (1986) Long-term normoglycemia in pancreatectomized dogs transplanted with frozen/thawed pancreatic islets. Cryobiology 23: 214–221

Lacy PE, Walker BS, Fink CJ (1972) Perifusion of isolated rat islets in vitro participation of the microtubular system in the biphasic release of insulin. Diabetes 21: 987–992

Leibo SP, Mazur P (1987) Methods for the preservation of mammalian embryos by freezing. In: Daniel JC (ed) Methods in mammalian reproduction. Academic Press, New York, pp 179–201

McKay DB, Karow AM Jr (1983) Factors to consider in the assessment of viability of cryopreserved islets of Langerhans. Cryobiology 20: 151–160

Rajotte RV, DeGroot TJ (1986) Effect of warming rate on slowly cooled isolated rat islets. Cryobiology 23:572

Rajotte RV, Stewart HL, Voss WAG, Shnitka TK, Dossetor JB (1977) Viability studies of frozen-thawed rat islets of Langerhans. Cryobiology 14: 116–120

Rajotte RV, Scharp DW, Downing R, Preston R, Molnar GD, Ballinger WF, Greider MH (1981a) Pancreatic islet banking: the transplantation of frozen-thawed rat islets transported between centers. Cryobiology 18: 357–369

Rajotte RV, Scharp DW, Molnar GD, Preston R (1981b) Feasibility of low-temperature banking for pancreatic islet cell transplantation. In: Federlin K et al. (eds) Islet isolation culture and cryopreservation. Thieme, Stuttgart pp 124–137

Rajotte RV, Warnock GL, Bruch LC, Procyshyn AW (1983) Transplantation of cryopreserved and fresh rat islets and canine pancreatic fragments: comparison of cryopreservation protocols. Cryobiology 20: 169–184

Rajotte RV, Warnock GL, Kneteman NM (1984) Cryopreservation of insulin-producing tissue in rats and dogs. World J Surg 8: 179–186

Rajotte RV, Warnock GL, Evans MG, Ellis D, Dawidson L (1987) Isolation of viable islets of Langerhans from collagenase-perfused canine and human pancreata. Transplant Proc. 19: 918–922

Rajotte RV, DeGroot TJ, Korbutt GS, Warnock GL (1989) Cryopreservation of isolated rat islets using slow cooling to −40°C and −75°C: percentage survival dependency on thawing rate. Cryobiology (in press)

Sandler S, Andersson A (1984) The significance of culture for successful cryopreservation of isolated pancreatic islets of Langerhans. Cryobiology 21: 503–510

Sandler S, Andersson A (1987) Cryopreservation of mouse pancreatic islets: effects of different glucose concentrations in the post-thaw culture medium on islet recovery. Cryobiology 24: 285–291

Sandler S, Nilsson B, Borg LAH, Swenne I, Petersson B, Hellerstrom C, Andersson A (1981) Structure and function of cryopreserved mouse pancreatic islets. In: Federlin K et al. (eds) Islet isolation, culture and cryopreservation. Thieme, Stuttgart, pp 138–151

Sandler S, Nilsson B, Petersson B, Hellerstrom C, Andersson A (1982) Functional characteristics of cryopreserved mouse pancreatic islets. Horm Metab Res 12: 71

Sandler S, Kojima Y, Andersson A, (1986) Cryopreservation of mouse pancreatic islets: effects of fast cooling on islet B-cell function in vitro and after islet transplantation. Transplantation 42: 588–593

Scharp DW, Lacy PE (1985) Human islet isolation and transplantation. Diabetes 34 [Suppl 1]: 19(5A)

Taylor MJ, Duffy TJ, Davisson PJ, Morgan SRA (1982) Slow cooling of isolated rat islets of Langerhans in the presence of dimethlysulfoxide or glycerol – effect upon the dynamic pattern of insulin release. Cryo Lett 3: 148–157

Taylor MJ, Duffy TJ, Hunt CJ, Morgan SRA, Davisson PJ (1983) Transplantation and in vitro perifusion of rat islets of Langerhans after slow cooling and warming in the presence of either glycerol or dimethylsulfoxide. Cryobiology 20: 185–204

Walsh TN, Alderson D, Farndon, JR (1987) Dispersed pancreatic graft cryopreservation in the dog: in vivo assessment of preservation protocols. Cryobiology 24:256–263

Warnock GL, Rajotte RV (1987) Effect of pre-cryopreservation tissue culture on the outcome of transplanted rat islets of Langerhans. Cryobiology 24:588–589

Warnock GL, Rajotte RV (1988) Critical mass of purified islets that induce normoglycemia after implantation into dogs. Diabetes 37: 467–470

Warnock GL, Rajotte RV, Procyshyn AW (1983) Normoglycemia after reflux of islet-containing pancreatic fragments into the splenic vascular bed in dogs. Diabetes 32: 452–459

Warnock GL, Gray DWR, Morris PJ (1986) Transplantation of cryopreserved isolated adult human islets of Langerhans into nude rats. Surg Forum 37: 334–336

Warnock GL, Rajotte RV, Evans MG, Ellis D, DeGroot T, Dawidson I (1987a) Isolation of islets of Langerhans following cold storage of human pancreas. Transplant Proc 19: 3466–3468

Warnock GL, Gray DWR, McShane P, Peters M, Morris PJ (1987b) Survival of cryopreserved isolated adult human pancreatic islets of Langerhans. Transplantation 44: 75–82

Weber C, Pi-Sunyer FX, Nilaver G, Reemtsma K (1983) Murine islet cryopreservation and corticosteroids: functional studies. Cryobiology 20: 219–225

Wise MH, Yates A, Gordon C, Johson RWG (1983) Subzero preservation of mechanically prepared porcine islets of Langerhans: response to a glucose challenge in vitro. Cryobiology 20: 211–218

Wise MH, Gordon C, Johnson RWG (1985) Intraportal autotransplantation of cryopreserved porcine islets of Langerhans. Cryobiology 22: 359–366

Islet Transplantation in Rodents

R. G. Bretzel, B. J. Hering, T. Linn, D. Strödter, S. Wiegand, M. Woehrle, and T. Zekorn

Zusammenfassung

Die Inzidenz an Typ I oder insulinpflichtigem Diabetes (IDDM) nimmt gegenwärtig in den westlichen Ländern, besonders in Finnland und dem übrigen Skandinavien, dramatisch zu. Diabetes ist vermutlich die am weitesten verbreitete schwere Erkrankung des Kindes und Heranwachsenden. In der Bundesrepublik wird etwa eines von 2500 Kindern unter 15 Jahren von Diabetes befallen und in der Regel benötigt der Patient ab dem Zeitpunkt der Diagnosestellung eine kontinuierliche Therapie für den Rest seines Lebens. Insulininjektionen können den Tod an akuten Stoffwechselentgleisungen verhindern. Sie vermögen aber langfristig nicht, das Auftreten von diabetischen Sekundärkomplikationen zu verhindern, die schließlich beim größten Teil der Patienten zu körperlicher Behinderung und Tod führen. Theoretisch kann ein Ersatz des erkrankten endokrinen Gewebes durch eine Transplantation einen Typ I-Diabetes heilen und vielleicht die Organfolgeschäden verhindern oder eingetretene Schäden gar noch zurückbilden. Unsere Untersuchungen wurden an fünf verschiedenen Diabetesmodellen bei Nagern durchgeführt. Besonderes Interesse galt dabei den Stoffwechseleffekten einer Inseltransplantation, dem optimalen Implantationsort für Inseln, der Konservierung und Langzeitlagerung von isoliertem Inselgewebe, Auswirkungen einer Inseltransplantation auf die verschiedenen Sekundärkomplikationen und auf das Empfängerpankreas, der Verhinderung einer homologen und heterologen Inseltransplantatabstoßung, dem Wiederauftreten eines Autoimmundiabetes nach Inseltransplantation, Untersuchungen zur Ausbeute und Viabilität von aus dem Pankreas höherer Säuger und des Menschen gewonnenen Inselpräparationen und den Möglichkeiten einer Inseltransplantation bei einem Typ II-Diabetes. Die in unserer Arbeitsgruppe in den vergangenen fünf bis zehn Jahren hinzugewonnene Erfahrung bestärkt uns, an die Zukunft einer klinischen Inseltransplantation bei Diabetikern zu glauben.

Introduction

Despite insulin therapy the leading causes of the high morbidity and mortality rate of type I and even type II diabetic patients at present are diabetic secondary complications such as peripheral, cerebral, and coronary vessel disease, nephro-pathy, neuropathy, retinopathy, and blindness. Therefore, the ultimate goal of attempts to transplant the pancreas or pancreatic islet tissue is to prevent or even reverse diabetic secondary complications. The discovery of collagenase digestion for islet isolation should, theoretically, enable total endocrine replacement ther-apy by grafting isolated islets of Langerhans via different routes into diabetic recipients. A variety of animal models of spontaneous and chemically or virus-induced diabetes mellitus with more or less similarity to type I und type II diabetes in humans have been reported on.

In our laboratory we have established five different diabetes models in rodents (mice, rats) each for studies concerning particular questions. Several years ago we started experiments in a chemical-toxic diabetes mellitus, streptozotocin dia-betes in rats. In that model we tested, physiological and with respect to immu-nologically privileged sites, various implantation routes, long-term storage of isolated islets by means of tissue culture and cryopreservation, methods of pre-venting islet allograft and xenograft rejection, and, of course, the rationale for islet transplantation, i.e., whether diabetic secondary complications are indeed preventable or reversible by this treatment. Using two models of autoimmunologi-cally induced diabetes mellitus – low-dose streptozotocin diabetes and the spon-taneously occurring diabetes in biobred BB rats – we studied factors influencing the onset and the course of symptoms and the effect of islet transplantation. Another question of great interest with respect to autoimmune type I diabetes in humans to be clarified was how to circumvent the recurrence of autoimmune diabetes after islet grafting.

A chemical-toxic diabetes mellitus induced in nonimmunocompetent nude mice served as a model for islet xenograft studies. The in vivo viability of mass-isolated islets from higher mammalian pancreas canine, bovine, porcine and from human pancreas was tested, particular consideration also being given to possible xenograft trials in diabetic patients in the future.

Finally, we, together with Dr. A. M. Cohen from the Hadassah University of Jerusalem, Israel, have established a model of a non-insulin-dependent (type II) diabetes mellitus, studying various topics in the spontaneously occurring experi-mental diabetes.

Materials and Methods

Diabetes Induction

Chemical-Toxic Diabetes Model. Male Lewis rats or BDII rats (ZTV, Hannover, FRG) weighing 200–250 g were rendered chronically diabetic by a single intra-venous injection of streptozotocin (65 mg/kg) via the tail vein.

Low-Dose Streptozotocin Diabetes Model. Male CD1 mice (Charles River, Sulzbach, FRG) at 6–8 weeks of age received daily intraperitonal injections of streptozotocin 45 mg/kg (Upjohn, Kalamazoo, USA) for 4 days.

Spontaneous Diabetes of the BB rat. Inbred BB rats (more than F_{20}) of the Philadelphia Colony (Department of Surgery, University of Pennsylvania) were used. The cumulative incidence of spontaneous diabetes mellitus ranged from 40% to 60%, with an onset of diabetic symptoms predominantly at an age of 60–120 days.

Chemical-Toxic Diabetes in Nude Mice. Male NMRI (*nu/nu*) mice (ZTV, Hannover, FRG) aged 6–8 weeks and weighing about or more than 30 g were rendered chronically diabetic by a single intravenous injection of streptozotocin 170 mg/kg (Upjohn, Kalamazoo, USA) via the tail vein. The animals were kept under sterile and constant environmental conditions (temperature 26°–28 °C, relative humidity 65%). They were fed sterile chow (Altromin, Lage, FRG) and were given sterile water (pH 2.5) supplemented with oxytetracycline 0.3 g/l and potassium sorbate 1.35 g/l ad libitum (Fortmeyer 1981).

Diabetes Model of Cohen's rats. These rats were bred at the Hadassah University of Jerusalem, Israel, by the group of A. M. Cohen (Cohen et al. 1972). By genetic selection based on glucose tolerance, Sabra albino rats are fed with a special saccharose-enriched and copper-deficient diet; this leads to an overt diabetes mellitus after about six generations. Animals of the diabetes-prone and the diabetes-resistant lines were shipped by plane to Giessen and were kept in animal houses under the original special diet.

Islet Isolation

Arterial Perfusion-Distension with Neutral Red, Collagenase, and Hand Picking. Pancreatic islets were isolated from adult donor rats weighing 180–250 g after in situ arterial perfusion-distension with cold neutral red solution (0.7%). Finely cut pieces were incubated with 15 mg collagenase (475 Mandl units/mg, Serva, Heidelberg, FRG) together with 7 mg bovine serum albumin per pancreas, as described in detail in Bretzel (1984). Purification was done by hand picking under a dissecting microscope.

Ductal distension, Collagenase Digestion, and Density gradient separation. In another series of experiments pancreatic islets from adult donor rats were yielded by ductal distension with collagenase (Serva, Heidelberg, FRG) and subsequent collagenase incubation at 37 °C (Lacy and Kostianovsky 1967). Islet purification was done by Ficoll density gradient centrifugation (Gotoh et al. 1985).

Mass Isolation of Higher Mammalian and Human Pancreatic Islets. Bovine and porcine pancreata were obtained from the local slaughterhouse. The organs were rapidly immersed and transported in cold (4 °C) Euro-Collins solution (Fresenius, Bad Homburg, FRG) to the laboratory. Surrounding fat and connective tissue were carefully dissected from the pancreas. After that, an 18-gauge angiocatheter was inserted into the exposed duct for distension of the gland by intraductal injection of Hanks balanced salt solution (HBSS) containing collagenase (Serva, Heidelberg, FRG), DNase type I, grade II (Boehringer, Mannheim, FRG), and heat-inactivated fetal calf serum (Gibco, Eggstein, FRG). Digestion of the gland was performed in a continuous digestion-filtration device similar to the automated method developed by Ricordi et al. (1988) for human islet isolation. Details of our method were published recently (Hering et al. 1989). Dog pancreata yielded by pancreatectomy from anesthesized dogs and cadaveric human pancreata sent to the laboratory from various university hospitals were processed similarly.

Culture and Cryopreservation

Culture. Isolated pancreatic islets were cultured in a free-floating manner at 37 °C or at 22 °/24 °C in humidified 95 % air and 5 % CO_2 in RPMI 1640 medium containing various supplements (described in detail in Bretzel et al. 1981a).

Cryopreservation. Freezing of isolated pancreatic islets was performed in a BV4 freezing chamber (Cryoson, Schöllkrippen, FRG) using 10 % dimethylsulfoxide (DMSO) as a cryoprotective medium. Various freezing rates from 0.25 °C/min to 2.0 °C/min were used, as described elsewhere (Bretzel et al. 1981b; Bretzel et al. 1986a). The frozen islets were stored in liquid nitrogen. Thawing was done in a water bath at 37 °C and the DMSO was rinsed by stepwise addition of Krebs-Ringer buffer.

Islet Transplantation

Intraportal and intraperitoneal islet transplantation was performed as described in Bretzel (1984). Islet transplantation under the kidney capsule was done as previously described (Woehrle et al. 1987; Reece-Smith et al. 1981).

Metabolic Studies

Indicators of glucose metabolism such as blood sugar, glycosylated hemoglobin (HbA_1), glucosuria, intravenous glucose tolerance tests, and serum concentration of insulin and glucagon were determined at regular intervals using methos previously described (Bretzel 1984).

Functional and biochemical studies with respect to diabetic nephropathy and cardiopathy included determinations of basement membrane antigens in the serum, analysis of the activity of the renal collagen-gucosyltransferase in kidney extract, and determination of enzymuria (alanine aminopeptidase, alkaline phosphatase and γ-glutamyl transpeptidase), proteinuria and albuminuria, and the content of high-oxygen phosphates in the heart muscle. Heart rate and hemodynamic parameters were studied in an ex vivo, in vitro working heart model. The methods used are described elsewhere (Bretzel et al. 1984a; Bretzel 1984b; Strödter 1987).

Morphological Studies

Numerous studies of the effect of diabetes and of the preventive and reversive effects of islet transplantation on diabetic secondary complications of the kidney, heart, retina, and peripheral nervous system were performed using histological, immunohistological (immunofluorescence and immunoperoxidase technique), and electron microscopic methods as described earlier (Bretzel et al. 1979b; Bretzel 1984a; Büscher et al. 1989; Strödter et al. 1987; Sharma et al. 1988).

Studies on pancreas morphology and on the morphology of isolated, cultured, cryopreserved, and grafted islets were performed using histological, immunohistological, and electron microscopic methods. For studies of islet immunogenicity represented by the expression of class I and class II antigens we predominantly used immunofluorescence techniques (Forsen et al 1984; Blum 1986).

Statistical Analysis

Tests applied were the Student's t test, the Wilcoxon rank sum test, and the non parametric U test of Mann and Whitney.

Results

Islet Transplantation in Chemically Induced (Toxic) Streptozotocin Diabetes in Rats

Metabolic Effects of Islet Transplantation. A single intravenous injection of streptozotocin (65 mg/kg) in adult Lewis rats induced a permanent, moderate, nonketotic diabetes mellitus with fasting blood sugar levels constantly above 300 mg/dl. Additional signs in this diabetes model are hypoinsulinemia, hyperglucagonemia, an increased percentage of glycosylated hemoglobin (HbA_1), polyuria, polydipsia, glucosuria, and weight loss. On intravenous testing (0.5 g glucose/kg body weight), decreased glucose tolerance with k values between 0.32 and 0.49 was found.

Syngeneic transplantation of islets (intraperitoneal 598 ± 74 islets per recipient vs. intraportal 667 ± 48 per recipient) was only partially effective when implantation was done intraperitoneally (11 cases), whereas diabetes was cured when

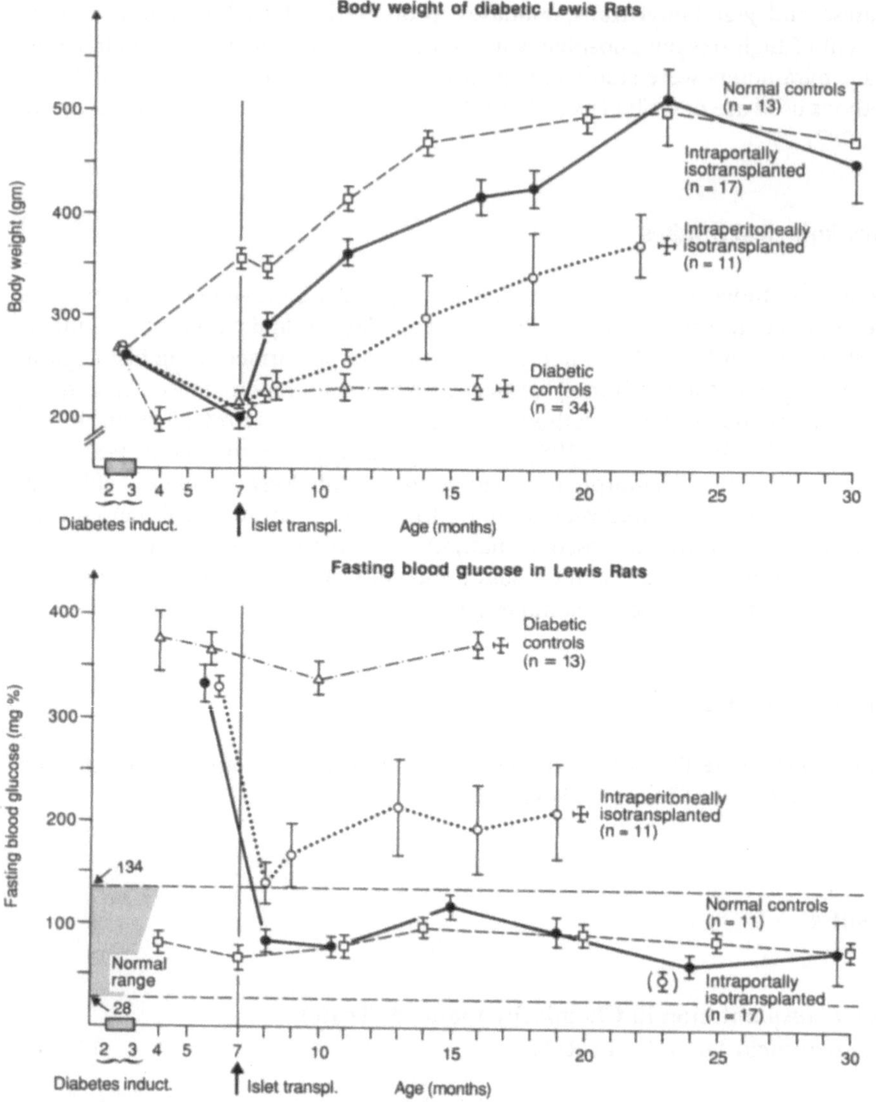

Fig. 1. Body weight (*top*) and fasting blood glucose (*bottom*) in syngeneic intraperitoneally or intraportally islet-transplanted rats, sham-operated diabetic controls, and normal controls

the same number of islets were embolized to the liver via the portal vein (17 cases). In all diabetic rats that received intraportal islet transplants the metabolic abnormalities were reversed, and this effect was long-lasting. Plasma glucose levels returned to normal (Fig. 1), circulating insulin levels became normal or slightly elevated, hyperglucagonemia gradually returned to normal within the following 6 months, the percentage of glycosylated hemoglobin normalized, polyuria, polydipsia, and polyphagia disappeared, and weight gain was restored. Glucose tolerance curves improved, with subnormal k values of 1.17–1.59 in intraportally islet-transplanted rats. Again, intraperitoneal transplantation was less effective, showing post transplant k values in the islet recipients of 0.72–1.14.

Following allogeneic islet transplantation across a strong histocompatibility barrier using strain combinations differing in the three main loci (BDII rat islets to Lewis rats), the blood sugar-lowering effect lasted only for 4–5 days and diabetes recurred afterwards. Morphological examinations of allogeneic islets implanted into the liver via the portal vein revealed strong lymphocyte and round-cell infiltration at that time. The intraportal route seemed not to be immunologically privileged compared with the intraperitoneal route.

Recent studies by our group revealed a minor immunological privilege of the renal subcapsular space for islet allografts in diabetic rats. But this route only becomes effective and allows islet allografting without immunosuppression of the host if the additive effects of a strong pretransplant immunomodulation and slow metabolic adaptation after transplantation (culture at 22 °C) are used (Woehrle et al. 1989).

Preservation of Isolated Islets by Culture. Isolated islets of adult Lewis rats were maintained in culture and followed for a maximum of 28 days. The morphological survival rate based on histological and immunohistological exminations ranged from 90% to 100%. The basal insulin production rate (immunoreactive insulin released into the medium during 24 h) averaged 70.7 ± 2.7 μU/islet but with a significantly lower value during the first 2 days (51.3 μU/islet). Static incubation with glucose (50 mg/dl and 300 mg/dl) and glucose (300 mg/dl) plus theophylline (10 mM) was done every 5th day on a representative number of cultured islets. After 5 days culture the stimulated insulin secretion in each test system was about 50% of that in freshly isolated islets. However, islets cultured for 10 or 15 days gained insulin secretory capacity and had insulin responses to glucose 300 mg/dl of 83.3% and 77.4%, respectively, compared with freshly isolated controls. The response levels to glucose (300 mg/dl) plus theophylline averaged 110.9% (day 10) and 103.7% (day 15). The preservation in vitro of insulin secretory capacity was confirmed by the sustained insulin secretion in vivo after syngeneic islet transplantation into diabetic rats. In detail, these animals ($n = 7$) gained weight, their blood sugar returned to normal, they showed hyper- or normoinsulinemia, the daily urine volume normalized, and glucosuria disappeared; these effects resembled those seen in rats ($n = 8$) transplanted with freshly isolated syngeneic islets.

Preservation of Isolated Islets by Cryopreservation. Rat, porcine, and human isolated adult pancreatic islets were frozen according to our initial freezing program at 2 °C/min to −35 °C and 6°–7 °C/min to −100 °C and were subsequently stored in liquid nitrogen for periods of up to 6 months. After rethawing, the survival rates in terms of histological integrity were about 80% in all experiments. Functional analysis in cryopreserved rat, porcine, and human islets showed that they had similar basal (50 mg/dl glucose challenge) and stimulated (300 mg/dl

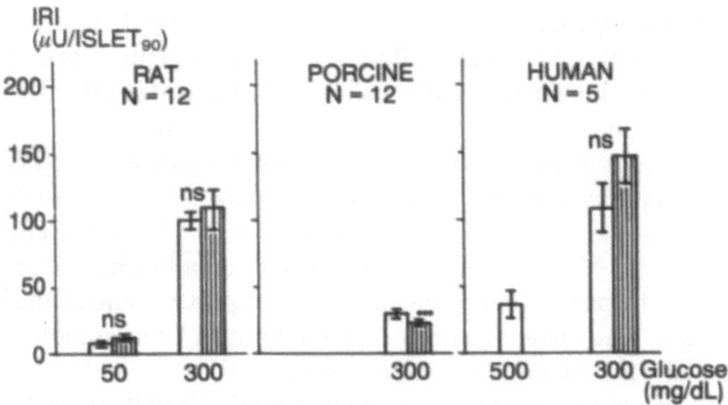

Fig. 2. Glucose stimulation of frozen-thawed (*shaded bars*) rat, porcine, and human pancreatic islets compared with freshly isolated islets (*open bars*). *** $p < 0.001$

glucose challenge) insulin secretion rates to freshly isolated islets (Fig. 2). However, the insulin biosynthesis rate of frozen-thawed rat islets was reduced to 20.3 % of that seen in fresh islets. On the other hand, proinsulin and insulin biosynthesis rates could be restored to 50 % by subsequent short-term (48 h) culture at 37 °C.

Intraportal transplantation of syngeneic cryopreserved adult rat islets resulted in sustained normalization of the fasting blood glucose and a permanent weight gain in the recipients similar to those seen in rats transplanted with freshly isolated islets. The number of cryopreserved islets needed to reach this goal, however, is about twice the number of freshly isolated islets.

The Effect of Islet Transplantation on Diabetic Secondary Complications. The renal lesions that develop in diabetic rats are similar, in some respects, to those associated with diabetes mellitus in humans. There is a progressive increase in mesangial matrix volume and in basement membrane thickness. Immunoglobulins and other macromolecules are nonspecifically deposited within the mesangium. Tubular vacuolization (Armanni-Ebstein cells) and hyalinization of arterioles occur.

In a series of experiments we showed that syngeneic transplantation of fresh or cultured islets could prevent or, if transplantation was performed not later than 3–6 months after onset of diabetes, even reverse these kidney lesions. Quantitative studies revealed a significant reduction in the number of affected glomeruli and in the mesangial enlargement, and a rewidening of the capillary lumen. Signs of diabetic tubulopathy also disappeared. Electron microscopy showed that the basement membrane thickening which took place to a large extent in nontransplanted diabetic controls was prevented.

In the context of our investigations, new markers of diabetic nephropathy were found. It turned out that structure-related markers of glomerular basement membrane collagen metabolism such as 7S collagen and laminin P2 can be found in raised concentrations in the serum in diabetic rats. After normalization of the disturbed glucose metabolism by syngeneic islet transplantation the serum concentration of these basement membrane antigens returned to normal. We found the same for the raised renal activity of collagen-glucosyltransferase in diabetic rats. Increased urinary excretion of brush border enzymes, alanine aminopeptidase, and alkaline phosphatase and decreased urinary excretion of the enzyme γ-glutamyl transpeptidase – both signs of diabetic tubulopathy – could no longer been found after successful islet transplantation. Studies in diabetic cardiomyopathy revealed a beneficial effect of successful islet transplantation on biochemical and functional signs of diabetic cardiomyopathy. The reduced utilization of carbohydrates found in diabetic rats accompanied by lowered production of ATP and the consequent reduced cardiac performance (cardiac output, aortic output) became normal after syngeneic islet transplantation. Utilization of triglycerides by the heart muscle cells also normalized following islet transplantation.

Very recently a modification of the digestion technique of Kuwabara and Cogan (1960) to yield preparations of the retina was established in our laboratory. Streptozotocin-diabetic Han-Wistar rats developed retinal changes which are similar to those associated with diabetes mellitus in humans: microaneurysms, hyperplasia of mesodermal strands and pericyte migration as signs of degeneration beginning after 2 or 3 months of diabetes, degeneration of acellular capillaries, loss of intramural pericytes on single capillaries, Ω-shaped capillary loops, and microthromboses after 5–8 months of diabetes. The most striking feature, which made quantification possible, was the diffuse and selective diminution of pericyte density. Compared to normal control retinas, the number of pericytes was already significantly reduced in the diabetics 1 month after diabetes onset and decreased further during the whole period of observation. Correspondingly, there was a steady increase in the endothelial cell/pericyte (E/P) ratio, which was approximately 1:1 in normal retinas.

"Early" syngeneic islet transplantation (after onset of the disease) and "late" syngeneic islet transplantation (6 months after diabetes induction) were comparmed in ten diabetic rats each. The retinas of islet-transplanted rats showed no pathological changes except some equivocal microthromboses in the early-transplanted animals and several severe forms of capillar degeneration (strand formation) in the late-transplanted animals. Quantitative analysis revealed that both pericyte loss and endothelial proliferation were completely prevented in the early-transplanted rats. Late-transplanted rats showed a partial restoration of the decreased pericyte density, still significantly different from normal controls. As a result, the increase in E/P ratio found in diabetic rats was completely prevented by early islet transplantation and significantly, but not completely, reversed by late islet transplantation (Fig. 3).

In another series of experiments lasting 12 months seven groups of Lewis rats aged 10 weeks were studied: one group at the start of the study ("onset" group); normal controls after 6 and 12 months; untreated streptozotocin diabetics after 6 and 12 months; and streptozotocin diabetics treated with syngeneic pancreatic islet transplantation after 1 ("early transplantation") and 6 ("late transplantation") months of diabetes. The number of myelinated fibers in the tibial nerve and their axonal areas were significantly greater in normal controls after 6 and 12 months than in the "onset" group. By contrast, at 6 and 12 months the number of

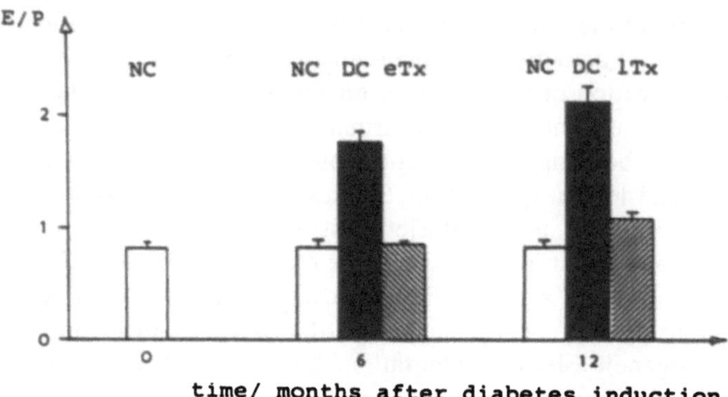

Fig. 3. Ratio of retinal endothelial cells (*E*) to pericytes (*P*) in early (*eTx*) and late (*lTx*) transplanted rats and diabetic (*DC*) and normal controls (*NC*). Mean ± SD

myelinated fibers and axonal areas were significantly lower in the diabetic animals than in age-matched normal controls but were not lower than in the "onset" group. These peripheral nerve structural abnormalities resemble those associated with diabetes mellitus in humans.

The reduction in myelinated fibers and axonal areas was prevented in early-transplanted diabetic animals, as the values were greater than in untreated diabetics and not different from controls. The reduction in fiber area was also corrected in the diabetic animals which were transplanted 6 months after the induction of diabetes; the values were greater than in untreated diabetics and not different from age-matched controls. Axonal area was also significantly increased in the late-transplanted diabetics compared with untreated diabetics but was not normalized. Thus, pancreatic islet transplantation prevented as well as reversed peripheral nerve structural abnormalities in experimental diabetes.

Table 1 summarizes the effects of metabolically successful experimental islet transplantation on secondary complications of diabetes mellitus.

Pancreatic Beta-Cell Restoration Following Islet Transplantation. A morphological and morphometric study on the remaining pancreas of untreated diabetic rats ($n = 8$), of islet-transplanted diabetic rats ($n = 8$; islet transplantation 2 months

Table 1. Effects of experimental islet transplantation or secondary complications of diabetes mellitus

---

Prevention of cataract

Prevention, delay, or reversal of:
  retinopathy
  nephropathy
  neuropathy
  cardiopathy
  skeletal disorders

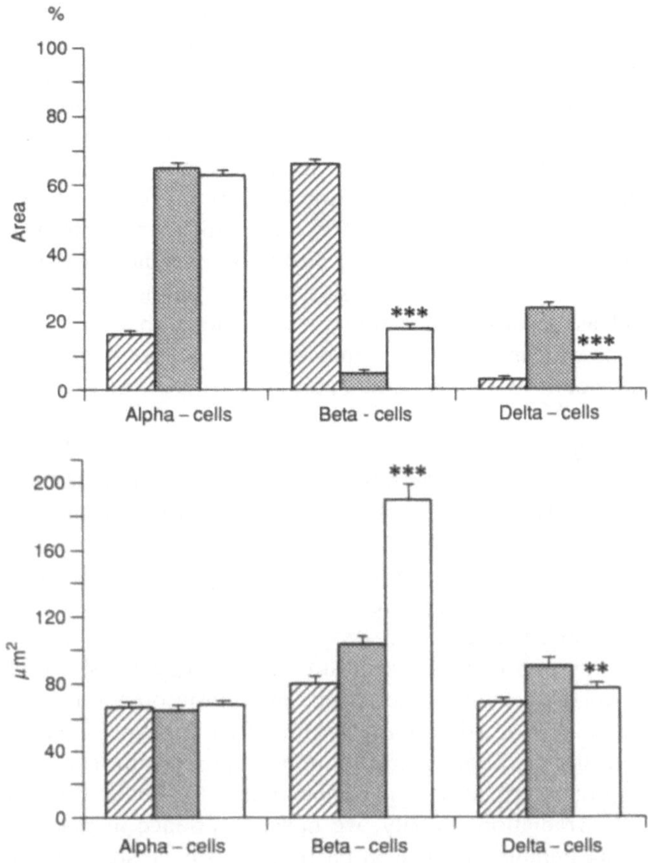

Fig. 4. *Top*, Area of endocrine cells in pancreatic islets of normal (*striped bars*), diabetic (*stippled bars*), and islet-transplanted (*open bars*) rats as a ercentage. Results expressed as means ± SEM. *** $p < 0.001$, DT vs. DC. *Bottom*, mean size of alpha-, beta-, and delta-cells in normal (*striped bars*), diabetic (*stippled bars*), and islet-transplanted (*open bars*) rats. Results expressed as means ± SEM. *** $p < 0.001$, ** $p < 0.01$, DT vs. DC

after diabetes onset), and of normal controls ($n = 8$) was done. In normal rat pancreas, islets of various sizes averaging 15 670 – 18 958 μm^2 were observed. Beta-cells comprised 66.2%, alpha-cells 16.2%, and delta-cells 2.9% of the islet area (Fig. 4). In diabetic controls both the number and the size of the islets were reduced to about 40% ($p < 0.001$). The islet area ranged between 6265 and 7623 μm^2. Most of the islets were composed of numerous alpha- and delta-cells. Beta-cells were markedly reduced and most of them were degranulated. Beta-cells were found in only 35% of the islets, comprising 3.7% of the area ($p < 0.001$ diabetic controls vs. normal controls) (Fig. 4). This resulted in a total beta-cell area per islet of 91 μm^2, compared with 10 767 μm^2 in normal controls ($p < 0.001$). After syngeneic islet transplantation, the mean islet area in the recipient pancreata was rather variable (5695 – 8158 μm^2) and did not differ significantly from untreated diabetics. No difference was found in rats killed 6 or 9 months after transplantation. In these islets we most frequently found clusters of hypertrophic beta-cells which were well granulated and contained large amounts of insulin. We observed numerous beta-cells in smaller islets, which were often found in very close connection to exocrine ducts. Morphometric analysis indicated a significant increase of the relative beta-cell area ($p < 0.001$, treated diabetics vs. diabetic controls), these comprising 17.2% of the islet area (Fig. 4). The total pancreatic beta-cell area per islet was around 975 μm^2, which was tenfold higher than in untreated diabetic controls ($p < 0.001$). From these studies we conclude that the restoration of blood glucose homeostasis and/or an unknown islet graft factor may stimulate at least partial regeneration or restoration of beta-cells within the islets of the host pancreas. In addition, it may give rise to neoformation of beta-cells, probably derived from pluripotential epithelial cells of the excrine duct system.

Attempts to Prevent Islet Allograft and Xenograft Rejection. Isolated pancreatic islets are definitely immunogenic and can be rejected very rapidly, within about 5 days, particularly if transplantation is across a strong histocompatibility barrier. Passenger leukocytes and dendritic cells are thought to play a major role in sensitizing a host to an allograft. They seem to stimulate recipient lymphocytes via class II antigen expression; these are then directed against class I antigens of the grafted tissue and destroy it.

Our own experience in attempts to prevent islet graft rejection is based on conventional and generalized immunosuppression of the recipient by various substances. Furthermore, we gained a lot of experience in prevention of islet graft rejection by altering graft immunogenicity with in vitro pretreatment by culture and/or cryopreservation, application of antibodies directed to class II antigens, or UV irradiation. Finally, we have experience in preventing islet graft rejection using immunomechanical barriers, and have studied multiple biomembranes in order to construct a device for macroencapsulation of isolated islets („bioartifical pancreas").

Using various protocols of generalized immunosuppressive treatment with azathioprine, imuran, cyclosporin A, ciamexon, or a preparation of gangliosides in diabetic rats we found only a partial but nut significant prolongation of islet allograft survival when transplantation was across a major histocompatibility barrier. Freshly isolated pancreatic islets of Lewis rats were found to contain 4.4 ± 0.8 (0–25) class II antigen-positive cells.

BDII rats ($n = 11$) transplanted with UV-irradiated isolated Lewis islets UV-C light of 616 J/m^2 [UV$_0$] and of 1032 J/m^2 [UV$_1$]) did not have a significantly longer mean graft survival time than rats transplanted with freshly isolated islets (7.9 vs. 5.2 days) (Table 2). Only a combination of UV irradiation with 24-h culture at 37°C and a single injection of antilymphocyte serum (ALS) to the recipient significantly prolonged islet allograft survival time (mean, 24.8 days with UV$_0$ and 25.3 days with UV$_1$) (Table 2).

Pretreatment of isolated rat islets with MHC Ia (class II) antibody and complement to lyse class II antigen-bearing cells significantly reduced class II antigen expression, 65.4% of the islets being totally negative for class II antigens after

Table 2. Effect of UV irradiation prior to transplantation on mean survival time (days) of allografted rat islets

Treatment	Survival (days)	n
UV_0	7.9	11
UV_1	7.9	11
$UV_0 + C_{24}$	7.0	12
$UV_1 + C_{24}$	8.4	10
$UV_0 + C_{24} + ALS$	24.8	11
$UV_1 + C_{24} + ALS$	25.3	9
UV_0 $\quad$ + ALS	8.6	9
UV_1 $\quad$ + ALS	8.2	10
C_{24}	10.5	10
$C_{24} + ALS$	8.8	8

UV-C light: UV_0, 616 J/m^2; UV_1, 1032 J/m^2; C_{24}, culture at 37 °C for 24 h; ALS, antilymphocyte serum; n, number of animals

2 days compared to 30.9% of islets also cultured for 2 days without MHC Ia antibody. Amongst freshly isolated islets only 6.5% were negative for class II antigens. Antibody treatment also reduced the total number of class II antigen-positive cells within the islet. By contrast, allotransplantation of these pretreated islets did not result in prolongation of graft acceptance (mean survival time 3.4 days vs. 4.2 days for rats grafted with freshly isolated islets).

Incubation of rat islets with ciamexon or a preparation of five different gangliosides (Cronassial) significantly reduced islet class II antigen expression but did not significantly prolong islet allograft survival.

Culture at 37 °C or 22 °/24 °C for 10–14 days was highly effective in minimizing or diminishing class II antigen expression; this could not be reinduced by adding interferon-γ.

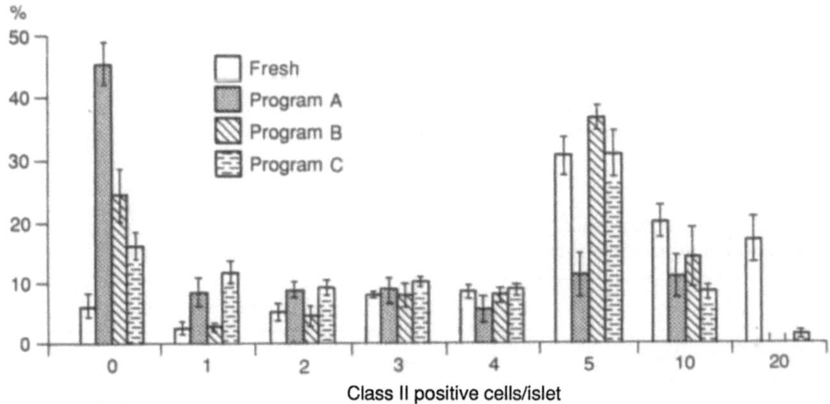

Fig. 5. Number of class II antigen-positive cells within frozen-thawed rat pancreatic islets cryoreserved by three different programs: A, 0.5 °C /min to −35 °C and 1 °C/min from −35 °C to −100 °C; B, 2 °C/min to −35 °C and 6 °C/min from −35 °C to −100 °C; C, 0.25 °C/min to −40 °C

Cryopreservation studies produced a freezing protocol (program A) that was optimal in deleting class II antigen expression whilst maintaining reasonable preservation of endocrine capacity (Fig. 5).

Allotransplantation of rat islets pretreated by culture or cryopreservation combined with a single injection of ALS to the recipient allowed long-term allograft acceptance (Table 3). A combination of cryopreservation with postcryoculture (Table 3) or 22 °C culture when implantation was under the renal capsule (Woehrle et al. 1987; 1989) even allowed permanent allograft acceptance without immunosuppression of the host in the majority of cases.

Immunomodulating pretreatment using cryopreservation of pancreatic microfragments derived from monkey or human cadavers resulted in islet xenograft acceptance in diabetic rats if a single injection of ALS was given at the time of operation (Table 4).

With respect to islet transplantation in humans, pretreating islets together with discontinuous immunosuppression of the recipient may enable successful islet allografting or even xenografting (e.g., pig to human) whilst avoiding the hazards of permanent and life-long immunosuppression of the diabetic patient.

Table 3. Success rates of intraportal islet allografts in diabetic rats in terms of islet endocrine function (normoglycemia of recipient) for more than 120 days following immunomodulatory and immunosuppressive treatment

Treatment	Success rate (%)
Fresh islets	0
Fresh islets + ALS	0
Fresh islets + CYA	0
Cultured islets	0
Cultured islets + ALS	90
Cultured islets + CYA	0
Cryopreserved islets	44
Cryopreserved islets + ALS	64
Cryocultured islets	80

ALS, Antilymphocyte serum; *CYA*, cyclosporin A

Table 4. Fasting serum insulin concentration in streptozotocin-diabetic rats ($n = 5$) following xenotransplantation of cryopreserved human pancreatic microfragments. Mean ± SEM

	Serum insulin (μU/ml)	$2p$
Before transplantation	14.2 ± 3.5	
After transplantation		
Day 3	47.6 ± 11.4	0.001
Day 8	25.7 ± 4.0	0.005
Day 15	34.3 ± 2.0	0.001
Day 22	44.1 ± 7.7	0.001

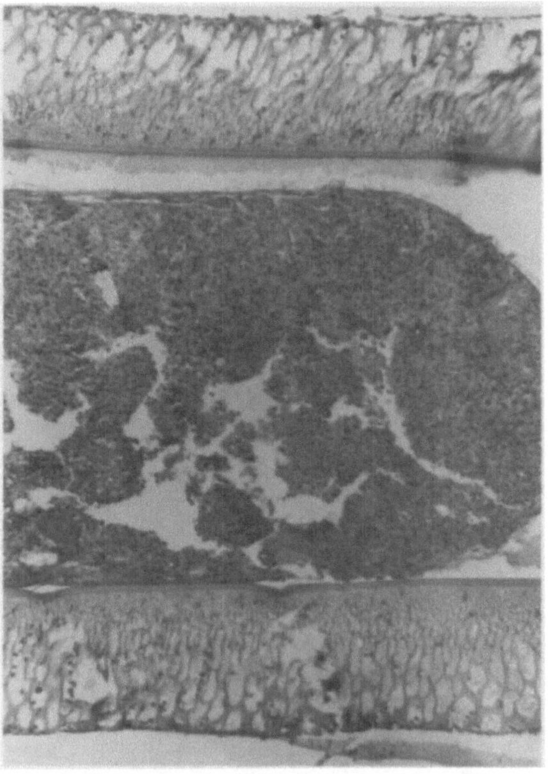

Fig. 6. Rat pancreatic islets encapsulated in an asymmetrical Hollow fibre device made from a
PEEK membrane at day 5 in 37 °C tissue culture. HE staining, x 200

Finally, detailed studies on numerous biomembranes for use in a Hollow fiber
device to immunoisolate and graft adult islets showed that specially prepared
polyether-ether-ketone (PEEK) membranes had superior diffusion characteristics. Now, basic principles and conditions such as the cut-off of the membrane,
the impact of the surface, the support of the membrane, the three-dimensional
architecture of the device, protein coating, and prevention of interleukin-1 (IL-
1) penetration are understood quite well. Questions of the biocompatibility of the
material and problems concerning supply of sufficient oxygen and nutrition to the
enclosed islets, however, still require intensive study (see also Fig. 6).

Autoimmune Diabetes Models

Low-Dose Streptozotocin (LDS) Diabetes of the Mouse. Diabetes was induced by
multiple subdiabetogenic doses of streptozotocin in CD1 and C57 B16 mice.
Streptozotocin injections were followed by hyperglycemia and mononuclear cell
infiltration of pancreatic islets (insulitis). Therefore, LDS diabetes is considered

to be a model of human type I (IDDM) diabetes mellitus. Ciamexon, a new immunomodulating agent with promising effects in experimental models of auto-immune diseases and practically no toxic side effects, delayed and reduced the islet destruction process if given before the administration of streptozotocin. Ciamexon does not exert the time- and dose-related beta-cell toxic effects seen with cyclosporin A.

Syngeneic grafting of isolated mouse islets during the initial period of diabetes onset was accompanied by an initial blood sugar decrease, but recurrence of the diabetes took place later on (Fig. 7). Late transplantation, however, was meta-bolically successful. Apparently, autoimmune destruction takes place in early-transplanted but not in late-transplanted islets.

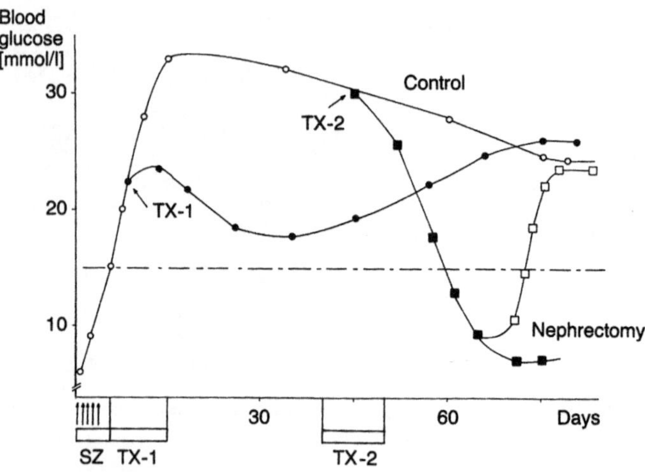

Fig. 7. Effect of early (*TX-1*) and late syngeneic islet transplantation (*TX-2*) in low-dose strep-tozotocin (*SZ*) diabetic mice on the blood glucose level of the recipients

Table 5. Survival of Wistar-Furth (WF) and Lewis rat islets transplanted immediately after isolation or after 14 days in tissue culture to BB rats

Donor strain	Islet treatment	Type of diabetes	Posttransplant normoglycemia (days)	Median survival time (days)
WF	None	Spontaneous	10, 10, 12, 25, 45	12.7 ± 0.35
WF	None	Streptozotocin	7, 14, 16, 17, > 90	13.0 ± 0.37
WF	Culture	Spontaneous	9, 12, 12, 14, 17	13.4 ± 0.21
WF	Culture	Streptozotocin	14, 14, 20, 55, 69	20.0 ± 0.46
Lewis	None	Spontaneous	4, 4, 5, 7, 8	4.7 ± 0.19
Lewis	None	Streptozotocin	5, 5, 5, 9, 12	5.6 ± 0.24
Lewis	None	Spontaneous	12, 16, 16, 18, > 20	14.6 ± 0.15
Lewis	Culture	Spontaneous	> 35, > 35, > 35, > 18	> 25.1 ± 0.38
Lewis	Culture	Spontaneous	23, 39, > 100 × 3, > 150	> 100
Lewis	Culture	Streptozotocin	> 100 × 3, > 125 × 2	> 100

Data from Woehrle et al. (1986, 1987, 1989)

Diabetes of the BB rat. Pancreatic islets maintained in tissue culture before transplantation into artificially induced diabetics are not rejected as shown above. In animal and human identical twin transplants, the autoimmunity of naturally occurring diabetes may destroy islets, even if rejection is avoided. Therefore, we studied whether autoimmune damage to islets can be avoided by pretransplant culture. We used the diabetes model of the BB rat, which resembles the type I diabetes of humans. Recipients were BB rats, donors were either Wistar-Furth (WF) (MHC identical to BB rats) or Lewis (MHC nonidentical to BB rats). Islets were inoculated into the portal vein, either immediately after isolation or after 14 days in tissue culture (95% humidified air, 5% CO_2, 24 °C). Recipients of cultured islets received a single injection of 1 ml ALS at the time of transplantation. Recurrence of diabetes after transplantation of freshly isolated MHC-incompatible Lewis islets occurred rapidly, due to rejection or autoimmune damage (or both) (Table 5). Precultured Lewis islets survived for longer or permanently. Freshly isolated MHC-compatible WF islets were destroyed, and no improvement was seen with culture (Table 5).

We conclude that autoimmune destruction of transplanted islets can be avoided by tissue culture, as can rejection. This is important because this strategy is effective only if recipient and donor differ at the MHC locus. Thus, islet donors may need to be selected on the basis of disparity of histocompatibility factors.

Xenotransplantation in Nude Mice

Recently, an automated digestion-filtration method was established in our laboratory for mass isolation of islets from canine, bovine, calf, porcine, and human pancreas which were further purified by density gradient centrifugation. Thymus-aplastic mice were rendered diabetic by streptozotocin injection. Because these animals are unable to reject grafted tissue this is an ideal model for bioassaying the endocrine viability of allogeneic and xenogeneic islet preparations.

A reasonable number of isolated higher mammalian islets were yielded (Table 6).

Xenotransplantation of porcine islets (800–1000 per recipient) reversed diabetes in all of seven diabetic nude mice within 1 day of transplantation (Fig. 8). These mice remained normoglycemic and gained weight until graft removal by nephrectomy on day 21 or day 100 post-transplant; this resulted in recurrence of

Table 6. Yield of isolated islets (mean ± SEM) from pancreas from various species by an automated digestion-filtration method established in our laboratory

	Dog	Calf	Cow	Pig	Human
Islet yield	2055 ± 496	6173 ± 1611	2099 ± 292	3288 ± 290	2241 ± 594
Number of pancreata	8	4	12	10	13

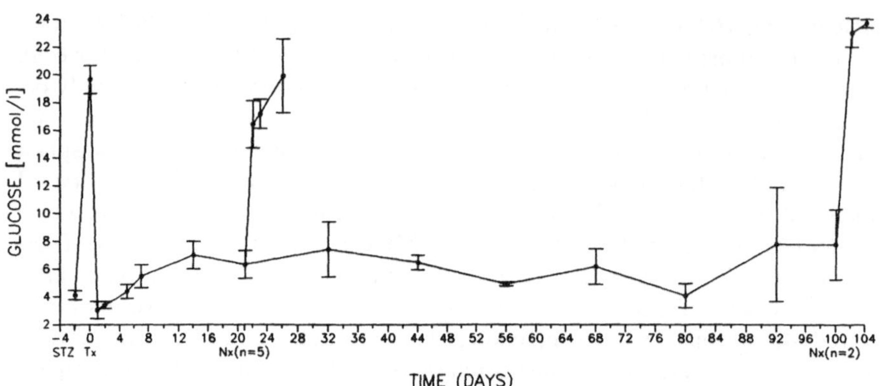

Fig. 8. Mean nonfasting plasma glucose after transplantation of 800–1000 porcine islets under the renal capsule of streptozotocin-diabetic nude mice ($n=7$). Normoglycemia was maintained until graft removal was performed by nephrectomy on day 21 ($n=5$) or on day 100 ($n=2$) after transplantation. *STZ*, induction of diabetes with intravenous streptozotocin; *Tx*, islet transplantation; *Nx*, graft removal by nephrectomy

diabetes in all of the animals and rapid weight loss, confirming that normoglycemia had been maintained by the porcine islet xenograft (Fig. 8).

Islet Transplantation in a Non-Insulin-Dependent Diabetes Model

Diabetes of Cohen rats resembles type II (NIDDM) diabetes of humans. Both have a similar genetic background, are triggered by extrinsic dietary factors, probably involve periods of hyperinsulinemia and peripheral insulin resistance, progress to hypoinsulinemia, have typical changes of the lipolytic and gluconeogenic enzyme pattern, and are associated with diabetic secondary complications.

Transplantation of about 1000 islets per recipient derived from the diabetes-resistant parental line decreased postprandial blood glucose levels (151 ± 7.8 vs. 274 ± 11.7 mg/dl), abolished glucosuria ($0.06 \pm 0.02\%$ vs. $2.6 \pm 0.75\%$), and increased the serum concentration of insulin (37.9 ± 3.5 vs. $30.2 \pm 2.3 \mu$U/ml). HbA_1 values returned to normal. As a consequence, the sevenrity of diabetic kidney lesions significantly decreased based on semiquantitative morphological examinations (Table 7).

Table 7. Incidence (%) of mild, moderate, and severe diabetic glomerular lesions in untreated and islet-transplanted diabetic Cohen's rats

Kidney lesions	Islet-transplanted rats	Untreated diabetic controls
None or mild	68.7	20.8
Moderate	57.4	28.0
Severe	3.2	22.0

From these studies we conclude that, at least in this type II diabetes model, abnormalities in insulin secretion in the beta-cells are of greater etiopathogenic importance than factors of peripheral insulin resistance.

Discussion

The results of vascularized pancreas transplantation in type I diabetic patients have improved in recent years, but the operation and the permanent immuno-suppression necessary continue to carry a significant morbidity and mortality. Since many of the problems encountered have been related either to surgical technique or to the exocrine portion of the transplanted pancreas, simple implantation of purified isolated pancreatic islets is an attractive alternative.

The majority of experience has been gained with experimental transplantations in diabetic rodents. Rodents were also widely used because the soft consistency of the pancreas in these species facilitates enzymatic digestion and separation of islet from exocrine tissue.

Our islet transplantation studies were performed in five different rodent diabetes models (mice, rats, nude mice). Four models resemble type I diabetes in humans: a chemical-toxic diabetes using the beta-cell toxin streptozotocin (Rakieten et al. 1963), the naturally occurring autoimmune diabetes of the BB rat (Rossini et al. 1979), low-dose streptozotocin diabetes in mice (Like and Rossini 1976), and a chemical-toxic diabetes in nude mice, a model which was introduced by Lake et al. (1988). Finally, a diabetes model which resembles type II diabetes in humans was established (Cohen et al. 1972).

An ideal site for islet implantation would be one that is safe and convenient to access, allows complete implantation of the transplanted tissue with optimal long-term metabolic function, and, if possible, is immunologically privileged. Comparing the intraportal and the intraperitoneal implantation routes in long-term studies following grafting of equal numbers of syngeneic islets in diabetic rats, we found the intraperitoneal route less effective. In other words, the intraperitoneal site seems to require larger quantities of islet tissue for reversal of diabetes (Kemp et al. 1973). Good metabolic function has also been achieved using other highly vascularized sites such as the spleen and the kidney capsular space (Koncz et al. 1973; Reece-Smith et al. 1981). From the point of view of metabolic efficiency, portal venous drainage seemed to be superior to systemic venous drainage and placing islets in the portal rather than systemic venous system requires implantation of less islet tissue to reverse diabetes and improve metabolic control (Reece-Smith et al. 1982; Brown et al. 1976). We showed further that the renal subcapsular space is to some extent immunologically privileged, at least in islet allografts in rats. A reliable technique for short-term preservation is necessary for clinical islet transplantation to be logistically practical. Long-term preservation would allow islets to be accumulated from various donors and islet banking, thus enabling metabolically successful islet transplantation and recipient selection on the basis of histocompatibility match or other factors. Two methods of islet preservation were investigated in our experiments: tissue culture and cryopreservation. The morphological integrity and the endocrine viability were well preserved in adult rat pancreatic islets maintained in culture for 28 days. Syngeneic transplantation of cultured adult rat pancreatic islets produced complete reversal of diabetes in the recipients (as had already been shown by Scharp et al. 1974; Bretzel et al. 1981a), confirming the preservation of islet viability. However, the relatively sophisticated equipment and fastidious conditions required for maintenance of islets in tissue culture make it difficult to store the quantities necessary for transplantation in large animal models or even in diabetic humans. Fortunately, cryopreservation has been found to be an optimal method, isolated pancreatic islets being stored in liquid nitrogen for weeks and years following programmed freezing. Despite some – reversible – loss of insulin biosynthesis capacity, but not of insulin secretory capacity, transplantation of frozen-thawed rat pancreatic islets completely reversed diabetes in syngeneic rats if the number of islets was doubled compared with freshly isolated islets (Rajotte et al. 1977; Bretzel et al. 1979b, Bretzel et al. 1982). In addition, pancreatic islets derived from higher mammals (dog, pig) and humans were successfully cryopreserved, showing preserved insulin secretory capacity in several experimental transplantations.

Minor abnormalities of blood glucose homeostasis, e.g., subnormal glucose tolerance and a loss of the cephalic phase of insulin secretion following islet transplantation, seem to exert no negative effect with respect to the ultimate goal of islet transplantation, the prevention and reversal of diabetic secondary complications. Indeed, one of the most exciting aspects of experimental islet transplantation has been the demonstration that the renal and other organ lesions associated with diabetes in animals are secondary to the diabetic state and that the early, but established, lesions either regress or stabilize following correction of the metabolic abnormalities by a transplantation. We demonstrated the influence of islet transplantation on established glomerular lesions, this leading to arrest or even reversal when a "late" isotransplantation had been done. On the other hand, „early" transplantation prevented kidney lesions. The influence of islet transplantation on the diabetic secondary syndrome was clearly demonstrated in the experiments presented here and in earlier studies (Mauer et al. 1974; Bretzel et al 1979a; Federlin and Bretzel 1984).

Another interesting aspect is the restorative effect that metabolically successful islet transplantation has on the remaining pancreas of the recipient. In the light of these findings, attempts to stop the decrease in the residual beta-cell mass in the early phase of type I diabetes or to treat subjects at risk of developing type I diabetes by immunomodulation or immunosuppression are becoming more rational.

The studies mentioned above were done in a syngeneic transplant system. Inbred strains allowed the multiple effects of islet transplantation to be evaluated independently of immunological factors. However, pancreatic islet allografts are subject to rejection, which takes place within only a few days, and no immunologically privileged site for islet allograft implantation has been found where these is also optimal blood supply to the islets and direct contact to the glucose-enriched portal blood flow (Reckard and Barker 1973; Reece-Smith et al. 1982; Brown et al. 1976).

Our attempts to prevent islet allograft and xenograft rejection revealed the most promising method to be immunomodulation by means of in vitro culture and cryopreservation prior to transplantation. This resulted in a quantitative and morphologically demonstrable depletion of antigen-presenting cells and a reduction in islet immunogenicity which enabled successful allografting and xenografting of pretreated islets with discontinuous immunosuppression, or even without immunosuppression, of the host. Other immunomodulatory methods aimed at diminishing islet immunogenicity prior to transplantation include application of antibodies directed against class II antigens or dendritic cells, UV light or γ-irradiation, and induction of tolerance (Bowen et al. 1980; Faustman et al. 1981; Lau et al. 1984; Gotoh et al. 1988; Kanai et al. 1989; Britt et al. 1982; Lau et al. 1983; Faustman et al. 1982; Faustman et al. 1984). However, we and others have had difficulty in reproducing some of the reported results; e.g., with UV irradiation or Ia antibody treatment of rat islets we did not obtain definite allograft acceptance. The conflicting results may be explained by species or strain differences and possibly by MHC restriction of some of these effects.

Another intriguing possible approach to the prevention of the rejection that would be applicable to islet allografts is the encapsulation of islets in a membrane. We tested several commercially available or specially prepared membranes and found ones that may prevent the entry cells, antibodies, and mediators such as IL-1, and yet have pores large enough to allow bidirectional diffusion of nutrients and insulin. There are four major devices for immunoisolation: extravascular diffusion chambers, intravascular diffusion chambers, intravascular ultrafiltration chambers, and microencapsulation by incorporating isolated islets into biocompatible spherical capsules using polylysine alginate membranes (Scharp et al. 1984). Transplantation studies using macroencapsulation and microencapsulation of islets initially gave frankly disappointing results. More recently, however, the idea has resurfaced with a report of reversal of experimental diabetes for up to 1 year using macroencapsulated human insulinoma tissue and microencapsulated islets in rodents (Altman et al. 1986; Taunton-Rigby 1986).

There is an emerging consensus that type I diabetes mellitus is an autoimmune disease and this gives rise to the question of whether autoimmunity might destroy transplanted islets in naturally diabetic hosts. This has been unequivocally demonstrated by the recurrence of diabetes in nonimmunosuppressed recipients of a vascularized pancreas graft from a nondiabetic identical twin (Sibley et al. 1985). However, recurrence of diabetes in such cases can be prevented by the use of immunosuppression (Sutherland et al. 1984). In our studies on islet transplantation in two different autoimmune diabetes models we indeed observed recurrence of the diabetes if MHC-compatible islets were grafted. We could further demonstrate that MHC-incompatible islets pretreated with tissue culture to reduce transplant immunogenicity are not affected and the recipient remains normoglycemic.

We conclude that to make clinical islet transplantation in type I diabetic patients a reality we must avoid two distinct immune responses: allograft rejection resulting from histocompatibility differences between donor and recipient; and recurrence of the autoimmune response initiating the disease and later directed against the transplanted beta-cells. Immunomodulation of islet tissue selected on the basis of disparity of histocompatibility factors prior to transplantation may resolve one of the two current major problems in clinical islet transplantation. Our experiments in isolating islets of higher mammalian and human pancreas have shown that the techniques now in use for islet isolation and purification have the potential to produce sufficient tissue to show a clinical effect, which until recently was the second major problem. The initial clinical trials of islet transplantation were unsuccessful and led to some disillusionment (Najarian et al. 1977; Sutherland et al. 1980; Kolb and Largiader 1980). It appears now that substantial progress in islet transplantation research has been made and so successful clinical islet transplantation in diabetes mellitus should be possible within the next few years.

Acknowledgements. This work was supported by the Deutsche Forschungsgemeinschaft (Br 944/1-1 and 944/1-2; He 1503/1-1 and 1503/1-2; Str 289/1-1) and by the Bundesminister für Forschung und Technologie (FKZ 07024806).

References

Altman JJ, Houlbert D, Callard P, McMillan P, Solomon BA, Rosen J, Galletti PM (1986) Long-term plasma glucose normalization in experimental diabetic rats with macroencapsulated implants of benign human insulinomas. Diabetes 35: 625–633

Blum B (1986) Homologe Transplantation Langerhans'scher Inseln nach Immunmodulation und Immunsuppression beim experimentellen Diabetes mellitus der Ratte. Dissertation, University of Giessen

Bowen KM, Andrews L, Lafferty KJ (1980) Successful allotransplantation of mouse pancreatic islets to non-immunosuppressed recipients. Diabetes 29 [Suppl 1]: 98–104

Bretzel RG (1984) Inseltransplantation und Diabetes mellitus. Pflaum, Munich

Bretzel RG, Breidenbach C, Hofmann J, Federlin K (1979a) Islet transplantation in experimental diabetes of the rat. VI. Rate of regression in diabetic kidney lesions after isogeneic islet transplantation. Quantitative measurements. Horm Metab Res 11: 200–207

Bretzel RG, Schäfer S, Schneider J, Dobroschke J, Federlin K (1979b) Cryopreservation of pancreatic islets for transplantation in diabetes mellitus. Excerpta Med Int Congr Ser 481: 32

Bretzel RG, Beule B, Federlin K (1981a) Function and morphology of adult rat islets after culture and transplantation. In: Federlin K, Bretzel RG (eds) Islet isolation, culture and cryopreservation, Thieme, Stuttgart, pp 96–110

Bretzel RG, Schneider J, Zekorn T, Federlin K (1981b) Cryopreservation of rat, porcine and human pancreatic islets for transplantation. In: Federlin K, Bretzel RG (eds) Islet isolation, culture and cryopreservation, Thieme, Stuttgart, pp 152–160

Bretzel RG, Merforth K, Maier V, Federlin K (1982) Kryokultur tierischer und humaner Pankreasinseln für die Transplantation bei Diabetes mellitus. Verh Dtsch Ges Inn Med 88: 824–828

Bretzel RG, Brocks DG, Federlin KF (1984a) Reversal and prevention of nephropathy by islet transplantation in diabetic rats. In: Shafrir E, Renolt AE (eds) Lessons from animal diabetes, Libbey, London, pp 425–435

Bretzel RG, Merforth K, Beule B, Federlin K (1984b) Effect of islet transplantation on biochemical variables in experimental diabetes. In: Shafrir E, Renold AE (eds) Lessons from animal diabetes. Libbey, London, pp 599–605

Bretzel RG, Blum BE, Höll E, Hering BJ, Federlin K (1986a) Rat islet allograft survival following different immunomodulative and immunosuppressive treatments. Excerpta Med Int Congr Scr 717: 181–185

Bretzel RG, Richardt M, Menden A, Federlin K (1986b) Perspectives from experimental islet transplantation: the retorative effect on the diabetic pancreas. Pediatr Adolesc Endocrinol 15: 398–403

Britt LD, Scharp DW, Lacy PE, Slavin S (1982) Transplantation of islet cells across major histocompatibility barriers after total lymphoid irradiation and infusion of allogeneic bone marrow cells. Diabetes 31 [Suppl 4]: 63–68

Brown J, Mullen Y, Molnar IG, Clark WR (1976) Importance of hepatic-portal route for control of diabetes. Diabetes 25 [Suppl 1]: 338

Büscher C, Weis A, Woehrle M, Bretzel RG, Cohen AM, Federlin K (1989) Islet transplantation in experimental diabetes of the rat. XII. Effect on diabetic retinopathy. Morphological findings and morphometrical evaluation. Horm Metab Res 21: 227–231

Cohen AM, Teitelbaum A, Saliternik R (1972) Genetics and diet as factors in development of diabetes mellitus. Metabolism 21: 235–240

Faustman D, Hauptfeld V, Lacy PE, Davie J (1981) Prolongation of murine islet allograft survival by pretreatment of islets with antibody directed to Ia determinants. Proc Natl Acad Sci USA 78: 5156–5159

Faustman D, Lacy P, Davie J, Hauptfeld V (1982) Prevention of allograft rejection by immunozation with donor blood depleted of Ia-bearing cells. Science 217: 157–158

Faustman DL, Steinman RM, Gebel HM, Hauptfeld V, Davie JM, Lacy PE (1984) Prevention of rejection of murine islet allografts by pretreatment with anti-dendritic cell antibody. Proc Natl Acad Sci USA 81: 3864–3868

Federlin K, Bretzel RG (1984) The effect of islet transplantation on complications in experimental diabetes of the rat. World J Surg 8: 169–178

Forsen JW, Blum BE, Bretzel RG, Federlin K (1984) Islet transplantation in experimental diabetes of the rat. IX. In vitro culture reduces Ia-bearing cells in rat islets. Horm Metab Res 16: 671–672

Fortmeyer HP (1981) Thymus aplastische Maus (*nu/nu*), thymus aplastische Ratte (*rnu/rnu*): Haltung, Zucht, Versuchsmodelle. Parey, Berlin

Gotoh M, Maki T, Kiyoizume T, Satomi S, Monaco AP (1985) An improved method for isolation of mouse pancreatic islets. Transplantation 40: 437–438

Gotoh M, Porter J, Monaco AP, Maki T (1988) Prolongation of islet xenograft survival by islet irradiation and ALS-treatment of recipients. Transplant Proc 20: 997–999

Hering BJ, Romann D, Clarius A, Brendel M, Slijepcevic M, Bretzel RG, Federlin K (1989) Bovine islets of Langerhans – potential source for transplantation. Diabetes 38 [Suppl 1]: 206–208

Kanai T, Porter J, Gotoh M, Monaco AP, Maki T (1989) Effect of gamma-irradiation on mouse pancreatic islet-allograft survival. Diabetes 38 [Suppl 1]: 154–156

Kemp CB, Knight NJ, Scharp DW, Ballinger WF, Lacy PE (1973) Effect of transplantation size on the results of pancreatic islet isografts in diabetic rats. Diabetologia 9: 486–491

Kolb E, Largiader F (1980) Clinical islet transplantation. Transplant Proc 12 [Suppl 2]: 205–207

Koncz L, de Lellis RA, Zimmermann CE, Franklin A, Davidoff F (1973) The spleen as transplant site for islets in diabetic rats. Diabetes 22: 437

Kuwabara T, Cogan DG (1960) Studies of retinal vascular patterns. I. Normal architecture. Arch Ophthalmol 64: 904–911

Lacy PE, Kostianovsky MA (1967) A method for the isolation of intact islets of Langerhans from the rat pancreas. Diabetes 16: 35–39

Lake SP, Chamberlain J, Husken P, Bell PRF, James RFL (1988) In vivo assessment of isolated pancreatic islet viability using the streptozotocin-induced diabetic nude rat. Diabetologia 31: 390–394

Lau H, Reemtsma K, Hardy MA (1983) Pancreatic islet allograft prolongation by donor-specific blood transfusions treated with ultraviolet irradiation. Science 221: 754–756

Lau H, Reemtsma K, Hardy MA (1984) Prolongation of rat islet allograft survival by direct ultraviolet irradiation of the graft. Science 223: 607–609

Like AA, Rossini AA (1976) Streptozotocin-induced pancreatic insulitis: new model of diabetes mellitus. Science 193: 415–417

Linn T, Becker M, Woehrle M, Zekorn T, Hering BJ, Bretzel RG, Federlin K (1989) Immune destruction of transplanted islets of Langerhans in a model of induced type I diabetes. Transplant Proc 21: 2685–2686

Mauer SM, Sutherland DER, Steffes MW, Leonard AJ, Najarian JS, Michael AF, Brown DM (1974) Pancreatic islet transplantation: effects on the glomerular lesions of experimental diabetes in the rat. Diabetes 23: 748–753

Najaran JS, Sutherland DER, Matas AJ, Steffes MW, Simmons RL, Goetz FC (1977) Human islet transplantation: a preliminary report. Transplant Proc 9: 233–236

Rajotte RV, Stewart HL, Voss WAG, Shnitka TK, Dossetor JB (1977) Viability studies on frozen-thawed rat islets of Langerhans. Cryobiology 14: 116–120

Rakieten N, Rakieten ML, Nadkarni V (1963) Studies on the diabetogenic action of streptozotocin. Cancer Chemother Rep 29: 91–98

Reckard CR, Barker CF (1973) Transplantation of isolated pancreatic islets across strong and weak histocompatibility barriers. Transplant Proc 5: 761–763

Reece-Smith H, Du Toit DF, McShane P, Morris PJ (1981) Prolonged survival of pancreatic islet allograft transplanted beneath the renal capsule. Transplantation 31: 305–306

Reece-Smith H, McShane P, Morris PJ (1982) Glucose and insulin changes following a renoportal shunt in streptozotocin diabetic rats with pancreatic islets isografts under the kidney capsule. Diabetologia 23: 343–346

Ricordi C, Lacy PE, Finke EH, Olack BJ, Scharp DW (1988) Automated method for isolation of human pancreatic islets. Diabetes 37: 413–420

Rossini AA, Williams RM, Mordes JP, Appel MC, Like AA (1979) Spontaneous diabetes in the gnotobiotic BB/w rat. Diabetes 28: 1031–1032

Scharp DW, White DJ, Ballinger WF, Lacy PE (1974) Transplantation of intact islets of Langerhans after tissue culture. In Vitro 9: 364

Scharp DW, Mason NS, Sparks RE (1984) Islet immuno-isolation: the use of hybrid artificial organs to prevent islet tissue rejection. World J Surg 8: 221–229

Sharma AK, Zimmermann O, Britland ST, Stracke H, Bretzel RG, Federlin K (1988) Ultrastructural nerve abnormalities in experimental diabetes: prevention and reversal with pancreatic islet transplantation. Diabetes Res Clin Pract 5 [Suppl 1]: 330

Sibley RK, Sutherland DER, Goetz F, Michael AF (1985) Recurrent diabetes mellitus in the pancreas iso- and allograft. A light and electron microscopic and immunhistochemical analysis of four cases. Lab Invest 53: 132–144

Strödter D (1987) Diabetische Kardiomyopathie – Tatsache oder Fiktion? Habilitationsschrift, University of Giessen

Strödter D, Schuster KR, Bretzel RG, Federlin K (1987) Der Effekt von Diabetes mellitus und Inselzelltransplantation auf Funktion und Stoffwechsel des isoliert arbeitenden Rattenherzens. Klin Wochenschr 65 [Suppl 9]: 207

Sutherland DE, Sibley R, Xu X, Michael A, Srikanta AM, Taub F, Najarian J, Goetz FC (1984) Twin-to-twin pancreas transplantation: reversal and reenactment of the pathogenesis of type-1 diabetes. Trans Assoc Am Physicians 97: 80–87

Sutherland DER, Matas AJ, Goetz FC, Najarian JS (1980) Transplantation of dispersed pancreatic islet tissue in humans. Autografts and allografts. Daibetes 29 [Suppl 1]: 31–44

Taunton-Rigby A (1986) Transplantation of encapsulated islets. Transplant Proc 18: 1841–1844

Woehrle M, Markmann JF, Silvers WK, Barker CF, Naji A (1986) Transplantation of cultured pancreatic islets to BB-rats. Surgery 100: 334–341

Woehrle M, Beyer K, Bretzel RG, Federlin K (1989) Prevention of islet allograft rejection in experimental diabetes of the rat without immunosuppression of the host. Transplant Proc 21: 2705–2706

Woehrle MF, Markmann JF, Armstrong J, Naji A (1987) Effect of transplant site on islet allograft survival in BB-rats. Transplant Proc 19: 925–927

Perspectives on Islet Cell Transplantation in Type I Diabetes Mellitus

R. Alejandro and D. H. Mintz

Zusammenfassung

Der stärkste Anstoß, nach einer sicheren und effektiven Methode der Transplantation von endokrinem Pankreas zu suchen, leitet sich aus der Notwendigkeit ab, erkrankte Inseln durch solche zu ersetzen, die auf physiologische Reize mit einer Signal-gekoppelten Insulinsekretion antworten und dadurch die Feinregulation des Stoffwechsels wiederherstellen. Die Transplantationsversuche in unserem Labor mit Hunden, die an einem spontanen oder durch Pankreatektomie hervorgerufenen Diabetes leiden, waren insbesondere deswegen so aufschlußreich, weil sie die für erfolgreiche Pilotstudien mit Inseltransplantationen beim Menschen wichtigen Grundvoraussetzungen klären ließen. Wir haben zunehmend Beweise dafür, daß funktionstüchtige Inseln in für eine erfolgreiche Transplantation ausreichender Zahl aus Pankreasorganen isoliert werden können, die für 24 Stunden (100% Transplantatüberleben), ja sogar 48 Stunden (60% Transplantatüberleben) in Beltzer's Lösung gehalten worden sind. Die alles andere überwiegende Voraussetzung, die letztlich die quantitative Ausbeute einer Inselisolierung von einem konservierten humanen Pankreas bestimmt, ist die Qualität und die Art des Enzymes, der Collagenase. Ein beachtlicher Fortschritt wurde auch bei den Methoden zur weiteren Aufreinigung und Anreicherung isolierter Inseln mit Hilfe von nicht-toxischen Gradienten unter Verwendung von Rinderalbumin unterschiedlicher Dichte erreicht. Andererseits mußte selbst zwei Jahre nach allogener Inseltransplantation noch ein Versagen der endokrinen Inselfunktion festgestellt werden, deren Ursachen noch diskutiert werden. Aber unsere tierexperimentell an Hunden gewonnenen Erfahrungen ermöglichten uns, klinische Inseltransplantationsversuche bei Typ I-Diabetikern zu beginnen. An unserem Zentrum erhielten vier Patienten intrahepatisch Inselallotransplantate, ein Patient wurde zweimal transplantiert. Bei allen Patienten ergaben sich Hinweise auf eine erhaltene Inselfunktion initial; in drei Fällen sistierte diese Funktion nach ein bis vier Wochen, ein Transplantat funktionierte über mindestens 26 Wochen.

Introduction

Although the life expectancy of patients with type I diabetes mellitus has considerably improved since the introduction of exogenous insulin, the quality of this life has been burdened by the unmasking of a chronic degenerative process characterized by retinopathy, neuropathy, nephropathy, and premature atherosclerosis. Largely circumstantial evidence can be marshalled in support of the notion that recurrent and/or sustained hyperglycemia are the key culprits responsible for the chronic degenerative disease. Resolution of this fundamental issue is so immensely important for the development of rational treatment strategies for patients and professionals that a national multicenter federally supported clinical trial to clarify whether intensive therapy retards, aborts, or prevents diabetes implications has been launched in the United States (Diabetes Complication and Control Trial, DCCT).

The major impetus for the development of safe, and effective transplantation of the endocrine pancreas is the need for a strategy to replace diseased islets with islets that respond to physiologic secretagogues with a signal-coupled insulin secretory response that enables fine regulation of metabolism to be reestablished. This requirement is intimately associated with the inadequacies of current insulin therapy, namely that intermittent subcutaneously administered insulin cannot achieve physiologic pharmacokinetics, and continuous subcutaneous or intrapertioneal insulin requires such vigilant and open-ended monitoring, that few patients can or should be expected to sustain such an effort over a lifetime.

A completely mechanical approach to the limitations of injectable insulin still awaits a sensing device that is capable of transducing physiologic signals to time and dose response curves that perfectly mimic pulsatile secretory activity of normal islets. The engineering principles inherent in design are known but our knowledge about the control mechanisms that govern secretory processes is still too limited to anticipate much more than a primitive prototype to evolve out of the current level of research.

Until now, attempts to transplant islet cells have been accomplished by transplanting the entire pancreas or a segment of it from cadaver or living related donor into a patient with diabetes who, in most cases, has already received a kidney transplant and is taking immunosuppressive drugs. As of March, 1988, 1394 cases had been reported to the registry, including 1129 cases since 1982. The overall 1-year patient and pancreas graft survival (insulin-independent) rates for all cases 1983–1988 were 82% and 46% respectively [1]. Technical problems, particularly related to the management of undesired exocrine secretions, and rejection problems still limit this approach. Transplantation of islets that have been isolated from a whole pancreas continues to be an attractive alternative for the reversal of diabetes.

Progress in islet transplantation in rodents over the past 10–15 years provides an impressive record of achievements that unequivocally demonstrates: the feasibility of isolating intact, functionally competent islets from the pancreas; the ability to modify the immunogenecity of the endocrine structure in vitro by culture at room temperature or in the presence of high O_2 and by treatment with cytotoxic monoclonal antibodies that are directed at antigens on antigen-presenting passenger cells within the islet; the ability to cryopreserve, store, and thaw islets with retention of their functional capacity in vitro and in vivo; that immunologic tolerance can be induced to islet allografts by immune modifications of islets, the recipients or both, so that continuous immunosuppressive therapies are not required to prevent rejection; that fetal pancreas can be a source of functioning islets, but unlike islets derived from adult tissues, a period of time is required for development in vitro and/or in vivo before the functional mass of developing islets is sufficient to result in a reversal of hyperglycemia; and that islet iso- and allografts can be transplanted into the liver, spleen, or beneath the kidney capsule of diabetic rodents and result in long-term reversal of hyperglycemia and prevention of cataracts, early retinal disease, delayed nerve conduction velocities, and mesangial hyperplasia. Thus, available data in rodents lends credence to the notion that islet allografts alone can induce near normal metabolism and prevent, abort, or reverse (early) complications in the eyes, peripheral nervous system, and kidneys of hyperglycemic rodents.

Studies in rodents have catalyzed similar efforts in other mammals (dogs, monkeys) in order to define the natural history of islet transplantation in large animals before embarking on larger scale clinical trials [2–6].

The experiments in dogs with either spontaneous or pancreatectomy-induced diabetes in our laboratory have been particularly instructive in clarifying issues that impact in important ways on the success of pilot studies of islet cell transplantation in man.

Organ Donation and Preservation

Our experience with canine pancreases indicated that islets have limited tolerance to cold ischemia (< 6 h). This finding imposed a geographic restriction for human donor organ procurement to a narrow catchment area or to the impractical option of transporting organs for research by chartered jet.

In the last several years, Beltzer's group at the University of Wisconsin developed a hyperosmolar colloid preservation fluid that also contains several agents that are theoretically beneficial, namely allopurinol and glutathione to protect against free radical damage and adenosine as a precursor for ATP synthesis during reperfusion, but this has still to be proven. They have shown, as have others, that vascular perfusion combined with cold slush immersion in this fluid will preserve canine pancreases for 72 h [7]. We have accumulated evidence that viable islets can be isolated in sufficient numbers for successful transplantation from glands that have been preserved in Beltzer's solution for 24 h (100% graft survival) and even 48 h (60% graft survival) [8].

The availability of this new preservation fluid that improves tolerance to cold ischemia prolongs the critical period between harvesting a gland and its transportation to an islet isolation facility. These results should radically expand nationwide access to donor pancreases for continued research, leading soon to multicenter clinical trials.

Islet Isolation

The overriding condition that ultimately determines the quantitative effectiveness of islet isolation from the preserved human pancreas is the quality and nature of the enzyme collagenase. This enzyme, currently a product of *Clostridium histolyticum*, is used to digest collagen bundles and other connective tissue structures in order to liberate islets that are deeply enmeshed in acinar and interstitial tissues.

Although it has been known for some time that batches of commercially available collagenase differ remarkably in their efficacy, it was not know whether these results were due to differences in connective tissue structures that were age and species dependent, or due to the purity and activity of the enzyme. It appears from ongoing work that each of these variables has important effects on the efficacy of collagenase. Moreover, until these issues have been addressed systematically, an ambiguity will continue to surface in human islet isolation laboratories, retarding progress toward a universally acceptable method for islet isolation.

A second important component of islet isolation relates to the need to develop rapid methods that will allow islets to be further enriched if not clearly separated from digest of residual tissue comprising nonislet pancreatic tissue. Considerable progress is being made in this area, as well, so that nontoxic gradients can now be constructed using different densities of bovine serum albumin (BSA) [8]. Moreover, islets can be layered in these BSA gradients by employing centrifugal devices that permit closed sterile separation of islet layers from the remainder of the pancreatic digest [9]. Thus, considerable progress in enrichment of human islet digest is now possible.

The need for islet enrichment is several-fold. The volume of the transplant should be kept as small as possible to: (a) minimize ischemic infarction at the transplantation site; (b) minimize inflammatory responses that are provoked initially by cells and cellular products at the transplantation site (inflammatory cells such as macrophages and polys are capable of releasing factors that can cause injury to islet cells by several possible mechanisms); (c) prevent intravascular coagulation that has been reported with relatively large volume cellular implants delivered intraportally; and (d) to theoretically minimize the antigenicity of the transplant by limiting the amount of nonislet tissue that is present.

Immunosuppression

Since isolated islets are avascular transplants, they are considered to manifest a heightened vulnerability to rejection. This notion gathered considerable support when it was demonstrated that immunosuppression regimens failed to protect islet allografts in rodents whereas protection was afforded to kidney and heart allografts from the same donors. The clinical experience with vascularized pancreatic grafts suggest that the function of intrapancreatic islet allografts was not adversely affected by conventional immunosuppressive agents administered in various combinations. However, the experiences with pancreatic allografts do not entirely dismiss the possibility that immunosuppressive agents may be cytotoxic to islets. We have administered cyclosporine to normal dogs in dosages required to uniformly prevent islet allograft rejection, and have demonstrated that islet secretory functions are irreversibly impaired after 1 month of continuous cyclosporin therapy [10]. Also, we have preliminary evidence that administration of cyclosporin is associated with premature failure of intrahepatic islet autografts in dogs.

These observations are particularly unsettling at this juncture since proper use of cyclosporin in dogs has consistently resulted in reversal of spontaneous and pancreatectomy-induced diabetes. Rejection has been encountered in only 2 of 38 consecutive islet transplants [5].

In view of these recent experiences, it is difficult to place the administration of cyclosporin in proper perspective as a sole effective agent for suppression of islet allograft rejection. It achieves this goal admirably in dogs, but it is possible that continuous administration of the agent may result in irreparable injury to the transplant so that islet mass ultimately declines below the threshold levels required to maintain fasting euglycemia despite effective immunosuppression.

If this prediction is correct, one can expect that islet allografts in recipients treated with continuous cyclosporin will all ultimately fail. This has been the finding so far in every islet transplant in dogs that we studied. Islet allograft failure has, in fact, been encountered as long as 2 years after successful transplantation [11].

There are, however, other mechanism(s) that might also contribute to late failures of intrahepatic islet allografts. Since islet autografts seem to suffer the same fate even in the absence of cyclosporin [3], the findings could reflect that heterotopic islets have a finite life span, that intrahepatic islets may be exposed to noxious factors peculiar to the portal venous system, or that the size of the islet mass that is needed to sustain normal metabolism over very long periods exceeds by many times the number of islets that are engrafted within the liver after transplantation. The later possibility would be consistent with conventional notions that chronic stimulation of an initially marginal intrahepatic β-cell mass could initiate a self-perpetuating and progressive metabolic deterioration and loss of β-cells.

Clinical Trial

The experiences gained in canine islet transplantation have allowed us to initiate clinical trials in patients with type I diabetes mellitus [12]. The current candidates for the clinical islet cell transplant trials include patients with previous kidney grafts and patients who will receive simultaneous kidney and islet allografts from the same cadaveric donors.

Four patients have received intrahepatic islet allografts in our institution; one of the subjects was transplanted on two occasions. Evidence for functional survival of islet allografts was obtained in each patient; three islet grafts failed to sustain this function after 1–4 weeks posttransplantation and one graft continued to function for at least 26 weeks. This patient received a second islet allograft that appeared to provide additional β-cell secretory capacity to the first graft, but both grafts eventually failed in temporal relationship to the substitution of azathioprine for cyclosporin A 18 weeks after the second transplant.

These pilot clinical trials highlighted the need for substantial improvements in two critical areas if progress was to be expected in islet transplantation in man. Limited yields of islets from a cadaveric pancreas and the heightened vulnerability of islet allografts to rejection seem to continue to slow advances in clinical application of this approach for treatment of insulin-dependent diabetes mellitus.

Since these initial trials, we have modified our technique for islet isolation and now obtain yields of islets that are several-fold higher than in the previous study. This is due partly to the availability of newer collagenase enzymes, as outlined earlier. Also, we now use a new density gradient separation system [11] to reduce tissue volume and increase islet purity rather than the crude separations performed at unit gravity that were used in the first clinical trials. The higher degree of purity and lower packed cell volumes should facilitate the application and effectiveness of protocols designed to delete or impair the function of antigen presenting cells in these newer islet preparations. These advances directly address, moreover, some of the limitations we uncovered in the clinical trial detailed here. A further extension of these pilot clinical studies seems to be warranted.

References

1. Sutherland DER (1988) Who should get a pancreas transplant? Diabetes Care 2: 681
2. Alejandro R, Cutfield RG, Shienvold FL, Latif Z, Mintz DH (1985) Successful long term survival of pancreatic islet allografts in spontaneous or pancreatectomy-induced diabetes in dogs: cyclosporine induced immune unresponsiveness. Diabetes 34: 825–828
3. Alejandro R, Cutfield RG, Shienvold FL, Polonsky KS, Noel J, Olson L, Dillberger J, Miller J, Mintz DH (1986) Natural history of intrahepatic canine islet cell autografts. J Clin Invest 78: 1339
4. Alejandro R, Latif Z, Noel J, Shienvold FL, Mintz DH (1987) Effect of anti-Ia antibodies, culture, and cyclosporine on prolongation of canine islet allograft survival. Diabetes 36: 269
5. Alejandro R, Latif Z, Polonsky KS, Shienvold FL, Civantos F, Mintz DH (1988) Natural history of multiple intrahepatic canine islet allografts during and following administration of cyclosporine. Transplantation 45: 1036

6. Gray DW, Warnock G, Sutton R, Peters M, McShane P, Morris PJ (1986) Successful autotransplantation of isolated islets of Langerhans in the cynomolgus monkey. Br J Surg 73: 850–853

7. Wahlberg JA, Love R, Landegaard L, Southard JH, Belzer FO (1987) 72-Hour preservation of the canine pancreas. Transplantation 43: 5–8

8. Zucker P, Bloom AD, Strasser S, Alejandro R (1989) Successful cold storage preservation of canine pancreas with UW-1 solution prior to islet transplantation. Transplantation (in press)

9. Lake SP, Bassett PD, Larkins A, Revell J, Walczak K, Chamberlain J, Rumford GM, London NJM, Veitch PS, Bell PRF, James RFL (1989) Large-scale purification of human islets utilizing discontinuous albumin gradient on IBM 2991 cell separator. Diabetes 38: 143–145

10. Alejandro R, Feldmann EC, Bloom AD, Polonsky KS (1989) Cyclosporine interferes with insulin C-peptide secretion in healthy beagles. Diabetes (in press)

11. Alejandro R, Bloom AD, Zucker P, Polonsky KS, Mintz DH (1988) The fate of intrahepatic islet allografts in dogs with spontaneous diabetes. Diabetes 38 [Suppl 1]: 246

12. Alejandro R, Mintz DH, Noel J, Latif Z, Koh N, Russell E, Miller J (1987) Islet cell transplantation in Type I diabetes mellitus. Transplant Proc 19: 2359–2361

Human Islet Isolation and Transplantation

C. S. McCullough, D. W. Scharp, and P. E. Lacy

Zusammenfassung

Inseltransplantation als eine zuverlässige alternative Therapie für Typ I–Diabetes Mellitus bleibt eine vielversprechende Möglichkeit. Es gibt aber keine gut dokumentierten Fälle von erfolgreichen klinischen Versuchen. Trotzdem wurden entscheidende Fortschritte gemacht, um die Isolation der menschlichen Langerhansschen Inseln zu verbessern. Inselautotransplantation nach vollständiger oder nahezu vollständiger Pankreatektomie macht eine Langzeitfunktion transplantierter Inseln wahrscheinlich. Anfängliche klinische Versuche mit allogenen Inseltransplantaten haben eine kurzfristige endokrine Funktion aufgezeigt.

Verbesserte Isolationstechniken haben zu verbesserten Ergebnissen bei Inseltransplantationsversuchen geführt. Diese Versuche haben ebenso wichtige Aspekte für die zukünftige Forschung ergeben. Zur Immunologie der humanen Inseltransplantationen ist noch viel aufzuklären. Ebenso bleibt die Interaktion der immunosuppressiven Therapie mit dem Angehen der Inseln nach Implantation und ihrer Funktion weitgehend unbekannt. Weitere Forschung und Fortschritte auf diesen Gebieten könnten eines Tages ein sicheres System schaffen für eine kontinuierliche Insulinversorgung, mit der sich die physiologische Glukosehomöostase erreichen ließe. Vielleicht könnten mit einer solchen Therapie im Anfangsstadium der Erkrankung eingeleitet, die krankmachenden diabetischen Sekundärkomplikationen verhindert werden.

Introduction

Short of prevention, the ideal therapy for human type I diabetes mellitus would provide, early in the course of the disease, a system for continuous insulin delivery which physiologically matches normal glucose homeostasis. Transplantation of functioning islet tissue has the potential to meet these criteria. Whole organ transplantation (discussed in another section of this book) requires continuous immunosuppressive therapy, with all of its attendant risks. Transplantation of purified isolated islets of Langerhans offers the possibility of achieving glucose control without the need for continuous immunosuppression. It is now possible to perform successful allotransplantation of purified islets in experimental animal model systems without long-term, continuous immunosuppression [1–5]. These animals have essentially normal glucose control by measurable parameters. Not only can control of serum glucose levels be achieved in experimental models, the complications of diabetes can be prevented or reversed as thoroughly presented by Federlin and Bretzel [6].

While the feasability of islet transplantation has been demonstrated in animal models there have been no well documented reports of long-term success with human allotransplantation. At least two factors have been identified as primary obstacles to successful human islet allografts: obtaining sufficient quantities of isolated, purified human islets and circumventing allograft rejection.

Despite these obstacles, sufficient progress has been made in the technology of islet isolation and in our understanding of the immunobiology of islet allograft rejection to allow for preliminary human trials.

Human Islet Isolation

The collagenase technique for isolation of islets from the rat pancreas was developed in the 1960s and 1970s [7, 8]. This technique allowed for the demonstration of the efficacy of islet transplantation in reversing experimental diabetes in animals. However, the collagenase technique, with the methods applied to rodents, does not yield large numbers of intact, viable islets from the human pancreas.

A major problem with islet isolation from the human pancreas is the large amounts of collagen present within the organ. Collagen in humans is primarily localized in the interlobular and intralobular septae, which would make the gland difficult to distend [9]. In addition, the large amount of collagen results in the formation of a gelatinous material during the collagenase digestion which entraps islets and prevents their isolation.

Consequently, various refinements of the rodent collagenase technique for application to human islet isolation have been reported. Gray and colleagues used collagenase in a distension and filtration technique followed by a Ficoll gradient separation similar to that used for the isolation of rodent islets [10]. Though the isolated islets were viable and functional the yield was only about 1000 islets/g pancreas with an overall purity of less than 30%. Kneteman and Rajotte used pancreatic duct perfusion with collagenase followed by hand teasing of the tissue and needle trituration. Islets were purified on a series of filters. The yield was greater than 80 000 islets/gland, with a purity of 20% –40% [11]. Viability and function were confirmed in vitro. Kuhn et al. [12] reported a technique of pancreatic duct perfusion with collagenase followed by the Velcro technique described by Lacy et al. [13]. The islet yield with this technique was approximately 80 000 islets per pancreas. Data regarding the purity and viability were not presented. Alderson et al. and Scharp et al. investigated the use of a tissue macerator for the dispersion of the digested human pancreas [14, 15]. The yield was over 100 000 islets/pancreas with a purity of greater than 50%. In vitro and in vivo experiments confirmed viability and funtion.

Unfortunately the number of transplanted islets necessary to reverse human diabetes is not known. In the human approximately 10% – 15% of the pancreatic mass is generally sufficient to prevent overt clinical diabetes following pancreatic resection. Clinical trials of islet autotransplantation after total or near total pancreatectomy for chronic pancreatitis have been performed in over 70 patients [16]. Long-term independence from insulin is rare. Morrow et al. [16] have reported on ten patients with autotransplantation following total ($n=1$) or near total ($n=9$) pancreatectomy for chronic pancreatitis. Four patients remained insulin independent for more than 3 months. The islet yield for these four patients was from 46% – 83% as calculated from the insulin content of the resected pancreas and the transplanted tissue. The purity ranged from 50% to greater than 90% based on the amylase content of the residual exocrine tissue. Three patients eventually reverted to insulin-dependent, nonketosis prone diabetes at 4, 5, and 15 months. The fourth patient was insulin independent until her death from cardiovascular disease 4 years after near-total pancreatectomy and islet autotransplantation via the portal vein. It should be noted that this patient had familial chronic pancreatitis hyperinsulinemia prior to near-total pancreatectomy, Islet hyperplasia was present on histologic examination of the resected gland. The possibility that the small pancreatic remnant remaining after near-total pancreatectomy was responsible for glucose homeostasis cannot be entirely excluded. These authors did show that plasma insulin levels were virtually undetectable following the pancreatectomy and returned to assayable levels following autotransplantation [16].

Cameron et al. in another series of eight patients with 95% pancreatectomy and "islet tissue" autotransplantation had six patients become normoglycemic [17]. Unfortunately, the amount of actual islet tissue transplanted was not clearly quantitated, nor was the purity. Three of these patients developed insulin dependent diabetes at 3, 6, and 8 months after surgery. Cameron et al. showed, with percutaneous catheterization of the hepatic and portal veins 4 months after islet autotransplantation, an increase in hepatic vein and peripheral vein insulin in response to an intravenous glucose challenge. The same studies showed no simultaneous rise in portal vein insulin, suggesting that the intrahepatic islet tissue was functioning and responsible for normoglycemia. In addition, glucagon was not detectable in portal venous blood but was detected in hepatic venous blood [18]. In the same study, Cameron et al. showed that their large-volume, relatively unpurified preparation frequently induced portal hypertension, with potentially fatal results.

The etiology of the failure of these autografts some months after apparently successful transplantation is not known. We have seen in our own laboratory a lack of durability of islet function in some rodent and canine autografts. This appears to be related to the quantity of viable islets transplanted (D. W. Scharp et al., unpublished results). The numbers of islets needed for successful human transplantation has been estimated as approximately 500 000 islets in a pure form with an insulin content of at least 100 units [27]. This laboratory has recently developed an automated method for isolating human islets [19]. This procedure yields approximately 3000–6000 islets/g pancreas. The range of yield of islets from a single human pancreas varies from 250 000–600 000 depending upon the amount of pancreatic tissue available and the state of the pancreas prior to digestion.

Pancreases used in our facility are either imported via NDRI (National Diabetes Research Interchange) or procured locally. While guidelines are made available to the retrieval surgeons, there is variability in the method of procurement, especially with imported glands. We prefer in situ cold perfusion and generous topical cooling with slushed saline. Adequate perfusion requires preservation of the splenic artery and vein, even in liver donors. This requirement is similar to that for whole organ pancreas transplantation. In the past, the majority of glands were preserved with Collins or Euro-Collins solution. Recently we have found the new University of Wisconsin preservation solution to give excellent results. In addition, removal of the intact gland requires preservation of the capsule so that subsequent distension with collagenase is possible. Detrimental effects of warm ischemia time on islet isolation has been well documented in experimental animals [20]. While similar effects can be expected in the human this has not been clearly shown.

All currently used techniques of islet isolation employ collagenase to enzymatically separate islets from acinar tissue. Collagenase is a mixture of enzymes produced by *Clostridia histolyticum*. There appears to be little consistency in the nutrients used in the fermentation process and there is consequently a large degree of variability from lot to lot of the same tpye of collagenase, even from the same supplier. The mixture of the enzymes required for optimal islet isolation is not known. The optimal temperature and pH for collagenase digestion of the pancreas are not known. A temperature of 37 °C may, in fact, be the optimal temperature. The rate at which a cold stored pancreas is warmed may also play an important role. An acidic pH has been shown to reduce islet yield [21].

Mechanical disruption of the islet-acinar interface by distension is a very important factor, as first emphasized by Lacy and Kostianovsky [7]. The most popular method of disruption is ductal injection or perfusion. The aim is to disrupt the islet-acinar interface, thus releasing islets. Disruption of larger ductules and ducts results in interlobular leakage of collagenase, loss of perfusion pressure and failure to disrupt intralobularly. Splenic vein distension with collagenase has been very effective in the dog but has not been effective in humans [22].

The digestion of the pancreas by collagenase can be enhanced, and overall damage to islets minimized, by appropriate selection of mechanical assistance of the digestion process. Shaking of the digestion vessel has frequently been used to enhance the digestion process. Addition of appropriately sized filters to the digestion process allows for removal of free islets and the retention of larger pieces of partially digested pancreas. Islets trapped in the larger fragments will be retained on the filter. Gross mechanical disruption of the gland increases the surface area for the enzymatic reaction and facilitates the dispersal of the gland. A disadvantage common to all techniques of mechanical disruption is increased trauma and fragmentation of the islets.

The technique currently employed in our facility [19] for human islet isolation combines a continuous digestion-filtration system with continuous shaking. Gross mechanical disruption is provided by glass spheres within the shaking device. Temperature is monitored and controlled. The pH is maintained by buffers in the perfusion solution. After islets and small fragments of pancreas leave the digestion circuit the digestion process is halted by dropping the temperature to 4 °C and quenching the enzymatic process with 10% serum albumin.

After digestion, islets are part of a heterogeneous mixture including acinar tissue, ductular elements, blood vessels, and lymphoid and neural tissue as well as islets. Various techniques have been introduced to purify the islets from the nonendocrine elements. Generally, an inverse relationship exists between the purity of the islet preparation and the islet yield after preparation. Simple filtering removes larger fragments (some of which may still contain entrapped islets) but still allows smaller fragments of nonendocrine tissue through. Depending on the mesh size, large islets may also be entrapped on the mesh.

Many investigators, including our own facility, use density gradients, such as Ficoll, to purify islet preparation. Alternative gradients include Percoll, albumin, and dextran. There are a multitude of variables affecting the efficacy of a gradient used for islet separation. Each gradient separation is probably species dependent. In addition, the overall quality of the islet preparation placed on the gradient will have a direct effect on the final purity and yield. Factors such as the selection of gradient compostion, densities, set up of the gradient, temperature, and centrifugation speed will usually have to be determined experimentally. The primary disadvantage of using density gradients is the potential for islet toxicity either from the gradient itself because of osmolar shock, or from the inclusion of impurities from the commercial processing of the gradient. Another disadvantage of density gradients, especially for the human pancreas, is the problem associated with the warm ischemia of the donor pancreas which depletes the exocrine enzymes, thereby making the acinar cells lighter in density and causing them to rise on the gradient to the islet level, and thus reducing their purification.

In our facility we use Ficoll density gradients of 1.058 g/cm^3 and 1.074 g/cm^3. Three milliliters of pelleted islet tissue is suspended in the 1.058 g/cm^3 solution and top loaded onto the 1.074 g/cm^3 gradient in specially constructed large-bore syringes. These are then spun at 800 g for 16 min at 4 °C. Purity of 90% is common and yield is usually greater than 60%.

A crucial factor when the goal is actual human islet transplantation is quality control of the isolation process. The entire process must be carried out under strictly sterile conditions. Cultures must be performed to ensure there is no contamination. In addition, the usual precautions taken with the donor regarding presence of transmissable diseases must be followed.

Another aspect of quality control involves the overall quality of a given isolation. We routinely assay for islet quantity by counting islets based on size and calculating an islet volume. Quality is assayed morphologically with phase contrast microscopy, light microscopy (aldeyhde fuschin and immunoperoxidase staining), and electron microscopy. Aliquots of the preparation are assayed for the contents of insulin, glucagon, somatostatin, and pancreatic polypeptide. Islet function is determined by glucose challenge in vitro with perifusion. Only those preparations which meet preestablished standards are considered for transplantation regardless of the number of islets obtained.

Human Islet Transplantation

Human islet allotransplantation to treat type I diabetes mellitus has been investigated by different groups using different isolation techniques and various implantation sites. At the Washington University Medical Center in St. Louis the first phase of clinical trials [23, 24] used the tissue macerator technique [14] for islet isolation with implantation via direct splenic pulp injection. The final preparation contained 20% – 25% islets, with an average of 240 000 islets. The diabetic patients all had had previous renal allografts (mean 4.5 years) and were on chronic immunosuppression. The average age of these six patients was 34 years with a mean duration of type I diabetes of 24 years. In three patients their basal immunosuppression (prednisone 10 mg/day and azathioprine 100 mg/day) was unaltered except for a perioperative increase in steroids on the day of transplantation. In the remaining three patients perioperative high-dose prednisone therapy was continued for 10 days: 1000 mg daily for 3 days followed by 100 mg daily for 7 days. There were no toxic reactions identified in relation to the islet transplantation procedure. One patient had a transient elevation of portal venous pressure to 40 cmH$_2$0. There were no adverse effects on the patients' renal allografts.

Prior to transplantation none of the six recipients had detectable levels of basal or stimulated serum C peptide. Three of the six islet allograft patients achieved measurable levels of C peptide for a period of 1–3 months posttransplant. None of the patients achieved normoglycemia without exogenous insulin. The three patients with detectable C peptide had lower insulin requirements than those patients with poor graft function.

In 1987 a second phase trial of clinical human islet transplantation was iniated at Washington University in St. Louis [25]. The second trial was based upon a broader approach to immunosuppression and on the more productive automated digestion-filtration method [19] of islet isolation.

Three recipients were chosen for the 1987 study. The average duration of type I diabetes was 20 years. As in the 1985 study, none of the recipients had detectable baseline or stimulated C peptide activity. As opposed to the 1985 study, none of the patients in the 1987 study had had a renal transplant for renal failure. Immunosuppressive therapy was begun 4 days prior to the actual transplant. This consisted of triple therapy with cyclosporin (8 mg/kg.day in divided doses to maintain a 12-h serum HPLC through of 200 ng/ml), azathioprine (2 mg/kg.day to maintain WBC > 3000), and prednisone (2.5 mg/kg.day in divided doses until the day of transplant, then 1.0 mg/kg.day in divided doses with a taper schedule.

In addition to the immunosuppressive therapy for the recipient, the islets were cultured at 24 °C for 6 days to try to reduce immunogenicity of the islet innoculum.

Using the automated method the average islet yield was 360 000 islets per transplant, versus 240 000 in 1985 (a 50% increase). In addition, there was a significant increase in purity from 25% in 1985 to 85% in the 1987 trial. This marked improvement in purity resulted in the entire transplantable islet mass to be contained in a volume of less than 1 cm^3. With this small volume of purified islet tissue, transplantation into the liver via the portal vein was now considered to be safe. Various studies have suggested that intrahepatic islet transplantation should give the most efficacious control of glucose metabolism [26]. Intrahepatic transplantation via the portal vein was performed in three patients in the 1987 trial. None of these patients demonstrated a rise in portal vein pressure during or after the injection.

All three of the recipients in the 1987 study demonstrated fasting and stimulated C peptide activity for up to 2 weeks posttransplant. Two of the three patients demonstrated stimulated C peptide levels into the low normal range. These patients rapidly and unexpectedly lost C peptide activity at 2 weeks posttransplant. They were treated for presumed acute rejection episodes with OKT3 (Ortho Pharmaceutical Corp., Raritan, NJ) at 5 mg/day for 5 days. This resulted in only minimal C peptide activity.

References

1. Lacy PE, Davie JM, Finke EH (1979) Prolongation of islet allograft survival following *in vitro* culture culture (24° C) and a single injection of ALS. Science 204: 312–313
2. Faustman D, Hauptfeld V, Lacy PE, Davie JM (1981) Prolongation of murine islet allograft survival by pretreatment of islets with antibody directed to Ia determinants. Proc Natl Acad Sci USA 78: 5156–5159
3. Faustman DL, Steinman RM, Gebel HM, Hauptfeld V, Davie JM, Lacy PE (1984) Prevention of rejection of murine islet allografts by pretreatment with anti-dendritic cell antibody. Proc Natl Acad Sci USA 81: 3864–3868
4. Gotoh M, Maki T, Porter J, Monaco AP (1987) Pancreatic islet transplantation using H-2 incompatible multiple donors. Transplant Proc 19: 957–959
5. Reese-Smith H, DuToit DF, McShane P, Morris PJ (1981) Prolonged survival of pancreatic islet allografts transplanted beneath the renal capsule. Transplantation 31: 305–306
6. Federlin KF, Bretzel RG (1984) The effect of islet transplantation on complications in experimental diabetes of the rat. World J Surg 8: 169–178
7. Lacy PE, Kostianovsky M (1967) Method for the isolation of intact islets of Langerhans from the rat pancreas. Diabetes 16: 35–39
8. Lacy PE, Walker BS, Fink CJ (1972) Perifusion of isolated rat islets *in vitro*, participation of the microtubular system in the biphasic release of insulin. Diabetes 21: 987
9. van Suylichem PTR, Pasma A, Wolters GHJ, van Schilfgaarde R (1987) Microscopic aspects of the structure and collagen content of the pancreas from the perspective of islet isolation. Transplant Proc 19: 3958–3959
10. Gray DWR, McShane P, Grant A, Morris PJ (1984) A method for isolation of islets of Langerhans from the human pancreas. Diabetes 33: 1055–61
11. Kneteman NM, Rajotte RV (1986) Isolation and cryopreservation of human pancreatic islets. Transplant Proc 18: 182–185
12. Kuhn F, Schulz HJ, Lorenz D et al. (1985) Morphological investigations in human islets of Langerhans isolated by the Velcro-technique. Biomed Biochim Acta 44: 149–53
13. Lacy PE, Lacy ET, Finke EH, Yasunami Y (1982) An improved method for the isolation of islets from the beef pancreas. Diabetes 31 [Suppl 4]: 109–111

14. Alderson D, Scharp DW, Kneteman NM (1987) The isolation of purified human islets of Langerhans. Transplant Proc 19: 196–197
15. Scharp DW, Lacy PE, Finke E, Olack BJ (1987) Lowtemperature culture of human islets isolated by the distension method and purified by Ficoll or Percoll gradients. Surgery 102: 869–879
16. Morrow CE, Cohen JL, Sutherland DER, Najarian JS (1984) Chronic pancreatitis: long-term surgical results of pancreatic duct drainage, pancreatic resection, and near-total pancreatectomy and islet autotransplantation. Surgery 96: 608–616
17. Cameron JL, Mehigan DG, Broe PJ, Zuidema GD (1981) Distal pancreatectomy and islet autotransplantation for chronic pancreatitis. Ann Surg 193: 312–317
18 .Cameron JL, Mehigan DG, Harrington DP, Zuidema GD (1980) Metabolic studies following intrahepatic autotransplantation of pancreatic islet grafts. Surgery 87: 397
19. Ricordi C, Lacy PE, Finke EH, Olack BJ, Scharp DW (1988) An automated method for the isolation of human pancreatic islets. Diabetes 37: 413:420
20. Corlett MP, Fonseca P, Scharp DW (1988) Detrimental effect of warm ischemia on islet isolation in rats and dogs with protection by oxygen free radical scavengers. J Surg Res 45: 531–536
21. Burghen GA, Murrell LR (1988) Factors influencing isolation of islets of Langerhans. First international congress on pancreatic and islet transplantation, Stockholm, 1988, abstract 15
22. Downing R, Scharp DW, Ballinger WF (1980) An improved technique for the isolation and identification of mammalian islets of Langerhans. Transplantation 29: 19–30
23. Scharp D, Lacy P (1985) Human islet isolation and transplantation. Diabetes 34 [Supl 1]: 5A
24. Lacy PE, Scharp DW (1986) Islet transplantation in treating diabetes. Ann Rev Med 37: 33–40
25. Scharp D, Lacy P, Ricordi C, Boyle P, Santiago J, Cryer P, Gingerich R, Jaffe A, Anderson C, Flye W (1989) Human islet transplantation in patients with Type I diabetes. Transplant Proc Vol 21, No 1 pp 2744–2745
26. Reckard CR, Franklin W, Schulak JM (1978) Intrasplenic versus intraportal pancreatic islet transplants: quantitative, qualitative and immunological aspects. Trans Am Soc Artif Intern Organs 24: 232–234
27. Scharp DW, Lacy P: Islet Transplantation: A review of the objective, the concepts, the problems, the progress and the future. In: Dubernard JM, Sutherland DER (eds.) Transplantation of the pancreas, Martinus Nijhoft Publishers The Netherlands (in press)

Summary and Prospects

E. F. PFEIFFER

It is not easy to summarize the proceedings of such a very full day, but some detailed analysis is necessary if only for the benefit of those who were not present throughout. We are grateful to Dr. Bretzel and Dr. Federlin for their careful analysis, starting with the immunologic aspects of insulin substitution and continuing with the dynamic aspects. Our preoccupation with the more immediate problems meant that we did not deal completely with the treatment of diabetes and with the significance of dynamic insulin substitution in the prophylaxis and treatment of secondary complications in diabetes, so important to the majority of us as clinicians. The symposium ended with islet and pancreatic transplantation, with the final paper by the Goodman group on transplantation and an early attempt at insulin gene transfer, now being studied by various research teams throughout the world.

I think that the first paper, given by Dr. Yoon on behalf of Dr. Notkins from Bethesda, gave a very clear message regarding the immunologic reasons for the development of diabetes, and we know that the message from this group is to concentrate on the viral genesis of type I diabetes. This is a matter which has aroused interest since a number of reports, including the paper of Dr. Yoon from Beth Israel Hospital referring to an encephalomyelitis, fulfilling all the postulates of Robert Koch. There was a viral lesion, the child was suffering from a diabetic condition and died of the diabetes, and the virus was isolated and transferred to mice, in which it reproduced the lesion. This was an extremely important paper. For those of us interested in this aspect, the type of virus was other than what we had expected, so Dr. Yoon had to bridge this gap and did so excellently.

Then there was a report from New York concerning mothers with rubella during pregnancy and the percentage of children who subsequently developed diabetes. This led to speculation about events in the beta-cell itself and to the two animal models, which suggested an interplay of the virus with some other factor. There is the model of monkeys suffering from Coxsackie B4 virus infection which subsequently develop diabetes. There are four types of virus; only one gives a positive result and the others are ineffective. Not to expand unduly on this topic, there was also the report of a child who contracted diabetes at the age of 13. There is also the very important idea that the CMV genome attracts the virus and subsequently also introduces the antibody information, which implies autoantibody formation to the virus and the affected tissues. There is also the important concept that the retrovirus actually selects the beta-cell for the supply of DNA information, leading to the formation of class II antigens which are substantially involved in antibody formation. Some of these parameters are necessary to satisfy the prerequisites for initiating the disease and its continuation.

Dr. Scherbaum of our own group drew attention to the fact that autoantibodies are found only in 50% of type I diabetics, and that it is only in a certain genetically identified group that we find the class II MHC antigens, acting as a kind of trigger mechanism, and on which cytoplasmic and surface antibodies can be easily demonstrated. This can be demonstrated initially and then it declines progressively. The complement-binding antibodies are of some importance because it has long been understood in immunology that complement is essential for lysis once the antibody has fixed the cell. This aspect can be found in the old textbooks of immunology of 40 or 50 years ago. The new thing is the 64 KD protein, which is used as an antigen, and the idea that has to do with sialyglyco-conjugation of the antibody, and that this can be demonstrated before diagnosis proper of the disease. There is a large ongoing study in Miami dealing with the screening of 5000 schoolchildren and a similar project of the German Research Council on German children, and some of the members of this group are with us today. Of course, we are all well aware of the fact that the CF-ICA antibodies can be found in 45% of the relatives of the affected cases, but positive results were found only for one of the other antigens and then only in two out of 665 relatives in our study. This indicates that this must be an islet-cell antibody, which may be helpful in selection and screening but perhaps no more than that.

Dr. Schernthaner reported on attempts of immunosuppressive treatment in type I diabetics. This was a European-Canadian study of some 200 type I diabetics in the first phase of the disease. It was a prospective study, and there was some selection on the basis that phase I of insulin secretion following intravenous glucose was lacking. They found that immunosuppressive treatment was a possibility, but that it was necessary to continue the treatment. Further, if treatment with cyclosporin-A is continued, it may affect the kidney tissue and probably also the beta-cell, which is also a problem of cyclosporin treatment in organ transplantation, and there were no real reports after the 12-month' follow-up period. There is really not much difference from cases given aggressive insulin treatment during the first few months, a treatment now more than 25 years old. I found it interesting that Dr. Schernthaner reported that children respond better than adults, which is entirely consistent with our own experience in Ulm a couple of years ago. We were then treating a number of juvenile patients very aggressively by means of the artificial pancreas and later with portable pumps, and it was notable that boys between 12 and 16 were the best responders and sometimes had remissions of up to two or three years. This was quite remarkable; there was much less success in the other cases.

But it is still not clear whether it is better to give a drug like cyclosporin in such a case rather than simply depending on insulin, in view of the side-effects. The general tendency throughout the world seems to be rather hesitant and reserved.

Dr. Andreani, of Rome, reported a historical review and told us that mono-component insulin has changed the picture, as has human insulin, but that the antibodies do not disappear when the patient is switched to human insulin, that hypoglycemia remains an important problem, and that antibodies are even found together with hypoglycemia in Japanese cases. Of course, this is something we discussed 20, 30 or even 50 years ago in connection with some kind of slow release of the antibody-bound insulin at the periphery. When we were discussing bound and free insulin 20 years ago this was something proposed as a possibly useful procedure, and some clinicians at that time emphasized antibody formation. Then came the report of the Eisenbarth group in Boston on finding autoantibodies in patients who subsequently developed diabetes. In 1956–1958 I was a Fulbright Fellow in Boston working with that group. Stewart Soeldner was the research fellow on my ward and was collecting sera at that time as instructed by Alexander Marble and E.P. Joslin, who were still practising then. These were the sera of patients attending the hospital, but nobody came to the Joslin Clinic who was not suffering from diabetes, so the sera kept there were those of a selected group. This was a one-community selection, and it must be borne in mind that the sera would not otherwise have been stored in the deep-freeze for such a very long time. It was not a pure selection as it now exists in the Miami study, and perhaps also in the study now under way in Germany.

We now move on to the reports of the dynamic aspects of insulin substitution. Dr. Waldhäusl reported on the significance of the finer changes. I would prefer to call these the "pin-point" changes in diabetes and to stress the importance of the contrainsular hormones and the pulsatility of insulin secretion. I am well aware that pulsatility is not absolutely necessary, but I believe that Dr. Waldhäusl is right when he says that by increase and decrease you can reduce the amount of insulin that has to be given. This is something which may be connected with the so-called combination therapy. He worked with clamp studies and by means of the biostator, and it is important that the contrainsular hormones really absorb insulin and give rise to insulin resistance. This happens not only in these cases and in his own studies, but also in patients who have received pancreas transplants, because one is forced to use immunosuppressive therapy. In these cases one has to give steroids and in this way one produces insulin resistance. As we have already stated in one of the discussions, we had no case with less than 15 micro-units of insulin in the fasting state after transplantation, with absolutely no need for insulin substitution. Certainly, the 60% reduction in daily insulin requirement shown in Dr. Waldhäusl's studies was good, but he was speaking of Schade's work with the primary algorithms which altered the circumstances. Our own work has been directly with the patient, and this has advanced recently since we have been able to determine the blood-sugar continuously with the portable apparatus.

Dr. Mehnert spoke of the dynamic aspects of food intake, and of course this is important and very relevant to the program. We are currently recommending less protein, and from the data he gave I calculate that the amount of meat allowed in future will be exceedingly small if his program is adhered to. I think this is a matter on which opinion may change from time to time. I very much liked the expression of "putting the diet on like a suit", and also the idea that the patient should be taught about diet, and it is quite clear that he can learn this. If you see the patient several times a year and he is in hospital several times, you will succeed in a proportion of cases. The most important point is to lose weight, at least in those who are insulin-dependent, and this can be done but the success rate is poor. Then for many male patients it is important to be careful with alcohol and perhaps we should stres this point more, though it is difficult in some parts of the country.

Dr. Schöffling reported on the 45-year history of the sulfonyl-ureas. But this has not become the "treatment of convenience" and this is true for many practitioners throughout the country. I feel that unfortunately type II diabetics are now worse off than type I cases. Everyone concentrates on the type I diabetics and does his best for them with care and substitution, but virtually nothing is done for the type-II patients. The blood-sugar swings up and down, and we have been told that there are more frequent complications in these cases, particularly vascular complications. Especially in type II cases, treatment has two aims: to control the blood-sugar and to normalize the blood-pressure, and this is more important than any kind of operation on these patients. Then we have been reminded of the UDPG study in 1971, with the rather syill idea of including all the sudden deaths in the mortality, an idea that has now revived in some circles. The secondary failure in a proportion of cases was first described by us in Frankfurt at that time, and this has not really greatly changed, and there is also the difference in the percentage of persons treated with these tablets in our area and other areas.

It is of course the case that the sulfonyl-ureas have had their ups and downs, and that it is time to have some new preparations. But of course, we have also learned more about diabetes from the sulfonyl-ureas than from anything else. It is now possible to differentiate clearly between the different types of diabetes and modern treatment is conducted very differently. I believe that the problem will solve itself because many persons are only remporarily treated with sulfonyl-urea substances. But it is a problem when they have to be changed over to insulin, and the strictness of the treatment regime outside the diabetes centers is problematic. But it is certainly true that many type II diabetics have had to die earlier than would normally be expected. My colleagues in the USA and elsewhere are agreed on this.

The last report in this session was that of Dr. Bottermann, on pro-insulin, which had a lot to do with mortality. The discussion on the insulin activities of pro-insulin was not conclusive. There is no convincing evidence that pro-insulin really aims at the liver as a target organ. Finally, there is the risk of mortality connected with pro-insulin, but I do not think that this is why the clinical trials were terminated. The commercial firm more or less gave up, not only because of the alleged increased mortality – again this question of mortality – but because there was no convincing proof of the need to use pro-insulin clinically.

The first of the three reports read in Dr. Teller's session was that of Dr. Beyer, dealing with the possibility of improving metabolic control with the aid of computers. Dr. Raptis spoke about treatment with insulin pumps and PEN systems, and finally there was my contribution on the glucosensor and the biostator. I feel it can be said that there is no question that the computer is at least as good as a check-list in an aeroplane, and we know that the pilot has to check this list point by point. Those enamoured of computers can show that we also have such a "diva computer". The dialogue between the doctor and the patient is far more intensive than before, when he was dealing only with superficialities. There is no doubt that the doctor is capable of this and must continue to be so, but we should not forget that we might compel other doctors with inadequate training also to talk more intensively with their patients, and to have feedback control. As long as we have nothing better, it is neither wasteful nor time-saving for the doctor; he will need more time to talk to the patient than he has usually had.

The report of Dr. Raptis dealt with insulin pumps, with special emphasis on injection systems. But there are some doubts as to whether the administration of insulin by a jet system has any advantages. On the other hand, the PEN systems are specially recommended by the patients. My own view is that the combined therapy is better than PEN treatment because it can be adapted to the patient, but there is no question that many patients desire the PEN therapy and that, because of this, the combined therapy emphasized by ourselves and Dr. Sauer has been somewhat relegated to the background.

I wish to emphasize Dr. Sauer's report, because it has two important aspects dealing with short- and long-acting insulin. The "old" insulin acts too slowly and "depot" insulin too rapidly. What we need is a long-acting "depot" insulin, a real basal insulin, an expression used before we discovered that basal insulin infused by pumps is not indentical with the long-acting insulin injected and falsely called "basal" by the pharmaceutical industry. At the same time, whoever now uses fixed combinations instead of individually planned combinations? We need a new insulin which is different from merely combining regular and "depot" insulin.

I shall not discuss my own contribution.

Dr. Standl told us about the problems of diabetic macroangiopathy, with special emphasis on the thesis that hyperinsulinism has an effect on the pathogenesis of macroangiopathy. He elaborated on the results of Ferrannini as regards insulin resistance and hypertension and their relationship. I am very interested in diabetic cerebral angiopathy, but this point was not discussed. Lundbaek always argued that there was a series of particularities, but after hearing Dr. Standl it may be thought that this is not the case. There is, for instance, the preferential cerebral type of angiopathy in women, and other instances besides.

Dr. Deckert, of Gentofte, spoke on diabetic retinopathy and nephropathy. The conclusion of the Oslo-Gentofte retinopathy study was that perfect control might improve in reducing the complications.

Dr. Gries spoke about diabetic neuropathy, which he thought due possible to vascular changes, though there was some controversy as to whether it is not really of metabolic origin. It is quite difficult to see how an isolated abducents or oculomotor paresis can be of vascular origin, since no other changes are seen and the condition disappears after a time if one is lucky.

Now, ladies and gentlemen, we come to the matter of pancreas and islet transplantation, the work of the Giessen group, which has laid good foundations and found many young persons to continue work in this field.

Dr. Barker, we are very grateful for your report on the Pancreas Transplant Registry, which really showed us the nucleus of three efforts. And the nucleus – I hope I can put it in this way – is that there is not much difference between using segmental pancreas or whole pancreas, or between draining the duct into the bowel or into the bladder. We also conclude that gross mismatches should be avoided for immunologic reasons, but that autoimmune diabetes may recur even in cases with lesser disparity. So there are two aspects to be considered, and we are really between Scylla and Charybdis as to which degree of matching to adopt. I believe this will be clarified in the future. There is the further problem about how to manage the kidneys. The generally accepted procedure is to transplant the kidney and pancreas together. There is the problem of organ procurement and viability, and we have about one in four cases which are successful with permanent endocrine function for up to 4 years. Afterwards, there is a steady decline in the success rate, but I think that we can obtain positive results for that period and, rather to our surprise, we have a 10% mortality from the figures presented. This remains something yet to be discussed in relation to the poor state of health of these patients when we are deciding and discussing pancreas and islet transplantation in general.

Dr. Rajotte reported on islets and cryopreservation, which is also being done here in Giessen in Dr. Bretzel's laboratory. The general strategy is accepted and the advantages of islet transplantation are clear. The renal subcapsular site allows repeated implantation of islets. I believe that under the influence of experience with transplantation of the entire pancreas, islet transplantation is having something of a renaissance, and this is significant. But, for general use in medicine, I would predict that some kind of animal islets should be available. We should have calf or pig islets abailable in quantity, and then perhaps repeat the islet grafting every six or eight months. Of course, this assumes that the metabolic situation is renormalized by pancreatic transplantation from the outset, which has not been the case with such transplantation so far. This aspect may have been somewhat overlooked by surgeons in the past in their zeal for a successful operation.

We then had various reports on aspects of islet transplantation.

Dr. Bretzel reported on the Giessen experience with islet transplantation in rodents: the transplantation site, the various preservation techniques such as cryopreservation, the selection of animal models, treatment with antilymphocyte serum and monoclonal antibodies to circumvent islet allograft rejection, and the question whether the diabetes recurs after the transplant and the question of reversal of the microangiopathy. This was discussed when we worked together in my department at Ulm, and it was clearly shown that if the point of no return has not been passed, it is possible to reverse the microangiopathic lesions in the kidney, the glomerulosclerosis, and this is a sustainable point of view. And, of course, the complicated mechanisms to do with islet graft rejection were also discussed.

Dr. Alejandro reported on experiments in the dog. In these cases he obtained the best results using monoclonal antibodies, cyclosporin and culture methods for preventing graft rejection. These three methods are likely to be most successful in the future.

Dr. McCullough from St. Louis reported on cases of adult human islet transplantation. Six cases were done in this institution. This was interesting, because last year, when I was in Shanghai in the People's Republic of China, I was shown many cases of fetal islet transplantation in man, and in Moscow there are many cases because of the large number of fetuses available. But in none of these cases was there any clear-cut record as to residual C-peptide secretion before transplantation, and evaluation of these cases is very difficult. We may conclude from the St. Louis experience that so far there is no cure for the patient.

Dr. Selden reported on the beautiful experiments at the Massachusetts General Hospital, where, induced by transfection, all cells in the transfected animal then bear the human insulin gene. After a certain period 70 % of the mice now survive with the human insulin, if I understand correctly, and after a couple of weeks this activity subsides and disappears. The same applies to the transfection and transkaryotic implantation of human growth hormone producing cells. Of course, from an ethical viewpoint it should be permissible to take tissue from a human subject to transfect it with the material we need to introduce the genome and to reimplant it into the patient. There is absolutely no obstacle, and no objection from all those various bodies and societies which make our life difficult at present. We are encouraged by this work. The first transplantation was done in L-cell (mouse fibroblast) transplantation in CBH mice. I wonder whether you can perhaps give us a short answer as to whether these nude mice suffer from hypoglycemia as long, and whether you have the hypoglycemic reaction in all of the animals or only in the nude ones.

Dr. Selden (answering): We had the hypoglycemic reaction in all of the animals.

Dr. Pfeiffer (continuing): This means that the feedback regulation for the islet cell is not active. So the transplanted material is not regulated by the general laws of endocrinology, which is a very interesting observation from a biologic point of view.

Thank you for your attention.

Subject Index